Assistive Technology for Blindness and Low Vision

Rehabilitation Science in Practice Series

Series Editors

Marcia J. Scherer, Ph.D.

President
Institute for Matching Person and Technology

Professor
Orthopaedics and Rehabilitation
University of Rochester Medical Center

Dave Muller, Ph.D.

Executive
Suffolk New College

Editor-in-Chief
Disability and Rehabilitation

Founding Editor
Aphasiology

Published Titles

Assistive Technology Assessment Handbook, *edited by Stefano Federici and Marcia J. Scherer*

Assistive Technology for Blindness and Low Vision, *Roberto Manduchi and Sri Kurniawan*

Multiple Sclerosis Rehabilitation: From Impairment to Participation, *edited by Marcia Finlayson*

Paediatric Rehabilitation Engineering: From Disability to Possibility, *edited by Tom Chau and Jillian Fairley*

Quality of Life Technology, *Richard Schultz*

Forthcoming Titles

Ambient Assisted Living, *edited by Nuno M. Garcia, Joel Jose P. C. Rodrigues, Dirk Christian Elias, Miguel Sales Dias*

Computer Systems Experiences of Users with and without Disabilities: An Evaluation Guide for Professionals, *Simone Borsci, Masaaki Kurosu, Stefano Federici, Maria Laura Mele*

Neuroprosthetics: Principles and Applications, *Justin C. Sanchez*

Rehabilitation Goal Setting: Theory, Practice and Evidence, *edited by Richard Siegert and William Levack*

Assistive Technology for Blindness and Low Vision

Edited by
Roberto Manduchi • Sri Kurniawan

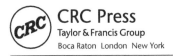

CRC Press
Taylor & Francis Group
Boca Raton London New York

CRC Press is an imprint of the
Taylor & Francis Group, an **informa** business

CRC Press
Taylor & Francis Group
6000 Broken Sound Parkway NW, Suite 300
Boca Raton, FL 33487-2742

First issued in paperback 2017

© 2013 by Taylor & Francis Group, LLC
CRC Press is an imprint of Taylor & Francis Group, an Informa business

No claim to original U.S. Government works

ISBN-13: 978-1-4398-7153-9 (hbk)
ISBN-13: 978-1-138-07313-5 (pbk)

Visit the Taylor & Francis Web site at
http://www.taylorandfrancis.com

and the CRC Press Web site at
http://www.crcpress.com

Contents

Foreword

Assistive technology has been an incredible force for equality of people with disabilities. With the right tools, people with a wide range of visual impairments have been able to engage in education, employment, and general society as never before. Alongside advances in civil rights, assistive technology has made much of these improvements practical.

As the creator of both successful and unsuccessful assistive technology products, I have learned through experience and observation about how to make new products and see them through to widespread adoption. This book will expose you to the full range of how technology is truly improving the lives of people with visual impairments. Written by world-class leaders in different segments of the assistive technology field, you will learn not only what is working today but also gain insight into what is next. Looking back over more than 20 years, it is amazing to see how much progress has been made!

Essential to these advances in assistive technology have been widespread technology advances, especially in the area of platforms and infrastructure. In testimony to the U.S. Congress in 1996, I described the personal computer (PC) as the "Swiss Army knife for people with disabilities," but it is now much more than the PC. The mobile phone, the tablet, and most of all, the Internet, have all created new opportunities. Powerful and flexible general-purpose technology and content can now be quickly adapted to the needs of people with disabilities, and this has greatly improved the capabilities and, even more importantly, the affordability of assistive technology.

Just as mainstreaming has become a core objective in education, mainstreaming with technology has been a key part of advancing the needs of people with vision impairments. To the greatest extent possible, people with disabilities would like to use the same applications, the same tools, and the same devices, and access the same content as their peers without disabilities. More and more mainstream vendors have seen the benefits of universal design in delivering value to a wider range of customers. Assistive technology has advanced quickly by exploiting the capabilities of new technology developed for the general market, and filling in essential missing pieces. More and more assistive technology will be built on top of general platforms like personal computers and mobile devices. However, Braille is a great example of an essential missing piece. There is no mainstream technology today that can effectively deliver Braille, but Braille displays, notetakers, and embossers connected to the Internet, smartphones, and PCs have made more Braille content available cost-effectively to today's blind Braille readers than ever before.

The assistive technology field has also followed the general computing device and software industries as they have shifted from technology-driven products to consumer-driven products to focus on solving the problems of real consumers with visual impairments. The most successful products, the largest improvements in quality of life, have come from carefully listening to user needs and responding to them. The field is littered with exciting technologies that did not lead to viable products, often because they were more gadgets in search of a problem.

The best way to learn is to observe the stories of today's successful products: the problems they solve, how they work, and how they have changed the lives of users. This book provides you with an unprecedented opportunity to understand the technologies that are improving the lives of untold numbers of people with vision impairments. Assistive technology has opened up a new world for people with disabilities, but the pace of change is increasing. I am excited about how future products will continue to remove even more barriers, enabling people with disabilities access to the same educational and employment opportunities as those without disabilities and fully realize the goal of social equality.

Jim Fruchterman
Founder, Benetech, Arkenstone and Bookshare
Palo Alto, California

Editors

Sri Kurniawan, PhD, is an associate professor of computer engineering, a faculty member of the Center for Games and Playable Media, and an affiliated faculty of the Digital Arts and New Media Program, at the University of California, Santa Cruz. Her research focuses on human-centered fun and enjoyable interactive systems for health and healthy living. Her current projects include formatting and layout of sociotechnical solutions for blind authors, a game to educate parents and clinicians on childbirth and labor as well as breastfeeding, a mobile application to motivate teenagers to exercise, and a game to motivate children who just underwent cleft lip and cleft palate surgery to perform speech therapy at home.

Roberto Manduchi, PhD, is a professor of computer engineering at the University of California, Santa Cruz. Before joining UC Santa Cruz in 2001, he worked at Apple Computer, Inc., and at the NASA Jet Propulsion Laboratory, where he conducted research on computer vision for autonomous navigation. His current research interest is in the application of computer vision and sensor processing to assistive technology for people with visual impairment. His research is supported by the National Science Foundation and by the National Institutes of Health.

Contributors

Billie Louise (Beezy) Bentzen, PhD, is a certified orientation and mobility specialist and experimental psychologist who has conducted, for more than 30 years, human factors research in wayfinding and mobility of people who are blind or who have low vision. Her research has included large print, tactile and electronic signs, audible signs, tactile maps, accessible pedestrian signals, visual contrast, detectable warnings, accessibility of roundabouts, and a variety of electronic wayfinding technologies. Results of her research are reflected in the American National Standards Institute A117.1-2009 Standard on Accessible and Usable Buildings and Facilities, the U.S. Department of Transportation's Americans with Disabilities Act (ADA) Standards for Transportation Facilities, draft ADA standards for accessible public rights-of-way, and the Federal Highway Administration's Manual on Uniform Traffic Control Devices. She is the founder of Accessible Design for the Blind, a company involved in human factors research and consultation in making the built environment more accessible to people who have visual impairments, where she continues as director of research.

Cristian Bernareggi, PhD, earned his PhD in computer science in 2006. Since 2007 he has worked as a research assistant at Università degli Studi di Milano, Italy. His primary research interest concerns assistive technology to support blind students in scientific education. From 2002 to 2006 he collaborated with European projects LAMBDA (Linear Access to Mathematics and Audiosynthesis) and TeDUB (Technical Drawings Understanding for the Blind). From 2007 to 2009 he was the coordinator of the European network @Science (Towards Accessible Science). Since 2010 Dr. Bernareggi has been a consultant for scientific education of blind students for the secondary school department of Milan, Italy. He has publications in international conferences (ICCHP, ASSETS, CHI, W4A) concerning multimodal access to mathematics, audiohaptic interaction for learning scientific diagrams, and nonvisual exploration of spatial representations.

Yonatan G. Breiter, BA, is a graduate student, enrolled in the Masters Entry Clinical Nurse Leader program, at the University of San Francisco. He is also a graduate research assistant working on the development of teaching strategies and technologies for persons with disabilities, and in particular testing devices for the blind for use in the study of mathematics.

Kim Casey, BA, has over a decade of experience working with accessible GPS systems at the Sendero Group. She has witnessed the advancement of accessible GPS over the years. She has expertise in testing and development, technical writing, and end-user training. Casey has written several successfully funded U.S. federal grants to advance accessible GPS systems and wayfinding technologies around the world.

Claude Chapdelaine, MA, completed a BA in computer science in 1984 at Université du Québec à Montréal (UQAM) and an MScA in human computer interaction at École Polytechnique de Montréal in 2000. Until 1996, she was involved in multimedia research at the Centre d'innovation en technologiques de l'information (CITI), where she mainly studied usability and navigational problems of large multimedia databases. Since 1997, she has been with the Centre de Recherche Informatique de Montréal (CRIM). She is a senior advisor on human factors issues for the design and evaluation of research works in the fields of speech recognition (real-time captioning) and vision. In 2006, she became involved in the design and testing of technology based on image detection algorithms to assist the production and broadcasting of descriptive video. She is responsible for the design and testing of an innovative accessible DVD player.

Mike Cole, BA, has worked in the fields of adult rehabilitation and special education for nearly 40 years. He attended college, beginning at a community college where he had a professor who was blind, a man who inspired him to study psychology, Professor H. G. (Jim) Burns. He received a BA from San Francisco State University. Cole taught for 10 years at what is now called the Hatlen Center for The Blind. He became the executive director of the center and in 1994 was made the administrator at the California Department of Rehabilitation's Orientation Center for the Blind, a state program for blind adults that Cole administered until his retirement in June of 2009. Cole has served in advisory roles with most of the nonprofits in the San Francisco Bay Area, and was an ex-officio trustee for the American Printing House for the Blind. Always active in access issues, he served on the Attorney General's Commission on Disabilities for John Van De Kamp. Cole has been awarded the Catherine T. (Kay) Gallagher Award from the American Foundation for the Blind, and the Lifetime Achievement Award from the Berkeley Chapter of the California Council of The Blind. Most recently, Cole was given the Fred L. Sinclair Award, the highest honor given by the California Transcribers and Educators for the Blind and Visually Impaired.

August Colenbrander, MD, was born and trained in the Netherlands. In 1971, he moved to San Francisco, where he was the medical director of the Low Vision Services at California Pacific Medical Center for 25 years and is an affiliate senior scientist at the Smith-Kettlewell Eye Research Institute. He was a founding board member of the International Society for Low Vision Research and Rehabilitation (ISLRR) and represents the subspecialty of Vision Rehabilitation on the Advisory Committee of the International Council of Ophthalmology (ICO). Because of his long-standing interest in classifications and definitions, Dr. Colenbrander worked with the World Health Organization (WHO) and International Council of Ophthalmology (ICO) in the 1970s to coordinate a thorough revision of the eye chapter in ICD-9. Presently, he co-chairs the WHO's Topic Advisory Group for Ophthalmology, which is preparing for ICD-11.

James Coughlan, PhD, received a BA in physics at Harvard University in 1990 and completed a PhD in physics at the same university in 1998. He is currently a senior scientist at the Smith-Kettlewell Eye Research Institute in San Francisco, California. His main research focus is the application of computer vision to assistive technology for blind and visually impaired persons, including systems to provide guidance at traffic intersections, find and read signs and other textual information, and detect terrain hazards for persons with combined vision and mobility impairments. He is also interested in probabilistic methods in computer and human vision, particularly the use of graphical models and belief propagation for visual search, segmentation, and 3-D stereo.

Bill Crandall, PhD, came to the Smith-Kettlewell Eye Research Institute in 1973 while pursuing his masters in physiological psychology at the University of Georgia. In 1981, he received a PhD in oculomotor neurophysiology and vision research. Dr. Crandall continued this laboratory research until 1990, moving to the Institute's Rehabilitation Engineering Research Center (RERC) where he began research in human factors utilization of disabilities access technology. He led the research, development, and technology transfer of Smith-Kettlewell's remote infrared audible sign system (Talking Signs®) for people who have print-reading disabilities such as blindness, low vision, or mental retardation. Dr. Crandall was recently a co-representative and voting member of the U.S. Delegation to the International Standards Organization ISO TC173/WG7 Committee on Assistive Products for Persons with Vision Impairments and Persons with Vision and Hearing Impairments, which set the standard for Audible Pedestrian Signals (APS) and is completing the standard for Tactile Walking Surface Indicators (TWSI). Dr. Crandall serves on the editorial board of *The Open Rehabilitation Journal*, and is an active member of the International Center for Accessible Transportation (ICAT) of Montreal, which acts to advise public and private entities.

Gislin Dagnelie, PhD, is an associate professor of ophthalmology at the Johns Hopkins University School of Medicine, and is the associate director of the Lions Vision Research and Rehabilitation Center, a division of the Wilmer Eye Institute. His work over the past 20 years, has been supported by grants from the National Institutes of Health, National Science Foundation, Foundation Fighting Blindness, and several companies developing ophthalmic devices and visual prosthetics. Dr. Dagnelie has been the center's principal investigator for clinical trials of the Optobionics Artificial

Silicon Retina (2004–2007) and the Second Sight Argus™ 2 retinal implant (2007–present). In addition, he studies signals in the retina of retinal pros-thesis patients and spearheads an effort to convert standard personal com-puters into precise tools for visual function measurement in the community and at home.

Yvonne Eriksson, PhD, holds the chair in information design at Mälardalen University. She obtained her doctoral degree in art history from Göteborg University in 1998 with the thesis *Tactile Pictures: Pictorial Representation for the Blind 1784–1940* and has been engaged in research and picture design for people with visual impairment for more than 20 years. She has worked at the Swedish Library of Talking Books and Braille and is a board member of the Swedish Braille Authority. In addition to research on tactile pictures and pic-torial representations for people with visual impairment, Dr. Eriksson has research interest in visual communication.

Eelke Folmer, PhD, is an assistant professor in the Department of Computer Science and Engineering, University of Nevada, Reno. His research interests lie in the area of human–computer interaction, specifically researching accessible interfaces for immersive 3-D applications such as video games and virtual worlds that accommodate the abilities of users with severe visual and motor impairments. Through extreme interaction design, Dr. Folmer and his research team try to solve interaction design problems for the most extreme gamer, with the potential to develop solutions that may benefit any user.

Duane Geruschat, PhD, is an associate professor at Salus University and a research associate in ophthalmology in the Johns Hopkins University School of Medicine. His work during the past 35 years has concentrated on low vision and orientation/mobility. This has included developing approaches to measuring mobility performance and studies that measure the visual behav-ior (eye movements) of low-vision pedestrians as they cross streets. More recently, Dr. Geruschat has worked with Second Sight, a privately held com-pany developing a retinal chip implant, to develop an assessment and instructional curriculum.

Nicholas A. Giudice, PhD, is an assistant professor of spatial informatics in the School of Computing and Information Science at the University of Maine, where he directs the Virtual Environment and Multimodal Interaction (VEMI) laboratory, and holds joint appointments in the University of Maine's Psychology Department and Intermedia program. Prior to his current appointment at the University of Maine, Dr. Giudice worked as a postdoctoral research fellow from 2005 to 2008 with Professor Jack Loomis at the University of California, Santa Barbara. Dr. Giudice attended graduate school at the University of Minnesota, where he was advised by Professors Gordon Legge and Herbert Pick. He received his PhD in cognitive and biological psychology in Fall of 2004. His VEMI lab at the University of Maine houses the university's first, and Maine's only, research facility combining a fully immersive virtual reality (VR) installation with augmented reality (AR) technologies in an integrated research and development environment. Research in his lab uses behavioral experiments to study human spatial cognition, to determine the optimal information requirements for the design of multimodal interfaces, and as a testbed for evaluation and usability research for navigational technologies.

William H. Jacobson, EdD, is chairperson of the Department of Counseling, Adult and Rehabilitation Education at the University of Arkansas at Little Rock, and professor of rehabilitation education. Dr. Jacobson has been the coordinator of the Orientation and Mobility (O&M) Program at the university since 1981. Prior to joining the faculty in 1978, Dr Jacobson taught children who are blind or visually impaired in Cleveland, Ohio, and taught O&M in Atlanta, Georgia and Albany, New York. Dr. Jacobson has consulted on O&M with the Jimmy Carter Foundation and the People's Republic of China, as well as with special education and rehabilitation centers in Guam, South Africa, Sweden, France, and Norway. In addition, Dr. Jacobson has written numerous articles, book chapters, and a textbook on orientation and mobility.

Arthur I. Karshmer, PhD, received his PhD in computer science from the University of Massachusetts at Amherst. Upon completion of his PhD he accepted a position in the Computer Science Department at the New Mexico State University where he was a professor of computer science and head of the academic department. In 2000, he moved to the University of South Florida where he was professor and founding chairman of the Information Technology Department. He now holds a position at the University of San Francisco. Since receiving his PhD, Dr. Karshmer has spent a postdoctoral year at the Einstein Institute of Mathematics, Computer Science Department at the Hebrew University of Jerusalem and held visiting positions at the University of York in England, The University of Pisa in Italy, Boston University, and the University of Kaiserslautern in the Federal Republic of Germany. He has received research grants from the National Science Foundation, the United States Air Force, the U.S. Army, Digital Equipment Corporation, AT&T, the U.S. Department of Education, the German Government, and the European Community to name a few. Dr. Karshmer has also worked at the U.S. National Science Foundation as the director for the Foundation's Program for Persons with Disabilities. Professor Karshmer has published numerous papers and regularly presents papers and delivers invited lectures in the United States, Asia, Europe, and South America.

George Kerscher, PhD, is dedicated to developing technologies that make information not only accessible, but also fully functional in the hands of persons who are blind or have a print disability. As secretary general of the

DAISY Consortium and president of the International Digital Publishing Forum (IDPF), Dr. Kerscher is a recognized accessibility expert. In addition, Dr. Kerscher is the senior officer of Accessible Technology at Learning Ally. He chairs the DAISY/NISO Standards Committee, the EPUB Maintenance Working Group and the W3C's Steering Council for the Web Accessibility Initiative (WAI). Dr. Kerscher also serves on the U.S. National Instructional Materials Accessibility Standard (NIMAS) Board.

Alasdair King, PhD, received his PhD from the School of Informatics, the University of Manchester, UK. Dr. King is an active practitioner of assistive technology software development, creating and supporting the WebbIE open-source assistive suite for screenreader users for 10 years. WebbIE is still one of the most widely used assistive suites by screenreader users in the United Kingdom. He is active in pursuing EU-funded and other research work at the University of Manchester, and is now running the international Claro Software assistive technology company in the United Kingdom. His other work has included the development of software for people with print impairments and dyslexia, deaf people, and people with physical impairments.

Roberta L. Klatzky, PhD, is professor of psychology at Carnegie Mellon University, where she is also on the faculty of the Center for the Neural Basis of Cognition and the Human–Computer Interaction Institute. Klatzky's work lies at the interface between perceptual and cognitive processes. She studies perceptually guided action, haptic perception, and spatial cognition. For over two decades she collaborated with Jack Loomis and associates on basic research in the area of spatial cognition, concerned with people's ability to represent and direct action toward spatial locations derived from sensory modalities and language. Over the course of a long-term research association with Susan Lederman, she studied how touch is used to recognize common objects and faces, along with their properties such as texture. Klatzky has had a longstanding interest in combining basic and applied research. A major aim of her collaboration with Jack Loomis was to develop a navigation aid for the blind. With Bing Wu and George Stetten, she conducted research on perception of distance in near space via multiple modalities, with the goal of developing an AR ultrasound display for image-guided surgery. Her research on touch has been applied to tele-operation using force-feedback interfaces.

Lynn Leith, BA, began working in the field of accessible materials in 1979 and has been involved with Digital Accessible Information SYstem (DAISY) since 1996. Since 2000 she has worked for the DAISY Consortium as international training & support coordinator, as head of information services, and is currently the editor of the Consortium's newsletter, the *DAISY Planet*. She played a key role in developing the DAISY production tool requirements, and coauthored the *DAISY Basic Training Manual* and *DAISY Structure*

Guidelines. She has published two articles in the *Institute of Scientific and Technical Communicators Journal.* Leith worked with the Canadian National Institute for the Blind (CNIB) Library for the Blind for 27 years, managing audio mastering. In 2008, she received CNIB's Grace Worts Staff Award, their highest employee award.

Jack M. Loomis, PhD, is professor emeritus in the Department of Psychological and Brain Sciences at the University of California, Santa Barbara, where he has been a professor since 1974. His early career focused on touch and color vision. In 1985, his interests turned to understanding complex behavior in three-dimensional space. Since then he has conducted research on a broad range of topics that include visual space perception, auditory space perception, navigation, visual control of driving and flying, multisensory spatial cognition, and analysis of perceptual experience in real and virtual environments. For over 20 years, he directed a project on nonvisual navigation with collaborators Roberta Klatzky and Reginald Golledge. The project was a combination of basic research on nonvisual spatial cognition and the development of a GPS-based navigation system. In the early 1990s, Dr. Loomis and Andy Beall began the development of visual VR technology for use in research. Joined later by Jim Blascovich, they and their colleagues used the technology to do groundbreaking research on perception, cognition, and social interaction. A legacy of this effort is WorldViz, a Santa Barbara-based company started by Beall and others, which is now a leading developer of VR technology.

Varju Luceno, MBA, is a marketing consultant, writer, blogger, and a digital technology enthusiast. She is convinced that all people, regardless of their ability or disability should have access to education and information. She earned a degree in library science from Tallinn University and an MBA from the University of Montana. Luceno's life experiences combined with her passion for technology, education, and information subsequently led her to DAISY. Luceno also speaks on technology and digital marketing–related topics and strongly believes in promoting innovative ideas and technologies.

James Marston, PhD, is a health research scientist at the Atlanta VA Medical Center's Rehabilitation Research and Development Center and the Atlanta Vision Loss Center of Excellence. He is also affiliated with the Center for Assistive Technology and Environmental Access (CATEA) and is an adjunct assistant professor with the College of Architecture, School of City and Regional Planning, Georgia Institute of Technology. He always had a strong interest in transit travel and urban exploration and after losing much of his central vision, decided to pursue a PhD in geography with an emphasis on cognitive science, with the pioneering behavioral geographer, Reginald Golledge at the University of California, Santa Barbara. His work focused on identifying barriers to independent travel for visually impaired people and examining how technologies could help overcome those barriers. He was awarded a U.C. President's Fellowship for research on making campuses more accessible to disabled travelers. Dr. Marston did postdoctoral research with Jack Loomis and Roberta Klatzky, helping to fine tune and conduct experiments on practical applications of the Personal Guidance System, a GPS system for the blind. He serves on the Transportation Research Board's Committee on Accessible Transportation and Mobility.

Mike May, MA, has been a pioneer in new product development since 1980. He has worked for the CIA, Bank of California, TRW, and Arkenstone. May is cofounder and CEO of Sendero Group, developers of the first accessible GPS for the blind in 1999 and distributors of various adaptive technologies. He has been the principal investigator on several U.S. federal grants and works with numerous organizations to advance wayfinding technologies around the world. May has been on the board of many nonprofits and currently serves on the board of The Seeing Eye. He holds the downhill speed skiing record of 65 mph for a totally blind person. Mike has met Presidents Carter, Reagan, Clinton, and Obama. A story of Mike's adventures is told in Robert Kurson's best selling book, *Crashing Through* and a movie by Stone Village Pictures is in the works.

1

Introduction

Roberto Manduchi and Sri Kurniawan

CONTENTS

Vision is by any measure the richest of human sensing modalities. Loss of vision has serious consequences in almost all aspects of human life: moving around, caring for oneself, social interaction, education, employment, leisure. Without vision, the world (the natural world and the urban world) suddenly becomes less accessible. Even partial vision loss (experienced by a large portion of the ageing population) can lead to significant changes in lifestyle: difficulty reading a book, recognizing people, driving. Yet, thanks to technology, blind and low vision individual can and do live active and productive lives, with a level of independence that was unthinkable only a few decades ago. They travel, on foot or using public transportation, knowing exactly where they are and how to get to destination, thanks to accessible GPS systems. They use computers, enjoying the powerful resources provided by the Internet (information access, communication, social networking). They increasingly use smartphones and their wide variety of mobile applications, including tools for recognizing colors, bank notes, objects.

This book presents a snapshot of the current state of technology for persons with visual impairment, with an emphasis on what we can learn from past experience and what the future holds in store. At the core of each chapter is the realization that any technological solution is doomed to fail if it does not consider all components of the problem, the human as well as the technological aspects. The field of assistive technology is rich with examples of prototypes that were never tested satisfactorily, or products that went into oblivion. Often, the reason lies with a lack of understanding of the very problem that the system is trying to address—in other words, with a technology-driven, rather than user-driven, design mentality. In other cases, the system did not work well enough, or was difficult to use, too cumbersome, with a poor interface, or just cosmetically unattractive. Sometimes an otherwise functional device was simply too expensive (and thus unaffordable by most), because the small size of the potential pool of users inhibits economy of scale. We should all learn important lessons from these failed attempts, and ensure that any new technological endeavor is sure-footed and directed at solving an actual problem with realistic potential to be adopted by the intended user.

This book strives to provide a holistic view of the different interconnected components that must be considered when designing assistive technology for persons with visual impairment. Its scope ranges from the physiological bases of vision loss, to the fundamentals of orientation, mobility, and information access for blind and low vision individuals, to technology for multiple applications (mobility, wayfinding, information access, education, work, entertainment) including both established technology and cutting-edge research. It was written for a broad audience encompassing designers, engineers, and practitioners as well as rehabilitation professionals and end users, and anyone who is curious about the reality, the promises, and the challenges of creating successful assistive technology.

Book Content Overview

Basics

Chapter 2 presents the medical (pathological and psychophysical) aspects of blindness and low vision. It provides an overview of the different stages of the vision process (the optical stage, the retinal receptor stage, and the neural stage) and analyzes clinical manifestations and practical consequences of various visual disorders. Chapter 3 discusses the basics of Orientation and Mobility using a long cane or a dog guide—the necessary techniques that a blind person needs to learn to be able to walk safely and purposefully to a destination. Several commercial Electronic Travel Aids (ETAs) are also presented, with a discussion of their benefits and shortcomings. Simple accommodations for living with low vision are discussed in Chapter 4. These range from basic tools for near, intermediate, and distance magnification, to more advanced camera-based systems.

Moving Around

Chapter 5 presents the state-of-the-art of accessible GPS. The potential of this technology for independent wayfinding and travel cannot be overemphasized, as first-person accounts of empowered blind travelers testify. A different wayfinding technology, Talking Signs, uses infrared beacons transmitting audible signals. Chapter 6 presents the evolution of the Talking Signs system, from prototype to world-wide deployment, emphasizing the importance of extended user studies. Chapter 7 addresses the important problem of how to test a given wayfinding technology. It discusses subjective and objective performance metrics, the design of unbiased evaluation experiments, and strategies for participants selection.

Accessing Information

Lacking visual access to the world, information can only be conveyed to a blind person via one of the remaining senses. Chapter 8 overviews the theory and practice of sensory substitution from the viewpoint of cognitive science and neuroscience, and provides useful guidelines for the designer. Chapter 9 discusses the issue of tactile access to graphical information, with a special emphasis on the design process of tactile storybooks for children. Visual information access by means of automated image analysis (or computer vision) is the topic of Chapter 10. Different applications of image processing and computer vision, from optical character recognition (OCR) to sign reading to modern mobile applications for object recognition, are considered.

Computer and Digital Media Access

Chapter 11 discusses access software for blind people (more specifically, screenreaders), explains how screenreaders work, and reviews some of the big challenges facing access software. Chapter 12 lays out the problems blind users face with inappropriately designed Web-based information and continues with the tools that can help Web designers and developers make their Web-based information more accessible for blind users. Chapter 13 starts with the history and scope of work of the Digital Accessible Information SYstem (DAISY) consortium. It then describes the different types of DAISY talking books and how to create accessible talking books. It closes with a discussion of accessible hardware and software that can be used to access DAISY talking books and files.

Education, Employment, Recreation

Chapter 14 discusses one of the most compelling problems for the education of blind children: teaching ad learning mathematics. Multiple technological solutions that stem from the baseline of Nemeth's extension to Braille are considered. Chapter 15 surveys existing work in the area of video game accessibility for users with visual impairments. It then discusses the specific barriers that users with visual impairments encounter when trying to play a video game and outlines several strategies to make video games accessible to users with visual impairments. Chapter 16 covers the state-of-the-art Description Video (DV) in North America and how DV is produced. It then reviews research done to understand this specific form of translation from visual cues to text and to find ways to assist the describers in making more effective DV for blind individuals.

Finally, Chapter 17 gives an account of the issues associated with employment for blind individuals. Assistive technology has a major role in providing access to jobs that would otherwise be denied to the community of the visually impaired. However, as discussed at length in the chapter, technology alone is not sufficient unless an adequate cultural, economical, and political infrastructure is in place to provide everyone with equal opportunities in the workplace.

2

Vision and Vision Rehabilitation

August Colenbrander

CONTENTS

Aspects of Vision Loss

Before discussing the use of Assistive Technology for vision loss, it is necessary to discuss the nature of vision itself and the consequences of vision loss.
Vision is by far our most powerful sense. The two eyes provide as much
input to the brain as all other senses combined. Although it is common to
think that we "see" with our eyes, most of the visual processing takes place
in the brain. Indeed, one hypothesis states that in the course of evolution
early brains may have evolved to process the input from primitive eyes (Ivan
Schwab 2011). An isolated eye cannot produce vision, but when we dream,
our brain can produce vivid visual images, without any input from the eyes.

    Vision is like a complex structure or sculpture, the essence of which cannot
be captured in a single snapshot; as we approach it from different points of

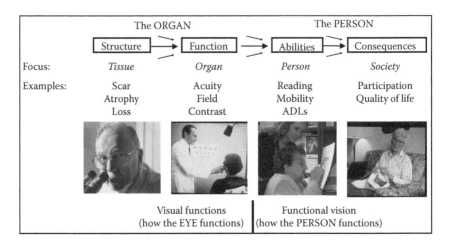

The ORGAN		The PERSON	
Structure ⟶	Function ⟶	Abilities ⟶	Consequences

Focus:	*Tissue*	*Organ*	*Person*	*Society*
Examples:	Scar	Acuity	Reading	Participation
	Atrophy	Field	Mobility	Quality of life
	Loss	Contrast	ADLs	

Visual functions (how the EYE functions)	Functional vision (how the PERSON functions)

FIGURE 2.1
A full discussion of vision loss requires consideration of many different aspects.

view, we may see very different aspects. To fully characterize vision, we must consider all of its aspects.

For this discussion, it is helpful to recognize four main aspects (Colenbrander 1977). Of these, two refer to the organ; two refer to the person as a whole, as shown in Figure 2.1.

As we proceed from left to right, the context in which we view each aspect widens, from the tissue, to the organ, to the person, and finally to the society in which that person functions.

- The first aspect is that of changes to the anatomical and structural integrity of the organ. Examples may include scarring, atrophy, or loss. We need a pathologist to study this aspect.

- Various structural changes may interact in their effect on the function of the organ. The next aspect therefore needs to describe how the *organ* functions. We need the clinician to measure various parameters, such as visual acuity, visual field, contrast sensitivity, and so on.

- Organ function alone, however, cannot adequately describe how the *person* functions. We need to consider the skills and abilities of the person. For this aspect, we want to measure the actual performance of Activities of Daily Living (ADLs). We need rehabilitation workers to help and train patients in various activities, such as reading and mobility.

- The last aspect places the person in a societal context and describes the societal and economic consequences of any functional deficits. Here we want to measure participation and Quality of Life and in economic terms: job loss or dependence on others.

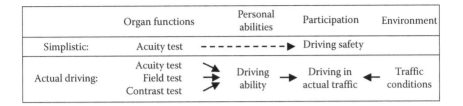

	Organ functions	Personal abilities	Participation	Environment
Simplistic:	Acuity test	- - - - - - - - - ▶	Driving safety	
Actual driving:	Acuity test Field test Contrast test	Driving ability	Driving in actual traffic	Traffic conditions

FIGURE 2.2
The degree of actual participation results from the interaction of many different aspects.

It should be clear that comprehensive rehabilitation cannot be the work of a single professional. To deal effectively with all aspects of rehabilitation we need a team, and the patient needs to be a part of that team.

These aspects can be applied to many health conditions. In the field of vision we will use the term *Visual Functions* to describe how the *eyes* and the visual system function; we will use the term *Functional Vision* to describe how the *person* functions in vision-related ADLs (Colenbrander 2003).

One practical example of the use of these aspects may be seen in Figure 2.2, where these aspects are applied to driving safety.

Most states and countries utilize a visual acuity test as an important criterion for obtaining a driver's license, but it is too simplistic to draw a straight line from visual acuity to driving safety. Factors such as visual acuity, visual field, and contrast affect the ability to drive. But so do many other factors that are less easily tested, such as attention and reaction speed. The safety of participation in actual traffic further depends on the interaction of driving ability with actual traffic conditions. The farther apart the aspects are, the less direct their interaction.

The four aspects are linked, but the links are not fixed. It is important to remember that how the eyes function does not automatically determine how the person will function. Helen Keller may serve as one example of how a person can function very well in society, even with total blindness and total deafness. The links are flexible, since various interventions can modify them. How this can work is shown in Figure 2.3.

Preventive interventions are aimed at preventing various external causes from causing damage. Their success can be measured in the absence of tissue damage.

Therapeutic interventions are aimed at preventing various organ changes from affecting organ function. They can range from the prescription of glasses to counteract refractive error to the surgical repair of a retinal detachment. Their success is measured in good organ function.

Rehabilitative interventions come into play when the preventive and therapeutic options have not been fully successful. They aim at restoring the abilities of the person, regardless of the level of organ function.

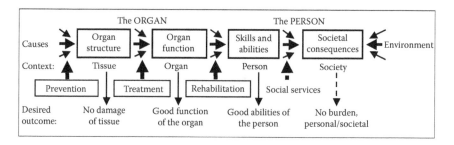

FIGURE 2.3
Different interventions affect different parts of the chain.

A final group of interventions is aimed at improving participation in society and at reducing the burden on the person, on the person's environment, and on society in general. These interventions are generally considered as social and public health services, rather than as medical ones. Providing a paraplegic individual with a wheelchair is the duty of the health care system; the provision of ramps and curb cuts to promote participation is a public health concern and the duty of the department of Public Works. Obviously, the two need to cooperate to assure the most effective solutions.

Ranges of Vision Loss

A term often used when discussing vision loss is the term *Blindness*. This term is confusing, since blindness is a black-and-white term. One is either blind or sighted; one cannot be "a little bit blind." The term blindness, therefore, should not be used for persons with residual vision. The most extreme example is the use of the term "color blindness" for even minor color vision deficiencies that can be detected only with special tests.

Actually, being blind and being normally sighted are the extremes of a continuous scale. Between these extremes is a large gray area, which is called *Low Vision*. The word "low" indicates that vision is less than normal; the word "vision" indicates that it is not blindness. Rather than using the dichotomy sighted/blind, we prefer to speak about *Ranges of Vision Loss* with modifiers, such as mild, moderate, severe, profound, and total, as is shown in Figure 2.4.

The visual acuity values in this table follow a logarithmic progression, as first advocated by John Green in 1868 (Green 1868), and now generally accepted since the National Eye Institute popularized it a century later by use on its ETDRS charts (Ferris et al. 1982). The ranges are those advocated in the ICD-9-CM classification (U.S. Public Health Service 1978).

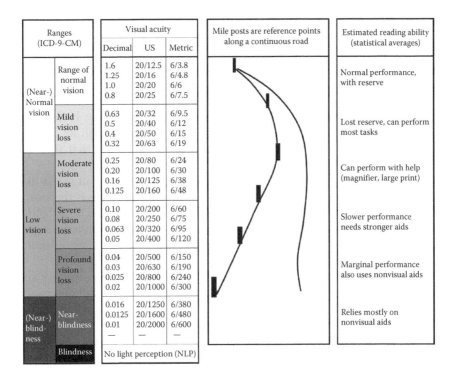

Ranges (ICD-9-CM)		Visual acuity			Mile posts are reference points along a continuous road	Estimated reading ability (statistical averages)
		Decimal	US	Metric		
(Near-) Normal vision	Range of normal vision	1.6 1.25 1.0 0.8	20/12.5 20/16 20/20 20/25	6/3.8 6/4.8 6/6 6/7.5		Normal performance, with reserve
	Mild vision loss	0.63 0.5 0.4 0.32	20/32 20/40 20/50 20/63	6/9.5 6/12 6/15 6/19		Lost reserve, can perform most tasks
Low vision	Moderate vision loss	0.25 0.20 0.16 0.125	20/80 20/100 20/125 20/160	6/24 6/30 6/38 6/48		Can perform with help (magnifier, large print)
	Severe vision loss	0.10 0.08 0.063 0.05	20/200 20/250 20/320 20/400	6/60 6/75 6/95 6/120		Slower performance needs stronger aids
	Profound vision loss	0.04 0.03 0.025 0.02	20/500 20/630 20/800 20/1000	6/150 6/190 6/240 6/300		Marginal performance also uses nonvisual aids
(Near-) blind-ness	Near-blindness	0.016 0.0125 0.01 —	20/1250 20/1600 20/2000 —	6/380 6/480 6/600 —		Relies mostly on nonvisual aids
	Blindness	No light perception (NLP)				

FIGURE 2.4
Ranges are like mileposts along a continuous road.

The *Range of Normal Vision* includes the reference standard for visual acuity (20/20), established by Snellen in 1862. Note that 20/20 does not indicate "perfect" or even average vision. Average visual acuity for young adults is one or two lines better than 20/20; average visual acuity drops with age and does not reach 20/20 until age 60 or 70 (Colenbrander 2011).

Also note that comfortable performance of daily living tasks requires an ability level where the task is "easy" and well above threshold. Only Olympic athletes perform at levels that are "just possible." Snellen described his 20/20 reference standard as a size that is "easily recognized" by normal eyes. In Figure 2.4, the distance in meters at which 1 M print (average newsprint) can be seen, can be read from the decimal visual acuity column. This shows that in the normal range average newsprint can be read at 1.6–0.8 m (160–80 cm, 60″ –32″), which leaves an ample margin for effortless performance of ADLs.

In the next range (*Mild Loss*) newsprint can be recognized at 60–30 cm (24″ –12″); this is still sufficient for most ADLs, but the reserve for small print is gone. Many other ability scales do not differentiate between these top two ranges; they start when tasks are "possible" or "not difficult." Tasks that are "easy" at the 20/20 level may reach the "possible" rating at 20/40. This may explain why 20/40 is often quoted as the level at which people start complaining.

For subjects in the range of *Moderate Loss* reading of newsprint requires an even shorter distance (25 –12 cm, 10" –5") and stronger than average reading glasses or the use of a magnifier. Note that 25 cm is the traditional reference point for the strength of magnifiers.

In the range of *Severe Loss* the reading distance becomes 10 cm (4") or less; this prevents binocular viewing and requires even stronger magnifiers. The smaller field of view of stronger magnifiers slows down reading. Note that in the US persons with 20/200 visual acuity are labeled "legally blind" and are eligible for various benefits. (The adjective "legal" indicates that the term "blind" is used improperly.)

In the range of *Profound Loss*, the reading distance for newsprint is less than 5 cm (2"); this makes visual reading performance marginal. This is the level at which the WHO and many European countries start using the term "blindness." Yet, people in this range are not blind; their residual vision is an important adjunct for mobility. In this range reading with a magnifier may be limited to spot reading; for recreational reading talking books may be preferred.

In the last range (*Near-blindness* and *Total Blindness*) the remaining visual acuity is insufficient for visually guided task performance; patients in this range must rely on nonvisual means (vision substitution), although any remaining vision can still serve as an adjunct.

Many ability scales also combine these lower ranges. This may be acceptable for eligibility criteria; for rehabilitation purposes the distinction is important. In the range of severe loss, the emphasis is still on vision enhancement, with vision substitution (Braille, long cane, talking books) as an occasional adjunct. In the range of profound loss, the emphasis shifts to vision substitution with use of residual vision as an adjunct. In the (near-)blindness range, the emphasis is entirely on vision substitution.

One should be aware that the sharp dividing lines in the table do not represent stepwise increments in visual ability. The numbers given are like mileposts along a continuous road. The landscape does not change suddenly when we pass a milepost; it changes gradually in between the mileposts. The listed reading abilities are estimates, based on statistical averages. The performance of any one individual may be better or worse than the statistical average.

Figure 2.5 gives examples from each of the ranges that were discussed. In this image the author demonstrates his 1-m acuity chart for low vision. In successive images the pixel count has been reduced to simulate different levels of visual acuity. Since the chart is part of the image, the visual acuity can be read from the picture. Note that different tasks with different details become difficult at different acuity levels. Reading the letter chart becomes harder in the top row. Counting the books in the book case becomes hard in the middle images. Not bumping into people becomes hard in the bottom images; yet, even 20/2000 visual acuity is not the same as total blindness (No Light Perception, NLP).

The unfortunate result of extending the term blindness to individuals with residual vision is that the emphasis is on the abilities that are lost (the glass is half empty), rather than on the abilities that are retained (the glass is half full);

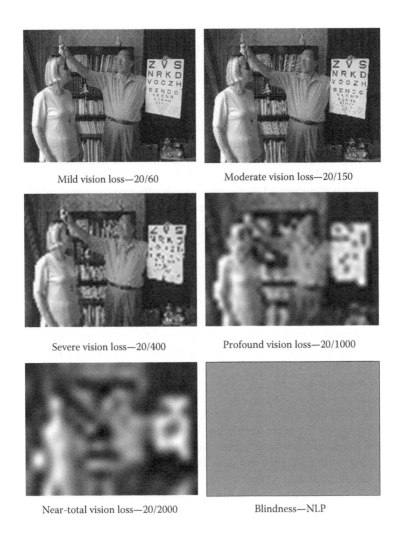

Mild vision loss—20/60   Moderate vision loss—20/150

Severe vision loss—20/400   Profound vision loss—20/1000

Near-total vision loss—20/2000   Blindness—NLP

FIGURE 2.5
Vision loss is a continuum, not a dichotomy between blind and sighted.

many believe that once a person has been declared "blind" there is *nothing more that can be done*. The reality is that only 10% of those who are labeled "legally blind" are actually blind; 90% have residual vision that can be used with appropriate aids.

The International Council of Ophthalmology (ICO) has proposed function-based definitions (International Council of Ophthalmology 2002):

> LOW VISION is to be used for those subjects who have residual vision, the use of which can be enhanced with appropriate *vision enhancement* aids.

BLINDNESS is to be used for those subjects who have no residual vision or so little residual vision that they must predominantly rely on *vision substitution* aids.

Although it may not be possible to change the anatomical or structural deficit, there is a lot that can be done to improve the person's Quality of Life. This requires attention to all of the aspects mentioned earlier. When designing technological solutions, the natural (and necessary) focus of the engineers will be on the technological aspects (the left side of the diagram). For a solution to be viable, however, the solution must also fit with human and ergonomic considerations. User acceptance is often more based on the ergonomic placement of knobs and switches than on the technology itself.

Vision Rehabilitation

Rehabilitation is the process of restoring normal functioning or of bringing a person as close as possible to that state. For children with congenital defects, the term *habilitation* is often used, since there was no prior normal functioning. In this book, the mention of rehabilitation will include habilitation, wherever appropriate.

In a broad sense, preventive care and medical or surgical interventions (the left side of the diagram) may be considered as leading up to rehabilitation. Usually, however, the term rehabilitation is used to refer only to the right side of the diagram, that is, to interactions that improve functioning beyond what is achievable with medical or surgical care.

In the development of vision rehabilitation, most attention has traditionally been given to the eye and its optics. Accordingly, traditional Low Vision Care deals primarily with magnification devices, illumination, and contrast. Figure 2.6 shows that comprehensive vision rehabilitation involves much more than the enhancement of strictly visual abilities.

Vision enhancement is the domain of traditional Low Vision care. Magnifiers of various kinds are the most obvious visual aids. Additionally, illumination and filters need to be explored. Details are discussed in Chapter 4 on Low Vision.

Vision substitution refers to the use of senses other than vision. Common examples include the use of Braille, a long cane, and of talking books and voice-output devices. Vision enhancement and vision substitution are not mutually exclusive. A patient may use a magnifier to read price tags, but may prefer talking books for recreational reading. A *Retinitis Pigmentosa* (RP) patient (with limited side vision and limited dark adaptation), who has normal mobility in the daytime, may need a cane (vision substitution) and/or a strong flashlight (vision enhancement) at night.

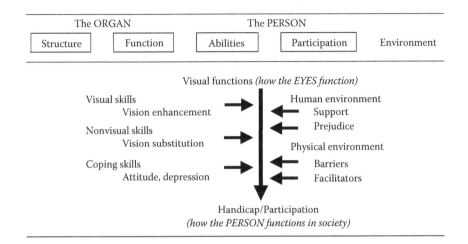

FIGURE 2.6
Comprehensive rehabilitation requires attention to many different aspects.

A special form of vision substitution involves using the eyes of others. Family members and caregivers should be trained to effectively assist visually impaired patients with minimal embarrassment. *Guide dogs* are also a possibility. Working as a team requires training of the dog as well as of the patient.

Coping skills also require our attention. Vision loss often causes a reactive depression. On the one hand, a depressed patient will be less receptive to rehabilitative suggestions. On the other hand, demonstration of rehabilitative success can be a powerful tool to lift a reactive depression and to motivate the patient for further success.

With regard to the *human environment*, an overprotective environment that deprives patients of opportunities to do things for themselves can be as detrimental as an overdemanding one that puts too much emphasis on the patient's shortcomings.

Finally, the *physical environment* needs to be considered. Good illumination of an uncluttered environment can facilitate visual functioning; poor contrast, such as when serving milk in a Styrofoam cup can be a barrier. Chapter 4 on Low Vision will discuss many of these factors.

From this listing it should be clear that successful rehabilitation needs to consider not only the "input," that is, vision itself, but also the "output," that is, perception, visually guided behavior and behavior guided by other inputs, as in vision substitution. All of these aspects contribute to optimal participation; none of them can be considered in isolation.

A simple technological example may illustrate the importance of human factors. Newer technology has facilitated the introduction of small handheld video-magnifiers. Early models had the camera next to the screen; newer models have the camera centered underneath the screen. The technology is the same, but the simple change of centering the camera made their use much more ergonomic and intuitive.

Stages of Visual Processing

Of all the factors mentioned, we must first concentrate on vision itself. The process that takes us from an object to the visual perception of that object has three distinct stages. Each stage may present its own distinct problems.

- The *optical stage* involves the optical apparatus of the eye. It should result in a clear image of the environment on the retina.
- The *retinal receptor stage* converts the light energy of the optical image into a pattern of neural impulses, which are transmitted to the brain through the optic nerve.
- *Neural processing* analyzes these impulses and leads to a perception, which eventually leads to visually guided performance. Early processing starts in the inner retina; higher order processing occurs in a wide variety of brain areas.

Stage 1: The Optical Stage

The main optical elements of the eye are the cornea and the crystalline lens. The cornea provides the larger part of the refractive power; its contribution is fixed. The crystalline lens provides a smaller, but variable, part. If their focus is not exactly on the retina, we speak of *refractive error*. The most common forms of refractive error are myopia, hyperopia, and astigmatism. A related condition is *presbyopia*.

Clinical Manifestations

In *myopia* the refractive power is too strong for the axial length of the eye, so that the image of a distant object falls in front of the retina. Only objects that are close are focused properly; hence the term near-sightedness. The correction is with a spectacle or contact lens of negative power. The degree of myopia is indicated by the dioptric power of the correcting lens. A –3 D myope needs a –3 D lens; without that lens the eye will be focused at 1/3 m (33 cm, 13″). A more technologically advanced way of correction is the surgical sculpting of the corneal surface with laser technology, as in LASIK and similar procedures.

In *hyperopia* the refractive power is too weak or the axial length is too short. Correction requires positive lenses. Young individuals with moderate hyperopia can provide compensation by accommodating, but this becomes more difficult as they get older (presbyopia).

In *astigmatism* the refractive power is not the same in all meridians. So it may be that when vertical lines are in focus, horizontal lines are not. The correction requires cylindrical or toric lenses.

Added to the basic refractive error is *accommodation*. This refers to the variable amount of power provided by the crystalline lens. As the lens gets older, its flexibility is reduced and its accommodative power is diminished. Young children may accommodate up to 10 D; a 40-year old may have only 3 D left. At 65 almost no accommodation is left. When the amount of accommodation is insufficient for a normal reading distance, we speak of *presbyopia*. Presbyopia requires correction with a reading addition (add). This can take the form of reading glasses (near vision only), bifocal lenses (near and distance focus), or progressive lenses (the focus changes continuously across the lens).

If the optical media of the eye are not optimally clear, light will be *scattered*. This will also result in a blurring across the entire image (Figure 2.8). The most common problem is a cataract (a partial or complete opacification of the lens). Today, the common solution is to replace the clouded natural lens with a clear artificial one. Most Intra-Ocular Lenses (IOLs) have only a single focus, so the patient has no accommodation (is completely presbyopic). Considerable technological efforts are being devoted to the design of accommodating or multifocal IOLs; however, to-date, no design can yet match the full amount of normal accommodation.

Visual Acuity

Whatever the optical problem is, the *sharpness* or "acuteness" of the retinal image is referred to as *visual acuity*. Clinical visual acuity is measured with a letter chart, as introduced by Snellen in 1862. Snellen defined as a reference standard (20/20) the ability to recognize letters that subtend 5 min of arc. If a subject needs letters that are twice as large, the MAgnification Requirement (MAR) is 2× and the Visual Acuity (VA) is said to be 1/2; if the MAR is 5×, the VA is 1/5; if MAR = 10×, VA = 1/10, and so on. This visual acuity value can be expressed in different ways. In the United States it is customary to standardize the numerator to 20, so that 1/2 = 20/40, 1/5 = 20/100, 1/10 = 20/200, and so on. In Europe decimal notation is common: 1/2 = 0.5, 1/5 = 0.2, 1/10 = 0.1, and so on. In Britain and former dominions (India, Australia) the common notation is: 1/2 = 6/12, 1/5 = 6/30, 1/10 = 6/60, and so on.

Originally, Snellen required that the numerator of the "Snellen fraction" reflected the actual testing distance; thus 20/... could only be used at 20 ft; at 18 ft the notation would be 18/.... Today, the standardized 20/20 "Snellen equivalent" notation has replaced the use of true Snellen fractions.

If a blurred image cannot be sharpened optically, the best solution is magnification. Clinicians estimate the required magnification using Kestenbaum's rule, which states that the magnification should be at least the reciprocal of the visual acuity value; this is a direct application of the formula: VA = 1/MAR or MAR = 1/VA as discussed earlier.

When testing optical lenses, the term MAR is often explained as *Minimum Angle of Resolution*; in the context of vision rehabilitation the interpretation as *MAgnification Requirement* is more appropriate.

Letter chart acuity measures only the performance of the small retinal area where the letter is projected; that is adequate for optical problems, since defocus of one area predicts equal defocus of other areas.

Stage 2: Retinal Receptors

At the retinal receptor level an entirely different set of conditions prevails. First of all, the receptor mosaic (rods and cones) in the retina is not homogeneous. The density is highest in the center (the fovea) and diminishes toward the periphery. This allows a more effective use of the receptors, since the high foveal density does not need to be maintained over the entire retina. However, it necessitates a complex oculo-motor system to always direct the fovea toward the object of regard. The function of the retinal periphery is to *detect* changes and to initiate an eye movement for fixation; the function of the center is to examine the area of interest and to *recognize* what it represents. This means that at the retinal level the topography of the functional losses, which was unimportant for optical problems, becomes very important. This topography is studied with *visual field tests*.

Clinical Manifestations

Peripheral field loss interferes with the detection of obstacles. Its primary functional effect is in Orientation and Mobility. To a limited degree compensation is possible with prisms (a technical solution) that deflect the image to a sighted part of the retina, but mostly compensation must come from *training* and *practice*, teaching the patient to make more frequent eye movements to the nonseeing area.

When the loss is severe, scanning alone may not be sufficient and the use of other senses may be needed. This can include the use of touch, as in a long cane, and/or the use of hearing to listen to traffic. Another solution is the use of another pair of eyes, either the eyes of a guide dog or the eyes of a sighted guide. Finally, there are hi-tech solutions where a computer-guided scanner presents an auditory or other warning when an obstacle is detected. One of the problems with these devices is that the auditory (or other) signal must not interfere with normal hearing and that the presentation must be so intuitive that its interpretation does not detract attention from other tasks. Thus, the human engineering aspects will be at least as challenging as the technical aspects.

Central loss can be of several types. Retinal changes are rarely diffuse; usually there are areas where the function is relatively good and other areas where it is worse. This means that adequate knowledge of the topography is essential for the design of the proper remedies.

When vision is lost in a limited area, we speak of a *scotoma* or blind spot. Scotomata may be *absolute* or *relative*. In a relative scotoma the sensitivity is reduced, but not absent. When given enough light, the cells in such areas can still contribute; with less light they fall silent. These are the cases where increased illumination can be most helpful.

A *Central Scotoma* is a scotoma that covers the original point of fixation (the fovea). The result is that when the detection of an object in the periphery elicits an eye movement to bring that object to the fovea, the object will disappear. In this situation the best way to see an object is to look past it, so that it can be seen beyond the edge of the scotoma. This is called *eccentric viewing*. Since the image now falls on a retinal area with a less dense receptor mosaic, the image will be less detailed; this effect can be countered by magnification.

Equally important, however, is that effective eccentric viewing requires a recalibration of the oculo-motor system. This recalibration cannot be done by any device, but is dependent on *practice* and *training*. When left to their own devices all patients will develop a new center of fixation, which is known as a *Preferred Retinal Locus* (PRL) (Fletcher et al. 1999). It has also been shown that they can be trained to adopt a different locus, a *Trained Retinal Locus* (TRL), which can sometimes be more effective than the spontaneously chosen PRL (Watson et al. 2006).

Para-central scotomata are areas of reduced or absent sensitivity outside the fovea. The central area of the retina is known as the macula; it covers about a 15^0 radius around the fovea, which has only a 1^0 radius. Since the macular area is the most highly developed area, it is also most at risk of deterioration. The best known condition is *Age-related Macular Degeneration* (AMD), which, due to an aging population, is the most frequent cause of vision loss in developed countries. This loss does not develop evenly and does not need to start in the very center. The result may be a central island of vision, surrounded by scotomatous areas. When this happens, a patient may be able to recognize a letter, but cannot recognize a word. Thus reading acuity will be much worse than letter chart acuity. An example is shown in Figure 2.7, where the word "wonderful" is projected on the retina; the small central island can only recognize one letter at a time.

For these patients reading of small print may be paradoxically easier than reading of headline print. In cases like these, *practice* and *training* will again be more important than magnification. Even minification can sometimes be helpful to fit the word into the remaining central area. Sometimes, using a more eccentric area combined with higher magnification may be effective.

A variety of retinal disorders can interfere with normal visual performance. As mentioned, AMD affects only the macula, never the periphery. So patients with AMD will never go blind (although they may qualify for "legal blindness" benefits). Their orientation and mobility (O&M) performance may be adequate, but because of their central loss reading will be severely affected. In developed countries with an aging population AMD is the single most common cause of vision loss.

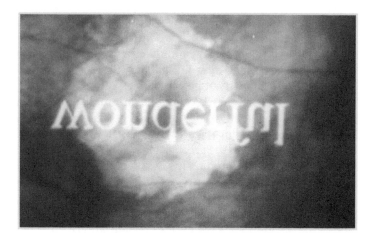

FIGURE 2.7
A ring scotoma may allow recognition of letters, but not of words. (Scanning laser ophthalmo-scope image, courtesy of Donald C. Fletcher, MD.)

Patients with *glaucoma*—another disease that is more common in older individuals—experience just the opposite. Glaucoma affects primarily peripheral vision; central vision is usually spared until late in the disease. These patients may experience O&M (Orientation and Mobility) problems, long before they experience reading problems. Since reading ability is maintained, glaucoma is often detected too late, so screening programs are very important.

Similar peripheral problems exist in *Retinitis Pigmentosa* (RP). This is a much rarer hereditary condition with different rates of progression in different variants. RP patients also have night vision problems.

As obesity is an increasing problem in developed and developing countries alike, so is the accompanying diabetes and *Diabetic Retinopathy*. It is the most important cause of vision loss among adults. Since the disease can affect the entire retina, it may present with central as well as peripheral losses. There may be scattered blind spots across the entire retina.

Figure 2.8 provides images that try to simulate these conditions. They are useful as reminders of the type of condition. However, still pictures cannot properly represent how patients see the world. Since the eyes are constantly moving, the blind spots are not stationary. Patients are aware that they see less detail, but they rarely experience this as discrete blind spots (Fletcher 2011).

Stage 3: Neural Processing

Once the optical image has been converted to neural impulses, the most important part of visual processing starts. This processing starts right in the inner layers of the retina.

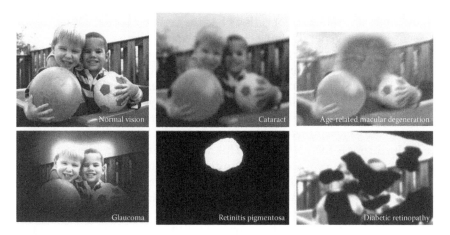

FIGURE 2.8
These images are not realistic, since they do not show the effect of eye movements. (Pictures courtesy of the National Eye Institute.)

At this point it is important to recall the structure of the eyeball. The outer support structure of the eyeball is the *sclera*; inside the sclera is the *choroid*, a vascular layer (not shown in Figure 2.9) which provides nutrition for the retinal receptors. Inside the choroid is the *retina*, which in embryology originates as an outpouching of the brain. The structure of the retina reflects its

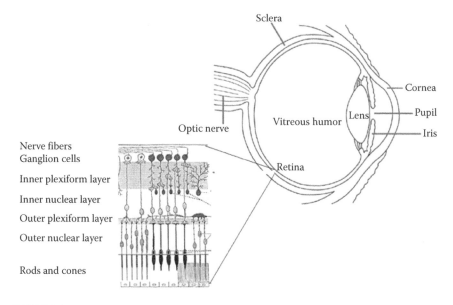

FIGURE 2.9
The retina already provides significant preprocessing of the retinal image.

origin; it has several layers of cells as has the cerebral cortex. Other peripheral sense organs generally have only one layer of cells.

Outermost in the retina are the *receptor cells*, the rods and cones. To allow for a dense packing of the rods and cones, the nuclei of their cells are in a separate layer, the *outer nuclear layer*. Inside that layer is a layer of nerve fibers, the *outer plexiform layer*, followed by another cell layer, the *inner nuclear layer*, and another layer of nerve fibers, the *inner plexiform layer*. These fibers finally connect to the *ganglion cell layer*, the nerve fibers of which will proceed toward the brain through the *optic nerve*. This whole structure is at most 0.5 mm thick; yet it already provides for a significant amount of processing.

Each eye has over 100 million receptors, but the optic nerve has only about 1 million nerve fibers. Thus, intraretinal processing must provide a 100:1 data compression. We know that there are some 60 different cell types in the various retinal layers, including some 20 different ganglion cells, but we have very limited knowledge about how the retinal information is actually coded (Masland 2011).

It is unlikely that the optic nerve conveys a pixel-by-pixel bitmap of the retinal image to recreate the same map in the visual cortex in the way a computer conveys an image to a monitor or to a printer. It is more likely that some nerve fibers convey information about edges, others about color and brightness and still others about movement and other parameters. This would be consistent with the need for data compression and with the general organization of the brain, where different attributes are often processed in parallel, rather than serially as in a computer.

One process, which probably takes place in the inner retina, is edge detection. While movement of the image across the pixel array of a digital camera results in a blurred image, this is not true for the retina. Indeed, experiments have shown that when the image position on the retina is completely fixed, perception quickly fades. Because of body and eye movements the retinal image is constantly moving; even when subjects try to stabilize their eyes, there are small micro-saccades, which sweep all image elements back and forth across several receptors. This provides a perfect mechanism for edge detection and also for data reduction. Receptors that are part of an even surface, or of a surface with a minimal gradient, will not signal change, but receptors under an edge will signal significant change. That edges are important for perception is evident from the fact that even young children can recognize line drawings, which reduce the complex information from a natural scene to edge information only. The static pictures of scotomata (Figure 2.8) that are often seen in the literature are misleading, because patients rarely "see" their scotomata. Since scotomatous areas provide no information at all, the brain is not aware of any edges and simply assumes that the area is filled with the same pattern or content as the surrounding area.

Other detectors will convey other parameters. It should be noted that motion detectors, whether in the retina or in the visual cortex, must be tuned to detect relative rather than absolute motion. During the relative quiet of a fixation, edges that move relative to their background draw our attention. During an eye movement all edges move, so nothing stands out.

As the information proceeds toward the brain, it initially maintains the topographic organization it had in the retina. We indicate this by saying that these cortical areas are *retinotopically* organized. In accordance with the principle of parallel processing in the brain, there are several retinotopically organized areas in the visual cortex; they probably perform different analyses in parallel. As the signals proceed to higher centers, the retinotopic organization is replaced with an organization that reflects perceptual concepts and ultimately intended actions. As this happens, the number of concepts is reduced, but their content increases. Consider looking at a picture of the house you grew up in; what started out as a 100 Mpixel retinal image, is reduced to 1 MB in the optic nerve and ends up as a single concept "my old house" that is connected to an enormous web of information and memories, almost all of which is not part of the picture you looked at.

What happens on this path is not a single, one-way connection. Electro-Encephalo-Graphic (ECG) recordings have shown that there is a constant interaction of top-down and bottom-up signals along a multitude of connections. Indeed, it has been suggested that these interactive streams are more characteristic of conscious awareness than is the mere location of active areas.

The advent of fMRI (functional Magnetic Resonance Imaging) has given us more insight into the location of various centers. Yet, our insights may be compared to looking at a government building at night. The lighted windows may indicate that the Africa desk is more active than the Asia desk, but we still do not know the details of the discussions (the activity of individual cells) behind each of these windows. We would have more information if we also knew the pattern of the telephone calls that go back and forth between the lighted offices.

One thing has become clear, namely that the higher cerebral functions are not just located in single brain areas. Most complex functions involve multiple interconnected areas in different regions of the brain. In the field of vision, a distinction has been made between the *dorsal stream* and the *ventral stream* (Goodale and Westwood 2004). The dorsal stream has been identified as *vision for action*; it works fast and mostly subconsciously and does not require memory. For instance: when asked to pick up an object, our hand will automatically open just wide enough and in the right orientation to grasp it; when walking, we place our feet reliably, without being consciously aware of every step. The ventral stream serves *vision for perception*; it does not work as fast, but the result is conscious perception and recognition of the object. The ventral stream also processes more details and connects them to stored memories. Patients with a lesion in the ventral stream may not be able to recognize an object, but may grasp it effortlessly. Yet, in normal operation the two streams do not operate independently; their actions are perfectly coordinated.

In this regard the remarkable flexibility of the brain should also be mentioned. It has been found that when the blind read Braille, areas of the "visual" cortex are activated. The question needs to be asked whether this represents a cortical "reorganization" from visual to tactile stimuli, or whether these areas are actually pattern recognition areas that are used for visual pattern recognition when visual stimuli abound, but in the absence of visual stimuli can be used for tactile pattern recognition.

The Mental Model

All of this makes it clear that visually guided action is not based directly on the content of the retinal image. There is an intermediary stage which we call the Mental Model of the environment.

The retinal image triggers and updates the mental model, but there are many important differences. The retinal image is constantly shifting; the mental model is stable. The retinal image is eye-centered; the mental model is anchored in the environment. When we walk around, we do not perceive the image of the environment moving across our retina, like the image in a moving video camera. Instead, we experience ourselves moving through a stable environment. The retinal image is made up of 2-dimensional images; the mental model is filled with 3-dimensional objects. Awareness of a third dimension is only added when the images from the two eyes are compared in the visual cortex. The retinal image is purely visual; the mental model incorporates input from other senses. Even the blind have a mental image of their environment. The mental model incorporates memory; that our perception of the room around us is sharp in all directions, is only because the mental model is stitched together from the memory of many previous fixations. The retinal image ends at the edge of our visual field and has gaps where there are scotomata; the mental model of our environment has no gaps and extends even behind us.

Clinical Manifestations

In the last decades vision problems that originate in the brain have increasingly asked our attention and will continue to do so for years to come. Such problems may arise from a variety of sources.

Strokes and *tumors* may cause localized lesions in the elderly. Depending on the location they may cause specific deficits that are generally known as *agnosias*, indicating the failure to recognize certain objects. Agnosias resulting from localized loss of previously established functions can sometimes be very specific, for instance failure to recognize numbers, but not letters.

Veterans from recent wars have drawn our attention to *traumatic brain injury* (TBI), which is often the result of severe concussions caused by Improvised Explosive Devices (IEDs). In previous wars IEDs were not as widely used and brain injuries were mainly caused by penetrating shrapnel. Today, vision problems are more common among veterans than amputations. Often the symptoms include problems with oculo-motor coordination. Symptoms may or may not include visual acuity loss; visual field problems may include actual field loss such as hemianopia, and/or *visual neglect*, indicating the failure to pay attention to part of the environment. Now that these symptoms have been recognized in veterans, the awareness of their existence has also increased for persons involved in car accidents or in contact sports, such as boxing and football. TBI is only one group within the broader category of *acquired brain injury* (ABI), which includes other causes such as stroke, tumors, and inflammations. The lesions from TBI are often diffuse and therefore more difficult to pinpoint than those of a localized stroke.

Today, as more premature infants are kept alive, *Cerebral Visual Impairment* (CVI) has become the most frequent cause of vision problems in newborns and infants. The abbreviation CVI is sometimes interpreted as Cortical Visual Impairment, but this term is too restrictive, since the lesions are often sub-cortical. The causes of CVI can be multiple, but often include birth-related ischemic incidents, which, again, may cause diffuse damage. The term CVI may be used if the results include a loss of visual acuity or visual field; the term *Cerebral Visual Dysfunction* (CVD) may be used when the visual information is processed inappropriately. In this case agnosias may exist, not because the function was lost, but because it never developed properly. This may include such problems as *simultan-agnosia* (inability to recognize objects that are close together, resulting in behavioral problems in a crowded environment) and *prosop-agnosia* (inability to recognize faces and/or facial expressions).

Distinguishing the symptoms of ocular visual impairment from those of cerebral visual impairment is important for rehabilitation, since the needed remedies are quite different. When a patient stumbles over a curb or a step because of poor contrast, vision enhancement (better lighting or a contrasting strip) may solve the problem. When a patient with CVI cannot decide whether a clearly visible line is a step or just a line on the ground, vision substitution (a workaround using other senses, such as a cane to feel the step) may be more appropriate.

Technological Implications

Knowledge of the complexity of the neural processing of visual information is important for the design of technological solutions that aim at replacing some of these steps. One area of current interest is the design of retinal implants for severe retinal degenerations. The aim is to replace the function of the retinal receptors by electrical stimulation. Some researchers design implants for subretinal placement; these implants replace only the receptor layer and can take advantage of whatever is left of the intraretinal circuitry. Others place their implants on top of the retina to stimulate the retinal ganglion cells directly; this solution bypasses the intraretinal processing. Still others try to stimulate the brain directly; they bypass even more preprocessing. Since different aspects of vision may be processed in different brain areas, stimulating in only one brain area also runs the risk of missing some aspects of the visual experience.

Some systems work with an external camera, which presents a stationary image to the retina. We saw earlier that the retinal image moves with each eye movement, but that the brain compensates for this movement. Conversely, when an eye movement does not cause image movement, the brain will interpret this as a movement of the object. Therefore, whatever form of external camera is used, the subject must learn to suppress all involuntary scanning eye movements and to scan only with voluntary camera movements. This requires more attentional resources, as discussed later.

Another problem arises from the fact that adjacent cells in the inner retina may process different visual attributes. Electrodes inevitably stimulate several cells at the same time, which may send confusing signals to the brain.

Figure 2.10 summarizes various problems we have discussed and the options for vision enhancement. It is clear that one size does not fit all.

Problems (Causes)	Effect	Vision enhancement options
Optical stage		
Refractive error (myopia, hyperopia, astigmatism)	Blurred retinal image	Magnification Refractive correction
Scatter (cataract, cornea opacities, vitreous opacities)	Blurred retinal image	Magnification
Receptor stage		
Peripheral field loss (glaucoma, RP, detachment)	Mobility problems	Training (travel skills, cane, guide dog)
Central scotoma (AMD)	Eccentric viewing	Magnification to compensate for reduced resolution. Training—to recalibrate the oculo-motor system
Central sensitivity loss	Contrast problems	Illumination, Environmental modifications
Para-central scotomata	Reading, scanning problems	Training (scanning skills)
Neural processing		
Inner retina (glaucoma)	Peripheral field loss	Training
Visual cortex, pathways	Cerebral visual impairment (with acuity, visual field loss)	Training, magnification
Higher cerebral centers	Cerebral visual dysfunction (no acuity, visual field loss)	Training

FIGURE 2.10
Different problems at different stages may require very different solutions. Note that various problems may coexist; for instance: cerebral visual impairment (lower centers) does not preclude cerebral visual dysfunction (higher centers) or vice versa.

Vision Substitution

So far we have discussed how residual vision can be enhanced. Another option is to use *vision substitution*. Vision substitution refers to the use of sensory systems other than vision to perform tasks that are usually performed using vision. Most prominent are the use of auditory and tactile input.

Talking books and voice output devices, although technologically complex, are simple at the perceptual level, since they use the auditory channels without any modification.

Reading Braille requires a new skill of recognizing Braille characters, but once this has been achieved, the speech and language systems process this information much like they process visually recognized characters.

A long cane serves as an extension of the arm. A remarkable aspect is that the user actually "feels" what is at the tip of the cane and does not need to go through a conscious conversion process. This is a normal feature of the tactile system; tennis players similarly experience their racquet as an extension of their bodily awareness. A long cane is a useful device, because the input is so intuitive. Listening to a beep and converting that to awareness of the presence and distance of an obstacle requires a more conscious conversion effort and more attentional resources.

Vision enhancement and vision substitution are not mutually exclusive. Computer users may use a screen magnifier for vision enhancement and a screen reader for vision substitution; sometimes they may use both simultaneously (see Chapter 11).

One problem for vision substitution is that the capacity of the visual channel is many times larger than the capacity of the auditory and tactile channels. Therefore, converting all potential visual input to auditory or tactile stimuli will quickly overwhelm those channels and hinder their regular use. This poses a challenge that is unrelated to the nature of vision itself, namely, how to filter the information so that only the most useful elements are presented. Under normal circumstances, the brain does a lot of this filtering before the stimuli enter into consciousness. One example is the well-known movie in which people who are asked to count how many times a ball bounces are completely unaware of a gorilla walking by in the background (Simons and Chabris 1999). This filtering is a function of attention, not of the visual stimulus. Two people, who are looking at the same scene with different interests, may filter the information differently. For example, one may follow the bouncing ball, while the other watches the background.

Unfortunately, the human brain has a limited amount of attentional resources, and those resources are shared across sensory modalities. When we perform a visual field test while asking the subject to simultaneously do a mental or auditory task, the field limits are narrower than when there is no additional task. A practical example may be that a GPS navigator with voice output promotes driving safety, because drivers do not need to take their eyes off the road. However, when carrying on a cell phone conversation, the larger amount of auditory input reduces safety, because attention is taken away from the driving task.

A special group of vision substitution systems combines features of two sensory systems by artificially projecting the structure of the retinal image to the tactile sense, originally to the skin (White et al. 1970), more recently to the tongue (Bach-y-Rita 2005). Those systems face a special challenge in that the tactile, kinesthetic perception of space is quite different from the retinal, visual perception. In the tactile domain a square is a square, no matter where it is or in what position. In the visual domain a square is a square, only when seen straight on. The visual size of the square changes with the viewing distance and when its angle changes, its shape becomes an irregular form, whose deformation may then be interpreted as a 3D spatial cue. To teach the tactile sense to process stimuli in the same way requires a considerable amount of training and practice.

Chapter 8 offers an extended discussion of the potential as well as the challenges and pitfalls of trying to substitute one sensory system for another.

We mentioned earlier that the ergonomic design of devices (placement of knobs and controls) is at least as important for general acceptance as are their technical capabilities. An intuitive design lessens the amount of attention needed to manipulate the device, thus increasing the amount of attention available for the task. High power magnifiers are usually stand magnifiers, to avoid the use of attention to keep the lens focused. It is sometimes thought that the blind have sharper hearing; the truth is that they have more attention available for auditory stimuli.

Related to the ergonomic design is the willingness to accept a device. Some people do not want to draw attention to their problem; hearing aid makers strive to make their devices as invisible as possible. Others wear dark glasses to alert others to the fact that they may have a vision problem. What may be acceptable for one person or one situation may not be acceptable for another person or for another situation. As a group, developers of technological solutions are at risk of overlooking such psychological problems.

Summary

Vision problems can have many causes and diverse consequences (see Figure 2.10). To provide effective vision rehabilitation one must not only pay attention to how the EYES function, but also to how the PERSON functions. Solutions often involve as much training and practice as they involve technology.

References

Bach-y-Rita, P. 2005. Emerging concepts of brain function. *Journal of Integrative Neuroscience*, 4:183–205.

Colenbrander, A. 1977. Dimensions of visual performance. In *Low Vision Symposium, American Academy of Ophthalmology, Transactions AAOO*, 83:332–337.

Colenbrander, A. 2003. Aspects of vision loss—Visual functions and functional vision. *Visual Impairment Research*, 5(3):115–136.

Colenbrander, A. 2011. Measuring vision and vision loss. Vol. 5, Chapter 51. In Tasman, W. and Jaeger, E.A. (eds.), *Duane's Clinical Ophthalmology* (updated and expanded in 2011 edition). Duane's Ophthalmology on CD-ROM. Lippincott, Williams and Williams, PA, USA.

Ferris, F.L., Kassov, A., Bresnick, G.H., and Bailey, I. 1982. New visual acuity charts for clinical research. *American Journal of Ophthalmology*, 94:91–96.

Fletcher, D.C., Schuchard, R.A., and Watson, G. 1999. Relative locations of macular scotomas near the PRL: Effect on low vision reading. *Journal of Rehabilitation Research and Development*, 36:4.

Fletcher, D.C. 2011. Patient awareness of binocular central visual field defects in age related macular degeneration (AMD). *ARVO 2011*, poster # 4236.

Goodale, M.A. and Westwood, D.A. 2004. An evolving view of duplex vision: Separate but interacting cortical pathways for perception and action. *Current Opinion in Neurobiology*, 14:203–211.

Green, J. 1868. On a new series of test-letters for determining the acuteness of vision. *Transact. Amer. Opth. Soc. 4th Meeting*, pp. 68–71.

International Council of Ophthalmology. 2002. Visual standards, aspects and ranges of vision loss with emphasis on population surveys. Available at http://www.icoph.org/standards.

Ivan Schwab, I.R. 2011. *Evolution's Witness: How Eyes Evolved*. Oxford University Press, USA.

Masland, R.H. 2011. Cell populations of the retina: The Proctor Lecture. *Investigative Ophthalmology & Visual Science*, 52:4581–4591.

Simons, D. and Chabris, C. 1999. *Selective attention test*. Available at http://www.youtube.com/watch?v=vJG698U2Mvo.

U.S. Public Health Service. 1978. *International Classification of Diseases*, 9th Revision—Clinical Modification (ICD-9-CM). Commission on Professional and Hospital Activities, Ann Arbor, MI.

Watson, G.R., Schuchard, R.A., De l'Aune W.R., and Watkins, E. 2006. Effects of preferred retinal locus placement on text navigation and development of advantageous trained retinal locus. *Journal of Rehabilitation Research and Development*, 43:761–770.

White, B.W., Saunders, F.A., Scadden, L., Bach-Y-Rita, P., and Collins, C.C. 1970. Seeing with the skin. *Perception & Psychophysics*, 7(1):23–27.

3

Orientation and Mobility

William H. Jacobson

CONTENTS

Introduction

Reverend Thomas J. Carroll noted in his seminal text, *Blindness: What It Is, What It Does and How To Live With It*, that "The loss of Mobility is perhaps the greatest of all the reality losses of blindness; it intensifies what might be considered the other great loss, that of social adequacy, both in its reality and its emotional aspects. Restoring mobility to the extent needed for normal life and work is necessarily one of the major objectives of a rehabilitation program, and modern developments have at last made it possible to achieve this objective" (Carroll 1961, p. 134). Since the publication of that text the profession of Orientation and Mobility instruction has emerged, which addresses how individuals who are blind or visually impaired can safely and efficiently travel in simple and complex environments. In this chapter we will learn who provides this expertise, how it is provided, and what are the special considerations that need to be addressed in order for individuals who are blind or visually impaired to travel effectively.

What is Orientation and Mobility?

The process of knowing where one is in space at any given moment in time is, for our purposes here, defined as *orientation* (Jacobson 1993). For a person who is blind or visually impaired this may mean knowing that one is standing in a hallway. For another, it may mean that one is standing in a hallway and facing north. Yet for another, it may mean that one is standing in a hallway, facing north, and is next to a water fountain. For a blind or visually impaired traveler, the preciseness of exacting one's location can mean the difference between being oriented and being lost. For such a traveler, as little as being one inch away from a tactile clue can cause disorientation. Further, orientation is necessary for purposeful movement. *Mobility*, then, can be defined as "the capacity or facility of movement" (Jacobson 1993, p. 3). One must have a need to move. The term, *Orientation and Mobility*, is generally defined as "the teaching of concepts, skills, and techniques necessary for a person with a visual impairment to travel safely, efficiently, and gracefully through any environment and under all environmental conditions and situations" (Jacobson 1993, p. 3). Hereafter, when the term, Orientation and Mobility (O&M), is used with capital letters, it will signify the teaching of the skill-set by a highly qualified professional Orientation and Mobility Specialist (see below).

Who May Benefit from Orientation and Mobility Instruction?

Orientation and Mobility instruction should start shortly after birth and once a diagnosis of blindness or visual impairment has been made (Jacobson 1993). As we will see later in this chapter, spatial, body and self-concepts play an integral role is the early formation of mobility skills. How well a child who is congenitally (born or shortly after birth) blind or visually impaired interacts with the environment is crucial to later, more advanced mobility skills. As children who are blind or visually impaired grow and develop they experience new impressions of their immediate environments. If they are allowed to explore, bump, and bruise themselves—like any other child—they can develop the necessary skill-sets and spatial understanding to navigate purposefully through a familiar or novel environment. For those who are adventitiously blind or visually impaired, that is, who become blind or visually impaired later on after birth through some disease, trauma or accident, Orientation and Mobility instruction can play a pivotal role in whether-or-not they will lead independent lives. Finally, as we age our remaining senses diminish. Our balance and stability become an issue—especially if we are blind or visually impaired. Orientation and Mobility instruction can offer a degree of independence and a sense of well being to individuals who are elderly and blind or visually impaired (Griffin-Shirley and Groff 1993). We would have to say, then, that nearly anyone who is blind or visually impaired would benefit from Orientation and Mobility instruction.

Who Provides Orientation and Mobility Instruction?

Some aspects of Orientation and Mobility instruction may be provided by a host of professionals. However, the primary instructor is the O&M Specialist. Depending upon the instructional setting, this professional may also be known as the O&M Instructor, the O&M Specialist or Instructor, or more recently, the O&M Therapist. Hereafter, we will refer to this individual as the O&M Specialist for continuity sake.

The O&M Specialist is educated in the theories and practices of teaching O&M skills to individuals of all ages and complicating conditions, for example, individuals who are blind or have low vision and who also have diabetes, multiple sclerosis, muscular dystrophy, brain injury, or other physical or cognitive impairments. Professional O&M Specialists receive their education and training at universities recognized through The Association for the Education and Rehabilitation of the Blind and Visually Impaired (AER), the only association of professionals that is exclusively dedicated to assist individuals who are blind or visually impaired. These university programs provide instruction to meet the standards and competencies of the O&M profession. University graduates of these programs are eligible to take the national O&M certification examination conducted through The Academy for the Certification of Vision, Rehabilitation and Education Professionals (ACVREP). Those who pass the examination become Certified O&M Specialists (COMS) and carry that credential for 5 years. The credential is renewable every 5 years by providing evidence of having participated in approved continuing education activities and the teaching of O&M skills. This is a national certification that is recognized in most states. Currently there are no states that license O&M Specialists, although licensing legislation is moving through the New York legislature as this chapter was being written.

O&M Specialists provide instruction to individuals of all ages who are blind or visually impaired in walking with a human guide, protecting oneself when walking alone in familiar indoor areas, orientation to an indoor environment, the prescription and teaching of long cane skills in indoor and outdoor settings, outdoor orientation systems, special travel situations such as escalators and revolving doors, public transportation systems, using accessible pedestrian signalizations, accommodating for quiet cars, and traveling in rural environments. O&M Specialists provide prescriptive long cane instruction, as well as orientation instruction for dog guide users, instruction with electronic travel aids and electronic orientation aids (see all below).

Other Professionals

In addition to the O&M Specialist, other professionals provide some aspects of orientation and mobility instruction. Certified Vision Rehabilitation Therapists (CVRT), formerly called Rehabilitation Teachers, are trained to provide basic O&M skills leading up to but not including indoor long cane skills instruction. They may teach some indoor mobility skills and orientation to daily living skills environments like the individual's home or office. Low Vision Therapists (LVT) may provide instruction in more efficiently using remaining vision and near and distance low vision devices like magnifiers and monocular telescopes and minifiers (see Chapter 4). They may show the individual with low vision how to use telescopes in the natural environments both indoors and outdoors. These two professionals are also certified through ACVREP. Certified teachers of children with visual impairments may also provide basic O&M skills and orientation to children who are blind or visually impaired in their schools and home environments. They are credentialed by their respective states.

When working with individuals who are blind or visually impaired, it takes an additional team of specialists to provide all of the education and treatment options. In addition to the O&M Specialist, the CVRT and/or the LVT, and depending on the setting, some of the professionals who may provide necessary support and services are social workers, rehabilitation counselors, counselor educators, occupational therapists, physical therapists, optometrists, and ophthalmologists. These professionals, however, should not provide O&M instruction but help bring a holistic approach to the education and/or rehabilitation service delivery.

A Brief History of the Orientation and Mobility Profession

As long as humans have existed blindness has occurred. In the earliest recordings of history there have been accounts of how people who were blind were treated by society. In some cultures people who were blind were ostracized and venerated. In other cultures people who were blind were given special status as seers and recorders of history. Mostly people who were blind were pitied and allowed to beg on the streets, which also became a special status of sorts. It was not until Valentine Hauy established the first school for the blind in Paris, France, in 1786, that people who were blind or visually impaired began to receive a formal education that took into account their special needs (Bledsoe 2010). Over the ensuing years more schools for the blind were established in England and in the United States.

It was during World War II that many blinded veterans were returning home to the United States and who required special treatment and rehabilitation. Dr. Richard Hoover and C. Warren Bledsoe established a training program in the 1940s at the Valley Forge Army Hospital and later the Avon Old Farms Home in Pennsylvania to provide them with skills so that they could return to their homes as productive citizens. The program was later transferred to the Hines Veterans Administration Hospital in Illinois (Bledsoe 2010).

Short, wooden canes painted white with a strip of red paint near the tip were the norm for travelers who were blind or visually impaired up to that time. Travelers would indiscriminately tap the cane as they walked along. Hoover and his colleagues established a revolutionary technique for swinging a long cane. Hoover's approach was to touch or tap down a longer, lighter cane where a person's next foot placement would be, rather than randomly tapping a short, wooden cane in front of the person. This was called the Hoover Technique or the Two-Point Touch Long Cane Technique (Bledsoe 2010), and it is still used today.

By giving the cane a new material, aluminum, and making it longer for greater forward preview, and by having the person touch or tap the cane where the next foot placement would be, the technique enabled travelers to concentrate on their orientation skills rather than worrying about whether-or-not they would step off of a curb into the street or fall over cracks or other hazards. Over time this revolutionary approach filtered down to the civilian population and eventually led to the establishment of university training programs in the 1960s and thereafter. For a more comprehensive look at the history of the O&M profession, the reader is referred to Bledsoe (2010) and Wiener and Siffermann (2010).

Systems of Mobility

How does a person who is blind or visually impaired travel through today's complex environments? There are five basic systems for negotiating simple and complex environments for today's traveler with a visual impairment or who is blind. They are the human guide; the long cane; the dog guide; electronic travel aids; and electronic orientation aids.

Human Guide

The human guide, once referred to as the sighted guide, is someone who assists a blind or visually impaired person to walk through a particular environment by having that individual hold onto his or her arm (Figure 3.1). The pair act as a team as they negotiate indoor and outdoor areas, doors, stairs and curbs, and the like. The human guide can be some significant other person in one's life or a total stranger. The human guide may act as a simple conduit to go from one location to another such that the person being guided need not be concerned with specifics about the environment they are walking through, or the guide might offer insights as to the travel environment. Such insights might include any landmarks that may trigger preciseness as to their location or any other information that may be useful for the person who is blind or visually impaired.

A properly trained human guide can be a useful and integral part of the travel process. One who is not properly trained to be a human guide, however, can put the person who is blind or visually impaired in a precarious or potentially injurious situation. Human guides learn to look ahead and provide preview information as to what will be occurring as they walk through an environment. For example, as the team walks down a hallway the guide

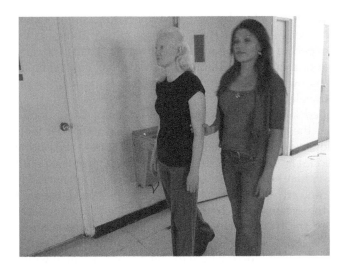

FIGURE 3.1
Walking with a human guide.

notices up ahead that there is a set of stairs they will need to negotiate. By alerting the traveler ahead of time and by slowing down and stopping at the top of the stairs, the guide keeps the traveler informed and wary so that when they negotiate the stairs they do so in a systematic, controlled and safe manner. Had the guide not done so, the traveler might have been unaware of the stairs and would have expected to find the floor when taking another step forward. The resulting loss of balance could imperil both the traveler and the guide!

While there is a degree of dependency in using a human guide, this system of travel is convenient in that the traveler need not be attending to all of the audible and tactile ambient clues and can simply rely on the guide to get to the final destination. A human guide is also expedient. For example, if people need to vacate an area quickly, a human guide can more quickly escort a person who is blind or visually impaired out of that emergency situation. More information about walking with a human guide can be found later in this chapter.

Long Cane

Travelers who are blind or visually impaired often use a long, white cane. This aluminum or graphite cane is lightweight and is composed of a long shaft coated in reflective, white tape with a five-inch strip of red reflective tape near the tip. The tip is typically made of composite plastic and can be shaped like a pencil tip, a teardrop or like a marshmallow or it can be a roller ball. The tip will wear down over time and need to be replaced. There usually is a putter-style golf grip at the other end. As mentioned previously, the long cane is prescribed by the O&M Specialist who considers such factors as: a traveler's length of stride and speed of walking; environmental conditions expected to be negotiated on a regular basis; and, any concomitant physical or medical conditions. The basic long cane, then, can be customized in many ways (by length and material) to meet the needs of the individual traveler.

As described later in this chapter, the Two-Point Touch long cane technique enables the traveler to preview the area where the next foot placement would set down (Figure 3.2). It takes a great deal of time and effort to develop the skills necessary to accomplish this seemingly simple task. Without visual input, the user may swing the long cane too widely or too narrowly from side to side (the cane arc width), or the cane tip may be raised (the arc height) too high off of the ground in between touch-downs. If any of these situations should occur, the traveler would receive false or incomplete information about the travel environment. For example, if the cane arc width is too wide, it will not be touching down where the next foot placement would be and it might unnecessarily touch down in areas beyond where the traveler is walking. Conversely, if the cane tip were to touch down too narrowly, it might not detect an object just off of the intended path of travel, like an overhanging bush or shrub. Finally, if the arc height is too high the cane might not detect in time an unexpected drop-off like a curb or stair step. The skilled O&M Specialist weighs all of these variables to develop an instructional program that meets the needs of each individual traveler. Adapted cane techniques like the constant contact long cane technique (see "Two Point Touch Long Cane Techniques" later on in this chapter) may be advised for travelers who

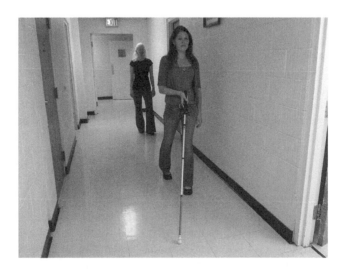

FIGURE 3.2
Walking while using the two-point touch long cane technique.

have difficulty keeping their arc height just off the ground. This technique eliminates the need to raise the cane tip off of the ground altogether.

The long cane technique is not a perfect technique. It does not detect objects above the waist, and only offers a modicum of orientation information. It does, however, offer a degree of safety that, when paired with useful orientation, will enable the traveler to negotiate unfamiliar environments in ways that were incomprehensible just 50 years ago. While the long cane technique does assist the traveler in walking a straight line, which is important when crossing streets and other wide-open areas, it does not ensure straight-line travel in all situations and conditions. Every state has enacted legislation, often called white cane laws, that requires safe passage for travelers using white canes as they cross streets at crosswalks.

An Orientation and Mobility program requires an inordinate amount of time and effort to learn how to maintain or regain one's orientation in various travel situations, conditions, and environments. The long cane skills are merely a means to that end.

Dog Guide

Formalized dog guide travel instruction began in the United States in the late 1920s when Dorothy Harrison Eustis established The Seeing Eye, Inc., in Nashville, Tennessee (Bledsoe 2010). Ms Eustis, along with Morris Frank, the first dog guide user, introduced the dog as a service animal for travelers who were blind with much awe and considerable resistance. However, as they were inundated with requests from people who were blind to assist them in becoming independent travelers, and for other reasons, they moved their facility to Whippany, NJ, and finally to Morristown, New Jersey, where it is still located to this day. It is currently the oldest and largest dog guide training program and facility in the world. Federal legislation mandates today that all public facilities allow dog guides.

Dog guide users (Figure 3.3) must be in generally good health, mature enough to care for and use a dog guide, and make use of traveling with a dog guide for constant and consistent periods of time. While dog guides do make useful companions and pets, they are primarily working animals and, as such, should not be interfered with while they are in harness and working. Dog guides are trained to assist users in getting from one location to another while it is up to the users to maintain their orientation. Dog guide travelers must determine when it is safe to initiate a crossing of a particular street; the dog guide will provide a safe and straight crossing. If the user makes a bad decision as to when to initiate the crossing, the dog is trained to provide intelligent disobedience, that is, the dog will stop and not let the user continue on into the path of an approaching vehicle.

Whereas with long cane travel the traveler must attend to every tactile and audible landmark along a particular route to maintain orientation, the dog guide traveler takes a broader view of travel and attends primarily to audible

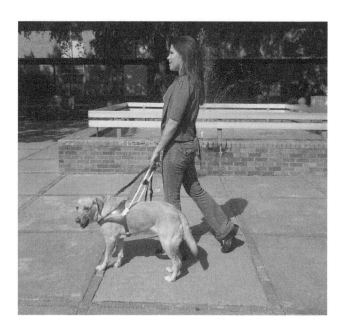

FIGURE 3.3
Walking with a dog guide.

landmarks. As the actual travel speed of dog guide travel is on average around 2.5 miles per hour, dog guide users must process incoming sensory information at a much quicker pace than would long cane travelers.

Electronic Travel Aids

There is an old saying that states that form follows function. This holds true for the electronic travel aids for the traveler who is blind or visually impaired. As engineers looked for ways to assist the traveler with a visual impairment, and as technology evolved over time, so did the proliferation and demise of certain electronic travel aids.

Sonicguide™

After World War II, and with the invention of the transistor, the very first electronic travel aid that reached the market place was the "Binaural Sensory Aid," which later became the "*Sonicguide*™." The Sonicguide™ (Figure 3.4) was a complementary or secondary travel device that was to be used along with either the long cane or a dog guide. It was a pair of spectacles with three transducers (two above one) in the bridge between the lenses and just above the user's nose. The bottom transducer emitted ultrasounds out into the environment. When these sounds bounced off of an object they would be

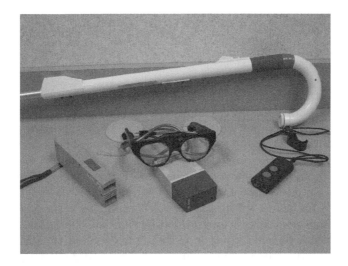

FIGURE 3.4
The Sonciguide™ (middle), Laser Cane™ (top), Mowat Sensor™ (lower left), and Miniguide™.

reflected back into either of two upper transducers. The top two transducers received ultrasounds reflected back from the environment from head height to the chest and from shoulder to shoulder. The ultrasounds would be translated into audible sounds as the signals traveled through the temples to either ear and then through ear flutes into the user's ear. If the signals were closer to the wearer's right side, they would be louder in the right ear. Thus, the binaural effect would provide the user with information as to the approximate location within the azimuth of the sound source by the signal's loudness in that ear. In addition, the pitch of the sound would determine the distance away from the user the object was located. The higher the pitch, the further away the object was, and, conversely, the lower the pitch the closer the object was to the user. Individuals could accurately determine how far away an object was within one-quarter to one-eighth inch—up to approximately 20 ft away at the furthest point of the signal. Finally, users could determine basic characteristics of the object in question by analyzing the tone of the signal. Humans shared basic tonal commonalities, trees shared basic tonal similarities with other trees, telephone poles shared the same tonal characteristics with other telephone poles, and so on. A user could develop a sonic vocabulary and be able to determine with great accuracy what it was that he or she was passing by, approaching or avoiding. The Sonicguide™ was, truly, the first environmental sensor for travelers who were blind or visually impaired. While it gave the user more information and confidence to travel in novel environments, it was bulky and required a special battery and battery pack in order to operate. Its complexity, expense and the small number of individuals who took advantage of learning how to use it led to it being discontinued in its manufacture several years ago (Jacobson 1993).

Laser Cane™

Another electronic travel aid that also gained popularity in the 1970s and 1980s was the Nurion *Laser Cane*™ (Figure 3.4). The laser cane was a primary or stand-alone device that emitted three laser beams: a high beam went about 3 ft in front of the user to head height; the forward beam went directly out from the cane approximately 18 feet about waist height at the closest to the cane to about 4–6 in. above the ground at its furthest point; and, the low beam extended out toward the ground about three feet in front of the cane tip. The invisible beams reflected off of objects and back to the cane to photo-diode cells that sent them through the cane shaft and up to the grip where they were translated into sounds and/or a tactile vibrator that lightly vibrated on the user's index finger. The lower channel beam did not signal the user unless its signal was cut off due to a drop-off or some object that impeded the signal from reaching the cane, for example, a table or a standing automobile and the like. As the device used laser beams the principles of light applied: beams would go through glass windows and doors or be absorbed by dark objects or reflected off of round objects. As such, there was a steep learning curve for using this device.

Mowat Sensor™

On the other hand, the Mowat Sensor™ was a secondary device that was easy to learn and use. It was akin to today's *Miniguide*™ (Figure 3.4). The Mowat Sensor™ was a small, hand-held device that emitted ultrasounds into the environment up to approximately 15 feet away from the user. When the reflected signals reached the device, they were translated into a vibration that could be interpreted roughly into two distances by the rate of vibrations: within 3 ft and from 3 ft to 15 ft. While the device was simple to learn and operate, it provided limited information: either an object was present in one's travel path, or it was not. The Mowat Sensor™, too, has suffered the same fate as its predecessors and has gone out of production.

There has been much discussion as to why electronic travel aids did not catch on with the consumers (Jacobson and Smith 1983, Jacobson 1993, Penrod and Smith 2010). It seems that the cart was created before the horse. That is, engineers created what they thought were useful devices for travelers who are blind, but with little input from potential users during the design process. Oftentimes the designs were too complicated or too expensive or did not provide the consumer with useful information—or provided extraneous information (Jacobson and Smith 1983; Penrod and Smith 2010). Further, Orientation and Mobility Specialists needed to have special training and certification in order to teach the devices to their consumers. This meant that fewer individuals were capable of teaching their consumers how to use the devices, and there were fewer consumers who were exposed to the capabilities of these devices. There was limited demand and, therefore, a very small niche market. For further information on these and other electronic travel aids, the reader is referred to Penrod and Smith (2010) and to the discussion at the end of Chapter 8.

Electronic Orientation Aids

The latest iteration of Orientation and Mobility systems is the evolution of electronic orientation aids (EOA). As voice output and recognition systems have evolved beginning with the Kurzweil Reading Machine in the late 1970s and early 1980s (Kurzweil 1978) and later into computers and mobile devices, so have the options and opportunities proliferated for the traveler who is blind or visually impaired. Electronic orientation aids are used for navigational and orientation purposes (Penrod and Smith 2010). They range from accessible signage like Talking Signs™ (described in Chapter 6) to accessible pedestrian signals that emit the familiar beeping, chirps, or clicks. In addition, numerous geographic positioning system devices have been introduced into the market over the past several years, and will be further addressed in greater detail in Chapter 5.

All of the devices mentioned above are simple navigation and orientation aids for the traveler who is blind or visually impaired. Travelers receive guidance from these devices but it is up to them to interpret the information to make it meaningful to their particular travel situations. For example, a Talking Sign might tell travelers that they are at Main St and Markham Boulevard but it might not tell them which street is which or which way they are facing. The Trekker Breeze™ (see Chapter 5) may tell travelers that they are on the north side of Main Street walking east but, in reality, they may have stepped off a driveway and were walking in the street, itself! Electronic orientation aids are not so precise that they can detect a gradual veering from the expected line of travel. They give information within a 25-foot radius of specificity. The traveler who is blind or visually impaired, therefore, must use an EOA as a complementary device and must rely on good orientation skills to augment the information received from the device.

Concepts Related to Independent Travel

When individuals who are blind or visually impaired travel through their immediate environments without the benefit of electronic travel aids or electronic orientation aids, they must understand the characteristics of the environment and how they, themselves, are positioned within it and how they must interact with it. (For expediency sake for this and ensuing discussions throughout this chapter, the traveler will be referred to in the feminine.) For example, when a traveler walks into a room, she is facing a particular compass direction and yet, by the time she moves within the room and in and around the various objects in her path, she may be facing a completely different direction. If the traveler thinks she is facing a particular direction but is not facing that direction in reality, her perception of the environment may be skewed such that she may erroneously believe, for example, that the entry door is to her left when it is actually behind her! One can easily see how this misperception could lead to disorientation.

Orientation and Mobility Specialists teach their students or clients the necessary concepts to maintain or regain their orientation as they move through various travel environments. In order to understand the immediate environment, travelers must understand their own positional relationship with objects within their travel paths (Hill and Hill 1980, Hill and Ponder 1976). This initial spatial understanding begins with understanding one's own body concepts. Once she understands her own body concepts, she can better relate to the environment spatially. As she relates spatially to the environment, she can become self-familiarized with it. We will discuss these principles and skills sequentially over the next several subsections.

Body Concepts

Body concepts do not just reflect what the different body parts are but also how these parts relate and interact with one another and with the environment. For example, one must not only know what the shoulder is, but, also, how it rotates and moves in and out from the body. This is important for more advanced travel skills, as when she swings the long cane her shoulder must work independently from the arm and wrist, for example (also see the discussion on long cane skills below). In another example, the arms must swing naturally as the feet move throughout the gait cycle such that the left arm swings forward as the right foot steps forward. Without the use of vision at early ages, the traveler would not automatically reproduce this seemingly natural movement (Jacobson 1993). In still another example, the traveler will inevitably veer off her intended path of travel if any of these conditions occur: the head is turned away from looking directly ahead; the head it tilted to one side; one shoulder is drooped below the other; one hip is lower than the other; or, one foot is out-toeing. Lastly, if the traveler walks at a very slow pace, veering is also likely to occur (Jacobson 1993). Some of the body parts that are integral for straight-line travel and the subsequent understanding of the environment are: head, shoulder, arm, forearm, wrist, hand, fingers, thumb, chest, waist, hip, thigh, leg, ankle, foot, and toes. Children, especially those who are born blind or visually impaired, must be taught their body parts and understand how they function. Without vision, these children do not necessarily learn these concepts and, eventually, they will grow up to be adults who do not understand these concepts. Ideally, they should be taught these concepts at a very early age so that the environment begins to make sense to them. Orientation and Mobility Specialists assist these young, future travelers in how to utilize their body parts for orientation purposes.

Spatial Concepts

For those who were born blind or visually impaired, there are certain concepts of space that must be learned. Basically, the following prepositional words and phrases are descriptors of space: in, under, around, beneath, up, over, beside, opposite, next to, in between, above, and below. These words and phrases relate the person with an object or objects: is the person next to the chair and is the chair next to the person? Is the ball under the chair and is the chair over the ball? Is the person next to the ball that is under the chair, and so on? When an object is outside the reach of a person, will she know that it is still there? As there is no other reliable verification for cues without vision (unless they produce a sound or odor), these concepts must be explored and learned. If they are not learned at age-appropriate times, the person will likely grow up with a misperception of the world around her. The Orientation and Mobility Specialist introduces these concepts at age-appropriate times and will, if necessary, reintroduce them to adults who are congenitally blind or visually impaired. As one can imagine, if these concepts are not understood it would be very difficult to travel independently, especially should one become disoriented.

Linear Concepts, Landmarks, and Compass Directions

Understanding the relationships among objects in the environment requires an understanding of linearity. One travels from point A to point B in the straightest line possible. It is far easier to understand object-to-object relationships if one thinks linearly. For example, the entry door to a room is directly opposite the chalkboard. If we add clock directions we can be even more specific without having traveled among the objects. When we enter a classroom, the chalkboard is directly in front of us at 12 o'clock and the television is at 1 o'clock. But there are limitations to these directions as once one turns right or left, these stationary objects are now located at different clock directions to the individual. But, if we add compass directions to the mix then there is more constancy in these relationships. Once we enter that room we are facing north and, as a consequence, the chalkboard is on the north wall and directly in front of us. Even if we turn right, and the chalkboard is now on our left, it is still on the north wall and, then, north is now on our left. We must understand the terms right and left, and the compass directions—and how each interacts with us as we move through the environment and turn to go down intersecting paths or around objects in our paths. Stationary objects that provide constancy at critical junctures are called *landmarks*. Landmarks must be available to be used. If one is walking from the classroom to the restroom, the traveler must be able to know when to turn down another hallway, for example. Perhaps the landmark is the water fountain, or the Principal's Office, or the supply room. Perhaps is it a particular bulletin board or set of lockers. Whatever will cue the traveler as to the correct time to turn—and will always be there—can become her landmark.

Route Patterns and Shapes

Travelers must conceptualize the environment and the objects within it in order to travel consistently through it. They must develop mental or cognitive maps. One method to traveling and visualizing the route through the environment is to utilize route patterns or shapes. Travel routes can be of four basic shapes: I, L, U, and Z (Jacobson 1993, La Grow and Long 2011). When paired with compass directions and street names, the traveler has a great deal of specificity about the route and can visualize herself walking along the route. For example, when going from her home to the grocery store, the traveler knows she will walk an L-shaped route going North and then West and crossing three streets along the way: she will go North along the West side of Main Street crossing 12th and 13th Avenues and then West along the North side of 13th Avenue crossing Center Street until she comes to the grocery store on her right-hand side. In order to return to her home, she will simply reverse that route and those compass directions. In this example she needed to have an understanding of laterality (right versus left), directionality (compass directions), street names, route shapes and how to reverse the route. This is referred to as "The Five Point Travel System" for orientation purposes (Jacobson 1993).

By using the Five Point Travel System, the traveler has a repertoire of concepts, skill-sets, and real-life objects in the environment at her disposal to use in order to travel in familiar and novel places. In essence, the traveler is creating a cognitive map or internal GPS, imagining where she is along the route, and where she needs to go to reach her destination. A seemingly complex set of environmental characteristics can be broken down into manageable parts and then reassembled into one holistic route. For example in a typical residential area, a traveler may have to walk 15 city blocks to get to her destination. This might involve a stair-step-like route (several connected Z-shapes) crossing numerous street corners along the way. But, by using the Five Point Travel System, the traveler can maintain her orientation. For example, she knows she is facing west and walking along the North side of a particular street. The next street corner she approaches will be on the NE corner of that new intersection. If she continues walking West, she will encounter the NW corner of that intersection, and then the NE corner of the next intersection, and so on, until she makes her first turn to go North. But, the pattern continues until she makes her next turn, and so forth. In essence, if she maintains her orientation, she already knows what her exact location on the next intersection will be—even though she has never before been there!

By keeping in mind certain geographical features like the terrain, slopes, traffic patterns and controls, the sun, and various landmarks, the traveler can reorient herself should the situation warrant it. The Orientation and Mobility Specialist creates a series of lesson units that places the student traveler into situations that challenge her to utilize her newly learned skill-sets in order to demonstrate to her that she has the knowledge and skills to maintain her orientation and reorient herself when necessary in all of the travel environments she may encounter. To accomplish all of this, the individualized Orientation and Mobility Program requires months, and sometimes, years of training.

Familiarization Processes

Orientation and Mobility Specialists teach their consumers how to self-familiarize to any environment. This is critical to becoming an independent or interdependent traveler. This process may begin with a simple room and culminate with the self-familiarization to an entire building, neighborhood or shopping mall. This familiarization process utilizes all of the concepts heretofore mentioned: body, spatial, directional and environmental concepts and route patterns. As such, as the consumer learns to negotiate indoor environments, she learns to self-familiarize to a particular room, floor and building. As she develops skills to traverse a residential area, she then learns how to self-familiarize with that environment. Thus, as each "unit" of instruction is mastered, the culminating lessons relate to familiarizations with that unit environment. For more information on familiarization processes, the reader is referred to Jacobson (1993), and La Grow and Long (2011).

Formal Mobility Skills

For purposes of clarification, it is necessary to describe and illustrate some of the basic orientation and mobility skills, as discussed earlier in this chapter. Some of the skills that need further elucidation include the Human Guide, Self-Protection (without a long cane), and some Long Cane skills.

Human Guide

As mentioned previously, the Human Guide technique is the basic and most accessible means of transportation for the traveler with a visual impairment. As such, it is important that the traveler not only masters the skills associated with it, but she must also learn to be able to teach it quickly to others and assist them to understand what other information about the environment is needed to maintain her orientation as they walk through it.

The basic Human Guide procedure is for the traveler to grasp the guide's arm just above the elbow with her fingers along one side of the arm and her thumb along the other side. She will stand one-half step behind her guide and maintain that position as they walk along, stop, or turn (Figure 3.1).

It may be necessary, on occasion, for the team to travel through narrow spaces. In this case, the traveler would step directly behind the guide and at arm's length (see Figure 3.5). Likewise, if they need to walk through a door-way, they will do so as a team with the guide first opening the door and the traveler taking hold of the door and holding it open as they pass through together (see Figure 3.6).

The traveler must quickly instruct a temporary guide on what she needs that person to do in order for them to traverse through an area. For more constant guiding, the traveler would provide more detailed instructions to the friend or significant other in her life such that most travel situations can be handled with minimal verbal information and more nonverbal cues,

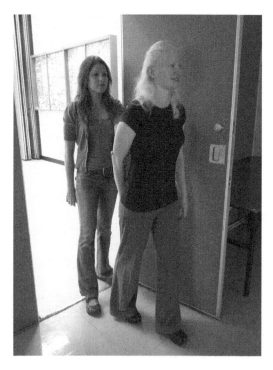

FIGURE 3.5
Walking along using the narrow spaces human guide technique.

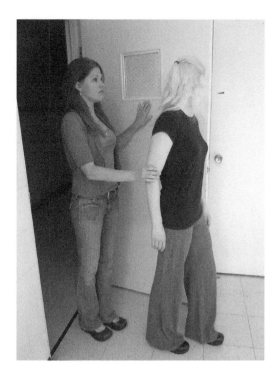

FIGURE 3.6
Walking through a door together as a team.

for example, a tensing of the guiding arm to indicate a stairway or curb, or a slowing down when approaching a door or elevator or escalator. In either case, the Human Guide technique offers the traveler a simple yet efficient mode of transportation—and one that she can control, herself.

Self-Protection Technique

Not all travel situations require a human guide or a long cane (or dog guide). When the traveler is in her home or any familiar, indoor area, it may not be necessary to use a long cane or human guide. In these instances, it may be helpful to use what is termed, the Self-Protection Technique. In this skill the traveler would simply raise one hand to chest height and then extend it forward, away from her body to nearly arm's length such that her arm crosses over her chest area and the forward hand is directly in front of her opposing shoulder (see Figure 3.7). In this manner, she is able to protect her chest and, sometimes, her head from obstacles, hazards, and obstructions. Imagine if you will, getting up in the middle of the night to go to the restroom in the dark. By using this technique one would avoid hitting one's head on the corner of the hallway or bumping into a lamp—or avoiding a collision with a

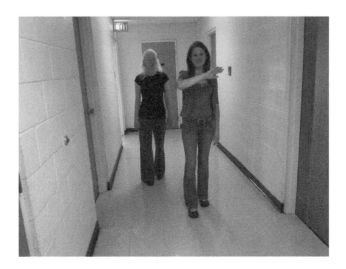

FIGURE 3.7
Walking using the self-protection technique.

closed door! This technique is especially useful when living with others who may forget to keep furniture or other objects in the same places all of the time!

Long Cane Skills

As travelers gain proficiency in the human guide and self-protection techniques, they become ready to expand and explore their environments in more complicated but familiar indoor areas and novel outdoor areas that pose additional challenges and hazards to safe travel. More complicated familiar and novel indoor environments might include protruding objects in the corridors like drinking fountains, benches and display cases, while stairs that descend to lower levels might be found at the end of corridors in some buildings. It becomes imperative, therefore, that travelers learn basic long cane travel skills that will afford them proper preview or warning before they reach such obstacles and hazards.

Diagonal Long Cane Technique

In this technique, the long, white cane is held diagonally across the traveler's body in a stationary manner while walking along familiar, indoor areas (see Figure 3.8). The long cane acts as a bumper for objects below the waist, but affords limited protection for objects above the waist or below the feet. As the environment is both indoor and familiar to the traveler, worrying about strange or unfamiliar situations or hazards is nearly inconsequential. There

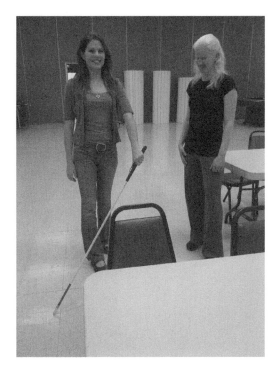

FIGURE 3.8
Walking while using the thumb grasp of the diagonal long cane technique.

may be those unexpected situations that could arise, but the traveler is not moving at a speed that is uncontrollable, should the unforeseen obstacle be detected (or go undetected) by the long cane. The Orientation and Mobility Specialist may offer the traveler other options for grasping the long cane while using this technique so that the skill may be more effective in various travel situations. For example, the traveler might wish to grasp the cane using a holding-a-pencil-like grasp when there are many people in a room or corridor—so that the long cane does not extend out and trip up unsuspecting individuals (see Figure 3.9).

Two-Point Touch Long Cane Techniques

The primary technique employed by the long cane user is the Two-Point Touch long cane technique. This skill will provide primary protection and preview in familiar and unfamiliar, indoor and outdoor environments. The traveler positions the cane hand at the midline, or just below the navel and just above the belt buckle, while pointing the cane tip to the ground. The cane is then swung to the left and then to the right side approximately 2 in.

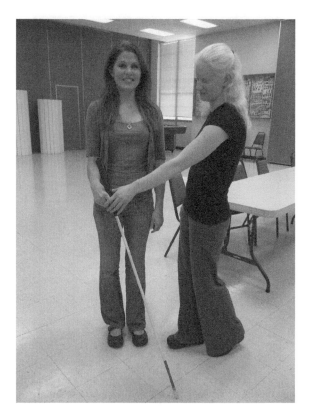

FIGURE 3.9
Using the pencil grasp of the diagonal long cane technique.

above the ground at midline (or in the middle of the arc) and then touches
down where the next foot placement will be. The cane tip, thus, previews the
location of the next foot placement. As the cane is swung from side to side,
the arm remains stationary while the hand remains at midline so that the
traveler can detect if the cane tip falls off into open space, or where the exact
location of an object is in the travel path (see Figure 3.2).

If the traveler is concerned about an upcoming drop-off, like a curb or
stair step, she can employ a modification to the technique called Touch and
Slide. When the long cane tip previews the next foot placement area, it glides
forward for 2 in. or so along the surface to provide additional ground contact to detect the drop-off. Another technique employed is called the
Constant Contact long cane technique. Instead of raising the cane tip
between touch-downs, the user keeps the cane tip gliding on the ground
the entire arc width (from side to side). There are other modified techniques
for the Two-Point Touch and Diagonal Cane techniques. For further

information the reader is referred to Hill and Ponder (1976), Jacobson (1993), and La Grow and Long (2011).

Street Crossings for the Traveler Who is Blind or Visually Impaired

As the traveler gains indoor travel proficiency she then becomes ready for outdoor travel. She learns to be acclimated to walking along residential street sidewalks while experiencing gradients, slopes, intersecting driveways, walkways and other sidewalks. Once she has become more comfortable with sidewalk travel she may then be ready for street crossings. For a traveler who is blind or visually impaired, it becomes imperative that she learns to listen for various traffic patterns and controls. For example, she can discern one-way from two-way streets simply by listening for traffic flow coming in only one or both directions. She can discern stop signs from stop light traffic controls by listening to what the traffic does when it reaches an intersection. She would ask herself, does the traffic stop (or slow down) each time vehicles get to the intersection (indicating a stop sign-controlled intersection) or do they go straight through and/or do they come to a complete stop (a stop light-controlled intersection)?

Once she determines the traffic pattern and control, she uses the sounds of the parallel traffic (the traffic along her side) to align her body so that she is facing directly across the street she wishes to cross and then ensures herself that she is within the crosswalk area. Over time, and through much guidance from the Orientation and Mobility Specialist, she learns to make judgments as to when it is safest to cross the street. She does so by analyzing the traffic patterns and initiates her crossing as close to the beginning of the cycle as feasible by using the surge of the parallel traffic.

Challenging Orientation and Mobility Travel Situations

Street crossings are extremely complex, especially with today's challenging traffic situations. Travelers learn to negotiate various intersection configurations (T or dead-end intersections, offset intersections, and plus sign intersections or through streets), various traffic-controlled intersections (actuated, self-actuated, no controls), and various geometries (traffic islands and roundabouts, split islands, and traffic-slowing devices). Additional challenges include quiet cars and other electric vehicles; terrains that can mask vehicular sounds like hills or bends in roads; and, objects that can create sound shadows such as bushes, signs, and parked vehicles that come between the vehicular sounds and the traveler.

Accessible Pedestrian Signals

For accessible pedestrian signals (APSs) to be useful for the traveler who is blind or visually impaired, there should be a locator tone that alerts to its presence, the push button should be within 10 ft of the curb line, and the audible signal should be intermittent or, ideally, a voice that indicates which street it is safe to cross (Barlow et al. 2010). City traffic engineers are required to follow the *Manual of Uniform Traffic Control Devices* (MUTCD) (Federal Highway Administration 2009) standards for placement of APSs. However, it is also true that these standards are guidelines that can be interpreted in different ways or may be applied only to new installations. For example, not all existing APSs have sound beacons. If there is no audible beacon present, it is difficult for the traveler to know if there is an APS at that corner and exactly where it is located. If the push button is indiscriminately located on an existing pole, for example, it may be too far away from the intended crosswalk for the traveler to locate, return to the curb or ramp, and then to align to the traffic in a timely manner. If the audible signal is the same sound for each street, then the traveler may have great difficulty knowing which signal indicates which crossing. Accessible pedestrian signals are not available at every intersection and are best installed at complex or very wide intersections. Although APSs may be available at a given intersection, the traveler must still utilize learned street crossing procedures (analyzing the traffic patterns, controls and flow, and auditorally aligning to the traffic in order to ensure a straight line of travel across the street and within the sidewalk) in case the signals are not working or unusual traffic situations occur.

Roundabouts and Traffic Circles

As roundabouts have become increasingly popular around the United States to direct traffic flow, they present particular challenges for travelers who are blind or visually impaired. With no traffic controls at crosswalks, roundabouts pose potential risks to the traveler. The traveler must identify the location of the crosswalk, align to turning traffic (rather than traffic that creates straight, audible sounds), and then must determine when there is an auditory gap in traffic sounds large enough to merit the initiation of a safe crossing (see Figure 3.10). If the roundabout is a novel one for the traveler, she must also determine if she has, indeed, completed the street crossing or if she is at a split island and still has another portion of the crossing to execute. The size of the roundabout does not determine the complexity or risk of the crossing in that some crosswalks at very large roundabouts are set back far enough from the circle of traffic that the crossing is less risky than those at

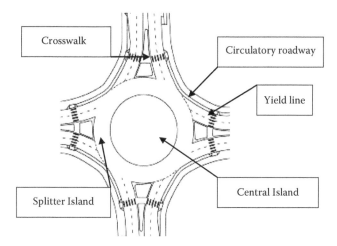

FIGURE 3.10
Selected features of a typical two-lane modern roundabout. (Reprinted with permission from Long, R. G. et al. 2005. *Journal of Visual Impairment & Blindness*, 99(10), Figure 3.1, p. 612. Copyright © 2005 by AFB Press, American Foundation for the Blind. All rights reserved.)

smaller roundabouts (where traffic enters or exits the roundabout right at the crosswalk). Time of day also plays a role in risk in utilizing roundabouts in that rush hour traffic may cause fewer auditory gaps in traffic sounds and, therefore, more risk for the traveler; whereas, nonrush hour periods of quiet time may allow the traveler to better discern when it is safer to make the crossing. Each roundabout, therefore, must be analyzed at varying times of the day or week. Traffic circles, for our discussion here, pose fewer risks than roundabouts as they usually have traffic signals for each incoming street. The traveler would treat each crossing as a separate traffic controlled intersection.

Public Transportation Systems

Travelers who are blind or visually impaired make use of the available public transportation systems in their communities. While the primary mode of transportation for these travelers is the city bus system, travelers also use taxis, subways, light and rapid rail systems, trains, and airplanes. Many larger city transportation systems are accessible for the traveler through online mobile and auditory maps, ticketing and schedules. Technology is moving toward fee payment through credit cards and smart phones, which would make travel even more accessible.

City Bus Systems

Orientation and Mobility Specialists teach travelers how to access buses, how to seek assistance on knowing when they have reached their destinations and what to do if they get off at the wrong bus stop. Travelers learn to read bus schedules and plan routes to and from bus stops. They learn where to stand and what to listen for in order to discern approaching buses. They learn to ask the driver for bus information, seat location, destination information and the location of the bus stop for return trip.

Taxi Cabs

Travelers are taught to ask for the approximate cost of the fare before going into the taxicab. Some taxi companies are offering customers fee payment through credit cards. Often, travelers will contact the cab company prior to their trip to get a fare estimate and then confirm that with the driver before entering the cab. If a particular cab driver appears to be courteous and reliable, the traveler may ask for his or her name and phone number in order to contact him or her directly for future trips.

Subways, Trains, and Rapid Rail (or Light Rail) Systems

Traveling on subways, trains, and rapid rail systems can seem a daunting task for the traveler who is blind or who has a visual impairment. However, if the O&M Specialist breaks down the task into small but meaningful parts, the lessons can be enjoyable and successful. Travelers learn how to purchase fare tokens or tickets, and proceed through turnstiles and escalators to find their way to the subway or train platforms. If necessary, they learn to locate a landmark to note exactly where their particular subway or train car will usually stop so that they ensure they enter the appropriate train or subway car. In addition, most subways have truncated dome detectable warning surfaces at the edges of platforms, which are on the same relative level as the subway car doors. Entry onto a subway car requires the traveler to ensure that she is not stepping in between the cars so good cane skills and effective use of landmarks are quite important. Finding a seat near a door is also important and, in some instances, it may be necessary for the traveler to stand and brace herself by holding onto a support rail as the subway or train moves to the next stop. Fortunately, subway trains stop at every stop along a route and conductors announce each stop so there need not be much guesswork to know when to exit the subway car.

As each subway, bus station, and airport terminal differs from another in terms of configuration and layout, travelers are taught basic information: entrances, baggage handling, security, and seeking assistance. Travelers are taught how to take a bus or taxi to the airport and how to get assistance once at the airport to check their bags, go through security and reach their gates.

For more information on accessing mass transit for the blind and visually impaired, the reader is referred to Uslan et al. (1990), Jacobson (1993), and La Grow and Long (2011).

Hybrid and Electric Vehicles

One of the most challenging technological developments to arise in recent years for travelers who are blind or visually impaired is the advent of quiet cars. As mentioned previously, travelers must rely on traffic sounds in order to assess traffic patterns and controls to determine when it is safest to make a street crossing and use those traffic sounds to maintain a direct line across the street in order to stay within the crosswalk area. Hybrid vehicles do not idle such that they are completely silent when not in motion. A traveler who is blind or visually impaired may not know a hybrid vehicle is present until it begins moving into the intersection, which could compromise her timing of when the cycle has commenced. With ambient sounds potentially masking the quiet sounds of the hybrid vehicle, the traveler might incorrectly judge exactly when it is safe to initiate the street crossing. As she makes her crossing, she may not be able to correctly gauge where that vehicle is as it passes alongside of her or as it crosses her path to turn around the corner.

Electric vehicles also do not make a sound when at rest. However, they also make little noise when in motion, and especially if there are other interfering ambient sounds present. As more electric vehicles make their way into society, it will become more difficult and challenging for the traveler who is blind or visually impaired to make judgments to minimize the risks for independent street crossings.

Working Together as a Team

As can be inferred from the previous section, it becomes imperative for all travelers, whether or not they are blind or visually impaired or have normal vision, that today's technological advances require a symbiotic relationship among various constituency groups. It does not matter if one has normal vision and hearing if more and more vehicles become quieter or silent. Every pedestrian can be put at risk when attempting to make a street crossing. What is good for the traveler who is blind or visually impaired, then, is good for everyone.

With this in mind, it is incumbent upon consumers, O&M Specialists, and engineers to work in concert with one another to develop technologies that complement the needs of all pedestrians. As one example, in an earlier discussion in this chapter it was noted that many of the electronic travel aids for blind or visually impaired travelers are no longer in production. This is in part due to devices being researched and developed with little to no input from either consumers who were blind or visually impaired or with O&M Specialists (Jacobson and Smith 1983). Once the aids were developed, consumers and O&M Specialists experimented with them, but most modifications had already been made. In another example, accessible pedestrian signals were developed in the early stages of usage with no consumer or O&M Specialist input. As a result, the early devices were put on poles too high to be useful, sounds were erratic and inconsistent, and the technology often broke down to be of little benefit.

Because of this disconnect among consumers, O&M Specialists and engineers, the O&M division of the Association for the Education of the Blind and Visually Impaired (AER) developed committees to consult with and assist engineers in the development of electronic travel devices and, later on, in accessibility issues. A good example of this symbiotic relationship is the development of electronic orientation aids in which consumers who are blind or visually impaired and O&M Specialists played integral roles with engineers in their development and subsequent usage.

Acknowledgments

The author gratefully acknowledges the help of Ms Nancy Jackman and of Ms Rebecca Missig, who posed as the O&M instructor and as the student traveler, respectively, in the pictures.

References

Barlow, J. M., B. L. Bentzen, and L. Franck. 2010. *Environmental Accessibility for Students with Vision Loss.* Edited by William R. Wiener, Richard L. Welsh and Bruce B. Blasch. Vol. 1. New York, New York: AFB Press.

Bledsoe, C. W. 2010. *The Originators of Orientation and Mobility Training.* Third Edition. Edited by Richard L. Welsh, and Bruce B. Blasch William R. Wiener. Vol. 1. New York, New York: AFB Press.

Carroll, T. J. 1961. *Blindness: What It Is, What It Does And How to Live With It.* Boston, MA: Little, Brown and Company.

Federal Highway Administration. 2009. *Manual on Uniform Traffic Control Devices for Streets and Highways*. Washington, DC: Department of Transportation, Federal Highway Administration.

Griffin-Shirley, N., and G. Groff. 1993. *Prescriptions for Independence: Working With Older People Who Are Visually Impaired*. New York, New York: AFB Press.

Hill, E. W., and M. M. Hill. 1980. Revision and validation of a test for assessing the spatial conceptual abilities of visually impaired children. *Journal of Visual Impairment and Blindness*, 74(10), pp. 373–380.

Hill, E. W., and P. Ponder. 1976. *Orientation and Mobility Techniques: A Guide for the Practitioner*. New York, NY: American Foundation for the Blind.

Jacobson, W. H. 1993. *The Art and Science of Teaching Orientation and Mobility to Persons With Visual Impairments*. New York, NY: AFB Press.

Jacobson, W. H., and T. E. C. Smith. 1983. Use of the sonicguide and laser cane in obtaining or keeping employment. *Journal of Visual Impairment and Blindness*, 77(1), pp.12–15.

Kurzweil, R. 1978. *Kurzweil Report: Technology for the Handicapped*. Edited by Raymond Kurzweil. Vol. 1. Cambridge, MA: Kurzweil Computer Products.

La Grow, S., and R. G. Long. 2011. *Orientation and Mobility: Techniques for Independence*. Alexandria, VA: Association for the Education and Rehabilitation of the Blind and Visually Impaired.

Long, R. G., D. A. Guth, D. H. Ashmead, R. W. Emerson, and P. E. Ponchillia. 2005. Modern roundabouts: Access by pedestrians who are blind, *Journal of Visual Impairment & Blindness*, 99(10), Figure 1, p. 612. Copyright © 2005 by AFB Press, American Foundation for the Blind.

Penrod, W. M., and D. L. Smith. 2010. *Adaptive Technology for Orientation and Mobility*. Third Edition. Edited by Richard L. Welsh, and Bruce Bl Blasch William R. Wiener. Vol. 1. New York, NY: AFB Press.

Uslan, M. M., A. F. Peck, W. R. Wiener, and A. Stern. 1990. *Access to Mass Transit for Blind and Visually Impaired Travelers*. New York, NY: American Foundation for the Blind.

Wiener, W. R., and E. Siffermann. 2010. *The History and Progression of the Profession of Orientation and Mobility*. Third Edition. Edited by Richard L. Welsh, and Bruce B. Blasch William R. Wiener. Vol. 1. New York, NY: AFB Press.

4

Low Vision: Types of Vision Loss and Common Effects on Activities of Daily Life

Duane Geruschat and Gislin Dagnelie

CONTENTS

Introduction

Chapter 2 provided a conceptual framework for understanding visual impairment, explaining how visual impairment affects function, describing the continuum of vision loss from (near) normal to (near) blindness with a brief description of the functional problems that occur through the progression of vision loss. This chapter will build on that conceptual framework, offering details on the demographics of low vision, describing the types of functional problems that are commonly experienced by persons with low vision, and offering the most common management strategies for addressing these problems. Keep in mind that many causes of low vision have no medical treatment or the medical treatments that are available will delay the progression of disease but not halt or reverse it. Therefore low vision habilitation for children and low vision rehabilitation for adults will take place in the context of lifelong adjustments to vision loss and changing ways to manage access to visually acquired information.

Demographics

Learning from Chapter 2 that blindness does not always mean total blindness, the demographics of visual impairment include the types of low vision and how many people have the various types of low vision. There are two main themes that actually summarize all of the specific details: (1) visual impairment is related to aging—the older you are the greater the risk of vision loss; and (2) very few people are totally blind. Now to the specifics: (1) The largest urban population-based study to date, covering well over 6000 individuals in Rotterdam, the Netherlands, found a steady increase of legal blindness with age, from 0.1% in the 55–64 year-old cohort to 5.9% in those 85 and over; for visual impairment the increase was from 0.1 to 29.9% (Klaver et al. 1998). Population-based studies in Australia (Taylor et al. 2005) and Wisconsin (Klein et al. 2006) found similar prevalence figures. (2) It is extremely difficult to obtain hard figures about total, or rather functional, blindness. Dr. William Feinbloom, decades ago, would tell students in his lectures that based on his estimation no more than 10% of legally blind individuals had no useful vision at all (Feinbloom 1935). Translated to today's approximately 1 million legally blind individuals in the US, this provides us with a rough estimate that around 100,000 Americans have no useful vision and conversely, that the visual impairment of millions of others is amenable to rehabilitation.

Low vision is commonly divided into two categories, central loss of vision and peripheral loss of vision, with central loss of vision caused by age-related macular degeneration accounting for most cases of low vision among Caucasians in the U.S., and peripheral (but in advanced cases also central) vision loss from glaucoma accounting for a large share of the disability among African Americans; both ethnic groups also show high prevalence of diabetic retinopathy among those with vision loss (Munoz et al. 2000; Rahmani et al. 1996; Sommer et al. 1991).

The most common pathology causing loss of central vision is age-related macular degeneration (AMD) (Congdon et al. 2004) which results in a central scotoma or blind spot. In functional terms, the loss of central vision means a reduction of visual acuity, or the clarity of seeing. People with central vision loss will not have 20/20 vision, they may have trouble seeing faces, reading books, watching television, and doing anything that requires good visual acuity. In the early stages of the disease they may complain of blurry vision, sensitivity to bright lights, and more difficulty than usual seeing in dimly lit areas. As the disease progresses they will notice difficulty with reading clocks, seeing faces, and seeing content on the TV.

People with loss of peripheral vision often have good visual acuity until late in the pathology. The most common causes of loss of peripheral vision are glaucoma and retinitis pigmentosa. People with peripheral field loss (and good visual acuity) will be able to read, watch television, and see faces without much difficulty. They will have problems seeing things to the side, resulting in challenges with mobility such as walking in a crowded shopping mall, difficulties playing sports and driving, and so on.

Effects of Low Vision on Daily Activities

It is important to understand that everyone with vision experiences limitations in vision and these limitations often cause a change of behavior. The difference between the limitations of vision for someone with normal sight and someone with low vision is the frequency with which the limitations are encountered and the amount of visual disability they cause. For example, when trying to read a book under dim illumination a fully sighted person may squint, pull the book closer, perhaps try to move the book closer to a light, and struggle with the text. Consider a candlelit restaurant. People in their 20s or 30s with 20/20 vision may have the ability to read the menu under dim illumination. Compare this to people in their 70s or 80s who also have 20/20 vision. The elderly person will most likely have a hard time reading the menu, either holding it very close to the candle flame or even pulling out a small handheld flashlight to read the print. The point here is that everyone with vision experiences limitations that occur because of environmental conditions and that these limitations are accentuated by the impact of age.

Now consider the person with low vision who wants to eat in the same restaurant. The same candlelight is available, the same printed menu is used but the person cannot adapt enough for the print to be visible, requiring that someone read the menu aloud. If there was enough illumination, if the print on the page had high contrast, and/or if the person was using their magnifier they could read the menu but these environmental and optical options were not available resulting in the inability to read the menu. Therefore, persons with low vision also experience limitations of vision. The difference is that they experience them with greater frequency, need to have much better visual conditions to complete visual tasks than the fully sighted, and they usually will benefit from optical devices that magnify the print. As the environmental conditions degrade, the person with low vision will quickly experience a degradation of performance, and of quality of life.

In the restaurant setting discussed here, the solution presented to a person with low vision can take three general forms: (1) a sighted person or the waiter provides assistance so the person with low vision does not have to read the menu; (2) a large print menu and better illumination are provided at some tables; or (3) the person with low vision carries an illuminated hand-held magnifier. In the first case, the person relinquishes his/her independence; in the second, an environmental modification is presented by the restaurant; and in the third, the use of technology provides full functionality. As their visual impairment progresses, more advanced tools are available for persons with low vision to maintain their independence. This chapter will be limited to mild and moderate visual impairment (the majority of the population with low vision) and the relatively simple adaptations available for these individuals.

Optical Devices

Optical devices can increase the access to visual information for those with low vision. Optical devices are made of lenses similar to what many people wear to correct for refractive error (near- and far-sighted). While the lenses are similar, they are prescribed for very different purposes—lenses for refractive error offer improved clarity of vision for near and distance viewing while optical low vision devices are for magnification and have a fixed focal distance for providing a clear image. Because of this difference, how optical devices are used and how they are experienced by the person with low vision is fundamentally different from the way in which a fully sighted person uses and experiences prescription glasses. For example, general viewing glasses or contact lenses are prescribed for continuous wear, increasing visual clarity for distance and near viewing. This is not possible with optical systems that magnify for low vision, because the magnified image is only clear at a fixed distance. As a general principle of magnification there is a relationship between the amount of magnification and the distance at which the magnifying lens will focus. For example, if you wear bifocals of 2.5 D, the bifocal lens focuses at 40 cm. If the power is doubled to 5 D, the focal distance is cut in half to 20 cm. Doubling again to 10 D halves the focal distance to 10 cm. As a general statement many users, especially readers with a life history of reading at 40 cm, do not like the requirement of holding reading material up close as the power of the magnification increases. An additional challenge is that magnification constricts the field of view leaving less of the peripheral field of view available for visual information that can be important: Imagine looking through a magnifying glass or binoculars and trying to walk around. If you have ever used a telephoto lens you will know that seeing finer detail within the field of view of the lens comes at the expense of seeing a narrower extent of the field.

Because of the effects of magnification, low vision devices are prescribed for specific problems so that many people with low vision will have multiple devices. For example, a person with low vision may have a device for reading the newspaper and their bible, one for looking at prices in the grocery store, another device for writing checks, and a fourth for watching television. Each task has unique requirements which can only be adequately addressed with a task-specific optical device.

Optical devices are generally divided into three categories based upon the distance where the device is in focus: near, intermediate/dual purpose, and distance devices. Each category can be further subdivided according to the type of housing that holds the lens. Specifically, near devices include hand-held magnifiers, stand magnifiers, and spectacles (microscopes). Intermediate/dual purpose devices are known as telemicroscopes because they can focus at a variety of distances from near to far, and distance devices are commonly known as telescopes. The relative advantages and disadvantages of the optical systems within each category are described in Table 4.1.

Reading is the most commonly requested goal for patients seen in a low vision clinic. Most people want to read newspapers, books, bibles, bank statements, utility and credit card bills, to name the most common. Because each of these may involve slightly different visual demands and slightly different viewing distances, different categories of devices are available to address these goals. The first category is hand-held magnifiers.

Hand-Held Magnifier

Hand-held magnifiers can be found in many stores for purchase over the counter without a prescription from an eye doctor (Figure 4.1). They range in power from just over 1× magnification to upward of 10× magnification. Because they have to be held, it is difficult for most users to maintain the proper focal distance for an extended period of time. If the proper focal distance is not maintained then the image will be blurry (held too far from the printed page) or the user will not obtain the maximum magnification (held too close to the printed page). In either case the user will have problems reading the print. Therefore most low vision clinics recommend the hand-held device for short-term reading tasks such as phone numbers, credit card statements, price tags, or looking at a photo. Higher-powered hand-held magnifiers often come with built-in illumination, since the short working distance causes the material to be shielded from ambient light by the user's hand and magnifier frame.

TABLE 4.1

Advantages and Disadvantages of Various Optical Devices

Advantages	Disadvantages
Near Device	
Hand-Held Magnifier	
Least expensive/most readily available	Must find the proper focal distance
Cosmetically acceptable	Both hands are not free
More variation in eye/lens/movement	Astigmatism correction is not included
More lighting control built-in	Motor control for elderly is a concern
Stand Magnifier	
Inexpensive and available	Book binding presents a problem
Flashlight-type good illumination	Can be large and cumbersome
Focal distance is set	Alignment of eye-lens is hard
Bar magnifier easy to use if low power	Illumination is a problem
Spectacle Microscope	
Looks like conventional glasses	High power—close reading distance
Both hands are free	May require more instruction
Field of view is wider	Maintaining focal distance is challenge
Low power may provide binocularity	High power requires monocularity
Available in high powers	
Intermediate Device	
Telemicroscope	
Both hands are free	More expensive than hand held
Allows for reading at varying distances	Not as readily available
Refractive correction can be included	Cosmetically unappealing
Near and distance in one device	May be heavy on nose
Binocularity may be possible	More head scanning
Distance Device	
Hand-Held Telescope	
Cosmetically inconspicuous	One hand to hold telescope
Less expensive than bioptic mounted	Hand movements affect fixation
Ocular lens can be held close to eye	Requires instruction on basic skills
Either eye can be used	Reduces field of view

Spectacle Microscope

Spectacle microscopes are glasses with powerful magnifying lenses that allow a person with low vision to read print (Figure 4.2). They come in varying powers (2 × –10×) which are prescribed according to the amount of vision loss of the individual user. As a general statement physicians prescribe the

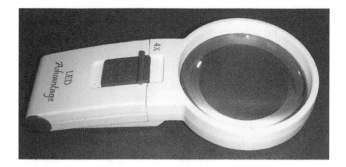

FIGURE 4.1
Hand-held magnifier. The user must hold the magnifier at the proper distance to benefit from a magnified image.

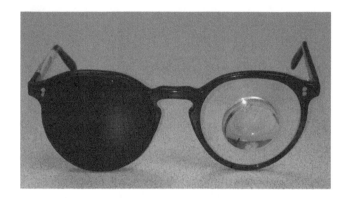

FIGURE 4.2
Spectacle microscope. The user holds the material close to the lens to focus the image.

lowest possible power to accomplish the reading task. The reason is that high-powered lenses have a reduced visual field and the material must be held very close to the face. The reduction of visual field from the higher power of the magnifier makes the device harder to use. The converse is also true. The lower the power, the wider the field of view, the greater the working distance, and the easier it is to use the device.

Stand Magnifier

Stand magnifiers are also available in many commercial stores and can also be obtained from low vision clinics (Figure 4.3). Stand magnifiers solve one of the biggest challenges of hand-held magnifiers and spectacle microscopes: they automatically set and hold the focal distance. All the user has to do is sit the magnifier on the page and it is in focus.

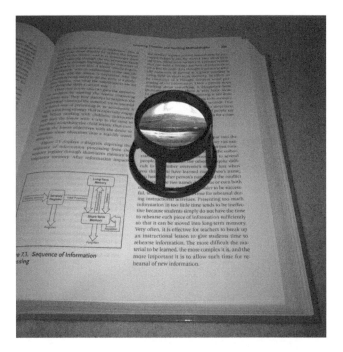

FIGURE 4.3
Stand magnifier. The stand magnifier rests on the page to be in focus.

The biggest problem with the stand magnifier is that it is hard to maintain a comfortable body posture while using the device, even with a reading stand. The second problem with the stand magnifier is that it blocks most of the ambient light; for this reason many low vision clinics will prescribe an illuminated stand magnifier (Figure 4.4).

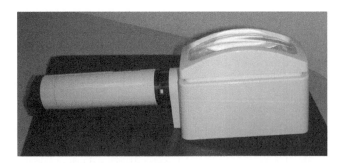

FIGURE 4.4
Illuminated stand magnifier. The illumination improves contrast and clarity.

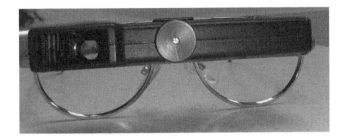

FIGURE 4.5
Telemicroscope. The telemicroscope allows for viewing at varying distances.

Telemicroscope

The final category of optical devices for near as well as distance activities is the telemicroscope. The word is very descriptive of the functionality of the device (Figure 4.5). Telemicroscopes have the distance viewing characteristic of a telescope and the magnification ability of a microscope. In practical terms, this allows the user to read small print at a viewing distance that more closely approximates the normal working distance of 15″ while reading. However, the opportunity to have a greater working distance comes at a severe cost. The depth of focus (meaning how precise the material has to be held from the lenses) is quite small, and the visual field is very narrow. From a functional point of view it can be very difficult to find and maintain such a precise focusing distance, and when combined with the small field of view, reading speed usually decreases.

Nonoptical Devices for Near Point Tasks

Ideally anytime an optical device is being used for near point activities, the user will also have nonoptical supports for the device. The most common nonoptical devices for near vision are flex arm lamps, colored filters, and a clipboard or reading stand. Lighting is critical to seeing as has been illustrated by the restaurant example. The reader may be familiar with the inverse square law, a concept well-known to illumination engineers. In functional terms the inverse square law means that moving the light closer to the page will provide a dramatic increase in illumination (squaring the available illumination), much more than would come from increasing the wattage of a light bulb. This law is why a single low power bulb built into an illuminated magnifier is adequate for reading. The bulb is so close to the page that it can use low power while yielding a high amount of light (Figure 4.6).

The type of light bulb can also impact on the quality of the visual response. Incandescent, fluorescent, LED, and halogen are the most commonly used bulb types. While each user will usually demonstrate a preference for a type of light, as a general statement fluorescent lights are not preferred because

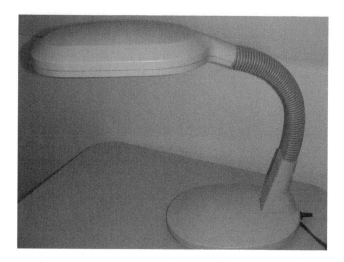

FIGURE 4.6
Flex-arm lamp. The flexibility of the lamp allows for increases in illumination.

some users will see a flicker, and halogen lights are not preferred because they generate a lot of heat and can cause a burn.

Any time you increase illumination you have the potential to introduce disabling glare. There is a constant struggle between increasing illumination and reducing glare. The use of a colored filter can assist with reducing glare.

This chapter has emphasized the challenges of finding and maintaining the correct focal distance when using magnifiers. Focal distance is so precise that even the indentation of the thumb/fingers when holding a newspaper or magazine can cause a blurry image which in turn will reduce the reading speed. The use of a clipboard and/or reading stand can ease the challenges of maintaining a flat surface (Figure 4.7). The key point is that to receive maximum benefit from an optical device the user needs to include nonoptical equipment such as flexarm lamps, clipboards, and filters.

Electro-Optical Systems

Another approach to providing magnification is through electro-optical systems. Commonly known as closed circuit television (CCTV) and more recently referred to as a video magnifier, all of these technologies have the same basic components: camera, lens, and display. The camera acquires the image, the lens allows for focusing and magnifying the image, and the display provides the user with the modified image. The first version of this technology became commercially available in the 1970s. These early desktop systems allowed for varying magnification, brightness control, contrast enhancement, reverse polarity, and a large field of view. Today these models also offer color. A significant advantage of the video magnifier is that the

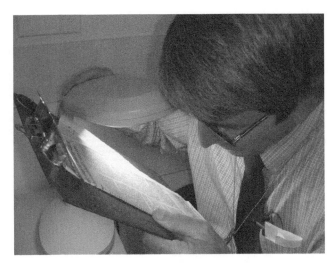

FIGURE 4.7
Multiple pieces of nonoptical equipment in use. To gain maximum benefit from an optical device, the use of non-optical equipment is usually required.

image can be seen binocularly (using both eyes at the same time). Another advantage is that the video magnifier does not constrain posture, allowing the user to sit comfortably while using the system.

CCTVs offer a range of magnification from 2× to 50× or 60× (Figure 4.8). Options include the ability to underline text as a marking system, and the ability to block or window text. Common uses of these devices are reading, writing checks, and viewing pictures. Computer compatible systems are a trend in which the CCTV is used in series with a computer displaying the computer information on the CCTV screen.

During the past 10 years, companies have introduced a variety of portable video magnifiers. As is true with all sorts of technologies, this is a rapidly changing approach to magnification which holds great promise for the visually impaired. These portable video magnifiers still have the basic components of a camera, lens, and display with many now featuring batteries for maximum portability. For example, because they are compact, lightweight, and with an integrated battery, it is possible to use them in a grocery store to read can labels (Figure 4.9). School children can use these in school and travel with the video magnifier in their backpack.

The biggest advantage of all electro-optical systems is the ability to magnify with a large field of view and a comfortable working distance (distance from the eye to the screen). The other main advantage is the ability to easily manage illumination and to enhance the contrast of the image. While these systems can be expensive when compared to other types of high-powered magnifiers (spectacle microscope, stand, hand-held magnifier), the electro-optical systems provide the user with all of the advantages

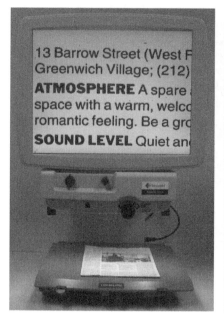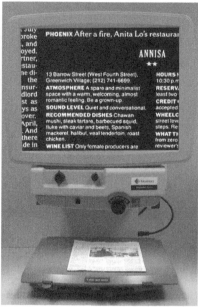

FIGURE 4.8
Closed Circuit Television: The CCTV can enlarge print, provide high contrast, as well as reverse the polarity of the image.

while minimizing the disadvantages of standard optical systems. The largest companies are Enhanced Vision, Optelec, Telesensory, and Humanware. Their websites offer information on their latest products and future developments.

Orientation and Mobility

Another important goal for many people with low vision is the desire to maintain independent mobility. This can include an interest to walk in the local community, traveling to a place of worship, medical appointments, grocery stores, or pharmacy, to name a few. In a majority of states it is possible to obtain a driver's license with low vision—in some states even up to legal blindness (see Chapter 2 for definitions).

Just as with reading and near point activities, independent travel with low vision is affected by the type and amount of vision loss. The three main functional challenges that have been identified via self-report are locating stairs/curbs, managing changes in illumination, and crossing the street safely. For example, a reduction of visual acuity typically results in difficulty

(a)

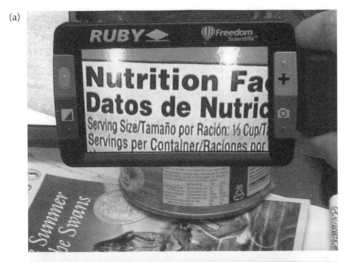

(b)

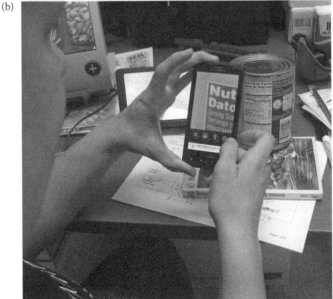

FIGURE 4.9
Video magnifier. The (a) and (b) images are of two different video magnifiers. They are portable and provide magnification without the need for extra lights.

with seeing changes in elevation specifically detecting the top step. Someone
with reduced acuity may also be more sensitive to changes in illumination
(light/dark adaptation) resulting in a temporary reduction of vision and fall-
ing because of not seeing the subtle change of elevation caused by the irregular pavement (Figure 4.10).

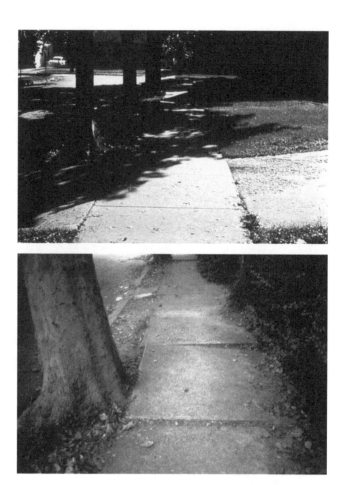

FIGURE 4.10
The effect of light adaptation on safe walking. A person who has trouble adapting to changes in illumination may not see the irregular sidewalk and fall.

The profession of orientation and mobility (O&M, see Chapter 3) provides instruction to people with low vision, including optical and nonoptical devices and instruction to enhance their safety and enable them to maintain some level of independent travel. O&M instructors utilize specialized equipment and techniques to address the challenges posed by loss of vision. To address the issue of changes in elevation, in the home or the neighborhood, the instructor may increase the contrast of edges by marking the edge with paint or tape (Figure 4.11). Increasingly, local jurisdictions—for example, public buildings, transit systems—are providing similar accommodations to the visually impaired.

For travel in less familiar areas of greater distances from the home, the use of the long cane (often associated with blindness but a valuable tool for

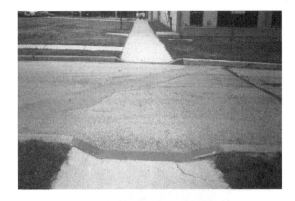

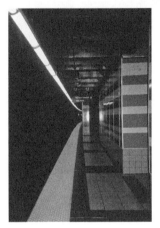

FIGURE 4.11
Modifying the environment to increase visibility. Increasing contrast can make travel easier and safer for the person with low vision.

the person with low vision) can be taught as a way to reliably identify curbs and stairs (Figure 4.12).

To address the issues of illumination, it is important to understand that the light that is most disabling is not the light that comes directly (perpendicular) to your pupil but the light that comes in "off-axis." The use of hats and visors and wrap-around sunlenses (Figure 4.13) either alone or in combination can increase comfort as well as maintain optimal visual acuity. These types of lenses come in a variety of colors and densities. Most people with low vision who have received professional services from a low vision clinic or an O&M instructor will be wearing these types of sunlenses. Polarizing lenses can be particularly effective if much of the off-axis light comes from reflections, since these tend to produce veiling glare that is polarized in a single plane. Similarly, photochromic lenses, that is, lenses

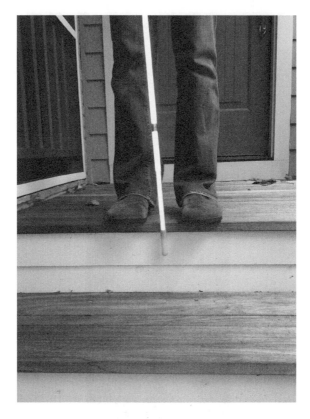

FIGURE 4.12
Cane and stairs. The use of the long cane, traditionally viewed as a device for the blind, can be used to increase safety for the person with low vision.

that reduce and increase transparency to compensate for changing light levels, can help people with adaptation problems, albeit the lenses do not respond instantly.

The third of the most commonly reported class of challenge with low vision and mobility is crossing the street. This includes identifying the type of traffic control, the location of the other side of the street, and monitoring the movement of vehicles and interacting with the drivers of these vehicles. From a technology point of view, hand-held telescopes are frequently provided for assistance with visually exploring the intersection to locate the traffic light, pedestrian signal, and to determine the size and shape of the intersection as well as to identify the location of the sidewalk for crossing. These telescopes vary in power from 2.5× to 10× and are prescribed based upon the visual acuity of the user (Figure 4.14). As the visual acuity decreases, the user requires a higher power of telescope. The problem is that

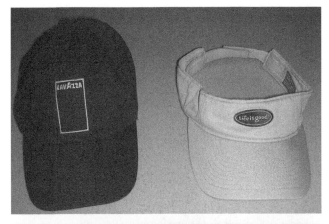

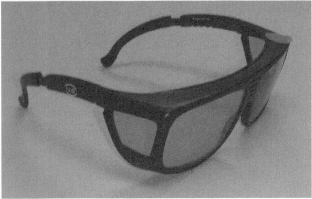

FIGURE 4.13
Hats, visors, and wrap-around sunshields. Control of illumination can enhance visibility and comfort.

that higher the power of the telescope, the smaller the field of view and the more difficult its use.

Driving with low vision is a topic of both interest and some controversy. A brief explanation of the idea that someone could drive safely with less than 20/20 vision is that everyone frequently drives with less than 20/20 vision. Driving at night, while it is raining, with the sun low in the sky and creating glare, are a few examples of times when people drive with low visual acuity and they drive safely by adjusting their driving behavior to fit the environmental conditions. However, there are times when 20/20 vision is important for maintaining safety. For example, when approaching a lighted intersection it is important to know the color of the traffic light well before you enter the intersection. Reading signs for the purpose of orientation or signs which indicate a change of traffic pattern during road construction may require

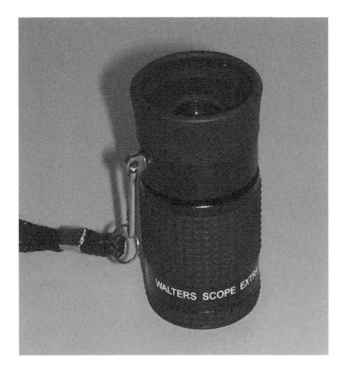

FIGURE 4.14
Hand-held telescope. This telescope is used to spot information such as street signs, traffic
lights, or bus numbers.

20/40 vision. Lastly, there are times when something unexpected may occur,
such as seeing a small brown object moving across the street and you want
to know whether it is a paper bag that you can drive over or a small dog
which would cause you to stop or veer. These situations do require good
visual acuity. The acuity requirement is addressed with a bioptic telescope.
A bioptic telescope is two optical systems in one spectacle frame. The carrier
lens is the regular eyeglass prescription, whose sole purpose is to bring distant objects into focus, with a telescope mounted in the superior (upper) half
of the glasses. As demonstrated in Figure 4.15, the user will tilt their head
back, looking under the telescope, using regular vision for the majority of the
driving task. When a situation arises where good visual acuity is required,
the user visually detects something through the carrier lens, lowers the chin,
and raises the eyes to look through the telescope which provides increased
visual acuity. With practice this can occur very quickly with the acquisition
of information being analogous to looking into the rear view mirror. The
point here is that while everything looks magnified and closer than it actually is, a similar phenomenon occurs when looking into the rear view mirror

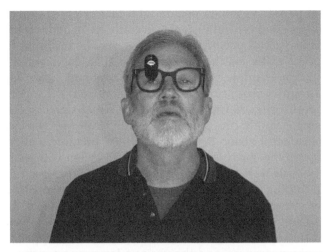

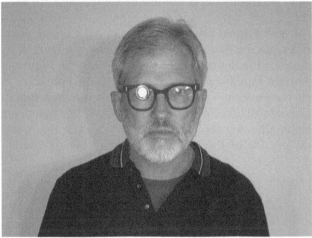

FIGURE 4.15
Bioptic telescope. This telescope can be used for a variety of purposes including reading, watching TV, and driving.

with everything being behind you and reversed. Instruction with the telescope and practice driving are obviously required.

Loss of Peripheral Vision

Keeping in mind that while the vast majority of people with low vision have a loss of visual acuity there is a subset of low vision that involves loss of peripheral or side vision. A person with loss of peripheral vision may have remaining good central vision, especially early in the course of their disease. The impact of peripheral field loss may be minimal for reading and near point tasks (assuming of course that good visual acuity is still present). For example, a person with peripheral vision loss may be able to read regular size print, watch television from a standard viewing distance, identity friends from far away, see street signs, and see pedestrian crossing signals in preparation for crossing the street. The impact of peripheral vision loss is in mobility. Imagine walking around looking through the core of a paper towel roll. When you see things you will see them quite well, but the challenge is finding things more than seeing them. Bumping into people in a crowded room and difficulty with crossing the streets are just a few of the major challenges with loss of peripheral vision. In terms of rehabilitation, the use of Fresnel prisms, increased scanning of the environment or inverse telescopes to increase peripheral field awareness, and the use of a long cane are the most effective strategies.

The concept with Fresnel prisms is to displace the image of objects in the far periphery by placing them in the near periphery (Figure 4.16). This is an efficient system for the detection of objects outside the normal visual field, but it comes at the expense of a "dead angle" at the boundary between the prism and the carrier lens. A system that effectively avoids this is essentially a narrow horizontal strip of prism material placed just below and/or above the line of sight, allowing the wearer to drop or raise the head in order to observe areas outside of the remaining field of view (Woods et al. 2010;

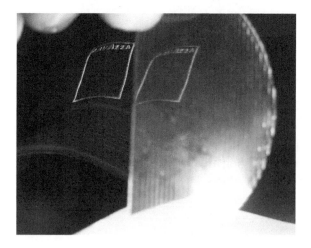

FIGURE 4.16
Fresnel prism. The prism is designed to displace the image of an object from an area of nonseeing to an area of seeing.

Bowers et al. 2008). This approach provides the user with constant visual feedback regarding objects to either side.

Summary

This chapter provided an overview of the demographics of the low vision population and described the functional effects of various types of low vision on daily life. Various types of optical and nonoptical equipment were presented to address the many challenges of having low vision. Near point activities such as reading are managed with various types of magnifiers (hand-held, stand, and reading microscopes) or with electro-optical systems like a CCTV. The importance of nonoptical equipment such as auxiliary sources of illumination, managing glare with filters, and the use of a clipboard when reading were described.

Mobility challenges include managing light adaptation, identifying and walking on stairs, and crossing the street. The use of hats/visors/sunglasses, the long cane, and telescopes were presented. For persons with good visual acuity but a loss of peripheral vision, Fresnel prisms may have the potential to minimize the impact of the loss of visual field.

References

Bowers, A.R., Keeney, K., and Peli, E. 2008. Community-based trial of a peripheral prism visual field expansion device for hemianopia. *Arch Ophthalmol*, 126:657–664.

Congdon, N., O'Colmain, B., Klaver, C.C. et al. 2004. Causes and prevalence of visual impairment among adults in the United States. *Arch Ophthalmol*, 122:477–485.

Feinbloom, W. 1935. Introduction to the principles and practice of sub-normal vision correction. *J Amer Optom Assn*, 6:3–18.

Klaver, C.C., Wolfs, R.C., Vingerling, J.R., Hofman, A., and de Jong, P.T. 1998. Age-specific prevalence and causes of blindness and visual impairment in an older population: The Rotterdam Study. *Arch Ophthalmol*, 116:653–658.

Klein, R., Klein, B.E., Lee, K.E., Cruickshanks, K.J., and Gangnon, R.E. 2006. Changes in visual acuity in a population over a 15-year period: The Beaver Dam Eye Study. *Am J Ophthalmol*, 142:539–549.

Munoz, B., West, S.K., Rubin, G.S. et al. 2000. Causes of blindness and visual impairment in a population of older Americans: The Salisbury Eye Evaluation Study. *Arch Ophthalmol*, 118:819–825.

Rahmani, B., Tielsch, J.M., Katz, J. et al. 1996. The cause-specific prevalence of visual impairment in an urban population. The Baltimore Eye Survey. *Ophthalmology*, 103:1721–1726.

Sommer, A., Tielsch, J.M., Katz, J. et al. 1991. Racial differences in the cause-specific prevalence of blindness in East Baltimore. *N Engl J Med*, 325:1412–1417.

Taylor, H.R., Keeffe, J.E., Vu, H.T. et al. 2005. Vision loss in Australia. *Med J Aust*, 182:565–568.

Woods, R.L., Giorgi, R.G., Berson, E.L., Peli, E. 2010. Extended wearing trial of Trifield lens device for 'tunnel vision'. *Ophthalmoic Physiol Opt*, 30:240–252.

5

Accessible Global Positioning Systems

Mike May and Kim Casey

CONTENTS

Defining the Navigation Problem

Without the ability to see surrounding location information, such as street signs and landmarks, it is difficult for a blind person to determine the accurate direction to travel and to efficiently move from place to place. Other common obstacles to independent travel for blind individuals are difficulty in determining when they have arrived at a particular destination and having limited access to information about the businesses and other features along the way. This can be contrasted with the vast amount of location information sighted people have access to when traveling by virtue of simply being able to look around.

To put this into a real-world scenario, imagine traveling on a bus to get to an important business meeting. You know the address of the building but cannot get your bearings because you do not know the exact address of the bus stop. As is common on many suburban streets, there is no one to ask and your guide dog, if you have one, is silent. The cell phone in your pocket has global positioning systems (GPS) and knows exactly where you are, but the trouble is without the ability to see the screen you do not have access to the map. You are now facing a barrier to location information that millions of individuals who are blind or visually impaired experience every day. The inability to know location information can often result in fear, reluctance to leave one's home or known routes, and a consequent withdrawal from major life participation in work, family, and community.

"One of the biggest challenges [for blind and visually impaired individuals] is lack of automatic information" (Weaver-Wyant 2010). A person with vision receives a constant wave of informational tidbits about the environment, such as traffic lights, construction zones, location of curb cutouts, driveway versus street crossings, what else is happening around us, nearby businesses, address numbers on buildings, what bus is passing, and the list goes on. It is this automatic information that people with sight use to avoid the barriers that would hinder successful travels.

Therefore, fundamentally, way-finding challenges for individuals who are blind or visually impaired can be considered problems of information access. While physical mobility and access to public transportation are important, perhaps the greatest unaddressed need of blind and visually impaired individuals is how to obtain, interpret, and use information in order to travel efficiently. Avoiding obstacles as well as detecting and negotiating changes in elevation are important mobility skills, to be sure, but modern techniques for using canes and dog guides have made obstacle avoidance less problematic for blind and visually impaired individuals compared with orientation and way-finding challenges.

Importance of Location Information

The term "location information" or "environmental information" refers to print that is on signs, on buildings, and any landmark that identifies a place in the environment. A person who can see accepts signage as part of life, so much a part, that they only notice it when the street sign is missing or obscured. For a blind person, location information has always been obscured, totally inaccessible.

"Knowledge is power," as stated by Sir Francis Bacon over 400 years ago (Bacon 1597), was considered a revolutionary statement, but the simple message behind this quote still applies today and more specifically it applies directly to this chapter. Justification for not traveling has been broken into three categories: (i) structural—barriers such as finances, abilities, time, or architectural; (ii) interpersonal—lack of travel partner or social interaction skills; and (iii) intrapersonal—lack of information or self-confidence (Crawford and Godbey 1987). For a person who is blind or visually impaired, all of these barriers equally thwart independent travel. However, in the following scenarios, the missing link in all of them is lack of information.

- A businessman who is blind frequently travels for work and often needs to plan business meetings in places he has never been to before. The popular mapping applications available on the Internet are graphic based and he has no way of visually navigating the map. The only way to pick a place is either calling the hotel concierge or asking a sighted colleague to provide him with a list of the potential meeting places.

- A Paratransit rider is late for a meeting and her driver is lost again. She wishes there was a way to help her driver find the way and get them both out of this mess.

- A college student who is blind is attempting to mentally map out his new campus. With all the meandering pathways and new buildings to remember, he wishes he could mark out the important places so that he could easily return to them. He feels like he is imposing by asking his guides to announce every building as they pass them, but he learns best through repetition.

What Mobility Tools and Traditional Maps Are Available for the Blind?

A blind individual who is learning basic mobility skills will initially be taught how to use a long cane or guide dog. These tools are essential to avoiding obstacles and staying safe while walking around. However, these tools are not useful in conveying the overall layout of a city.

In the days before accessible maps and GPS, blind individuals had two sources of information available to them, tactile maps or sighted guides. Tactile maps (introduced in Chapter 9) could provide a small-scale map of a specific location, but typically, due to size restrictions, they lack detail. Sighted guides greatly vary in ability to convey an environment. Consequently, orientation and mobility techniques (discussed in detail in Chapter 3) are founded and taught based upon the blind person not having location information. Specific routes are memorized, including the occasional landmark, to remind the blind traveler where to turn or conclude the route. Good travelers will learn how to cut corners or explore alternatives along the general route. The exceptional blind traveler will go exploring or create their own routes but the fundamental techniques and orientation tools have been limited in the past by the lack of a blind person's independent access to ubiquitous location information.

Alternatively, consider the travel experience of a sighted person. Forget that they can drive. While traveling, a sighted person processes a constant barrage of environmental cues such as street names, building signs, construction warnings, and landmarks. It is having access to this information, regardless of how much they use it, that plays a significant role in helping them navigate. Being able to see keeps them from running into obstacles, but having all this location information to provide constant feedback and choices is the key ingredient in successful travel.

Solving the Navigation Problem

"Accessibility for persons with vision impairments is usually a matter of having the right information at the right time. Having information means having choices and the ability to make the correct choice the first time" (Bentzen 1997).

Accessible GPS eliminates an enduring travel barrier experienced by individuals who are blind and visually impaired, the lack of location information. Every square foot of the earth essentially has an electronic label. These electronic labels begin in the form of a numeric latitude/longitude label. Every square foot on the planet has a "lat/lon." There are several commercial companies that focus on mapping out and naming these lat/lon coordinates. It is because of these companies that we have extensive databases of street names, addresses, and points of interest—everything from museums and restaurants to boat dealerships, and hospitals. If something stands still long enough, these companies will likely tag it and include it in the database.

Accessible GPS systems have millions of points of interest along with the street maps. Think of it like electronic yellow pages with locations attached to each of those points. With this tool, a blind person can conduct geographic research for a place to live, to go to school or to work, completely on his or her own.

The benefit of GPS for outdoor way-finding has been formally researched by Paul Ponchillia of Western Michigan University. This research consisted of three studies using Sendero GPS in different scenarios. One study measured 19 participants' ability to locate a 25-foot chalk circle from 150 feet away with and without a GPS. The participants using GPS located the circle independently in 53 of 57 trials, while only doing so 7 of 57 times without it (Ponchillia et al. 2007a). Three additional studies measured GPS effects on (a) a novice user's ability to reorient in a familiar neighborhood, (b) a novice user's ability to locate a house target in a familiar neighborhood, and (c) an experienced user's ability to utilize two levels of intervention to locate a house target in a familiar neighborhood. Those using GPS technology reoriented in 100% of the trials compared to 80% when using no GPS and they became reoriented in approximately 17% of the elapsed time taken in the no GPS trials. Additionally, GPS users located house targets 100% of the time, while only doing so 25% of the time when not using the device. The GPS users traveled a mean distance of about one-half as far as the nonusers did to locate the house targets and they did it about twice as efficiently (in terms of target distance vs. travel time). Another experiment demonstrated that a user could be more efficient at house target location using a simple GPS function (street address), than with natural way-finding skills, and even more efficiently with a higher-level GPS function (waypoint marking and following) (Ponchillia et al. 2007b).

Additional research has indicated that fear of stranding, disorientation, or in simply appearing confused is a barrier of such significance that many individuals who are blind or visually impaired do not and will not travel independently (Golledge et al. 2004). Additionally, it is our experience that when such individuals get specific travel and location information, they are far more likely to explore. For example, participants from a previous Sendero accessible way-finding study indicated that they currently travel to a new destination roughly once a month. If given a device that would provide orientation information and information about surroundings, the participants indicated that they would increase their travel frequency to once a week (Golledge et al. 2004). It is hard to overstate the importance of expanding the safe travel horizon for a blind or visually impaired person by even a few blocks; in most cities, such an expansion makes available new bus routes, transfer options, new access to goods, social functions, and healthful groceries.

History of Accessible GPS

A quiet revolution has changed the way sighted people learn about where they travel. With little fanfare, graphical handheld GPS devices seem to be everywhere. GPS technology has matured into a resource that goes far beyond its original design goals. These days, scientists, farmers, soldiers, pilots, surveyors, hikers, delivery drivers, sailors, dispatchers, firefighters, and people from many other walks of life are using GPS in ways that make their work more productive, safer, and sometimes even easier (Trimble 2011).

One can readily understand why the lure of GPS has long attracted research interest for the blind and visually impaired market. The idea of using GPS to assist with navigation by the visually impaired goes back to the mid-1980s (Collins 1985; Loomis 1985). The first evaluation of GPS for this purpose was carried out by Strauss and his colleagues (Brusnighan et al. 1989). Because their research was conducted during early deployment of GPS, the poor positioning accuracy available to them precluded practical studies with visually impaired subjects.

Starting in 1985, taking that initial research further, Jack Loomis and his colleagues, Reginald Golledge and Roberta Klatzky, began the personal guidance system (PGS) project that lasted for over two decades. Beyond providing basic GPS tracking, the PGS explored the feasibility of virtual auditory displays and speech recognition. Due to the complexity of the PGS and amount of technology needed to operate it, it never evolved into an end-user product.

Recognizing the need for an end-user product with input from actual blind consumers, Mike May and Charles LaPierre began working on the first accessible GPS prototype at Arkenstone in 1994. Their aim was to develop efficient, accessible, and blind-friendly user interfaces using the key feature of sustained blind user feedback. The resulting product was called Strider and was terminated in 1997. A related talking map product called Atlas was released for the PC in 1995 and was sold through 2001.

The first commercial GPS-based system was GPS-Talk, which was produced and sold by Sendero Group. GPS-Talk was a laptop-based system that used detailed digital street maps covering the United States as well as selected locations in other countries. A synthetic speech display provided both information about the locations of nearby streets and points of interest and instructions for traveling to desired destinations. The limited success of GPS-Talk can be attributed to the high expense of the system components, inefficiency due to short battery life and slow start-up times, and lack of portability.

A year later, Sendero teamed up with HumanWare with the first accessible GPS on a portable digital assistant (PDA), the BrailleNote. Sendero GPS for BrailleNote offered longer battery life, instant access to information, and lighter weight. Development on Sendero GPS has continued over the past decade. Some of the features now offered to blind consumers by BrailleNote GPS version 2011 include (a) a description of the nearest or next intersection; (b) heading and distance to a destination as defined by entering an address or by picking from millions of points of interest; (c) hearing the heading and distance to the nearest school, business, or other points of interest; (d) browsing streets and cross streets; and (e) following an automatic route to a destination.

After the initial success of the BrailleNote GPS system, two other companies endeavored to develop competitive accessible GPS products. The resulting products were "Trekker" from Visuaide, now HumanWare, and "StreetTalk™" from Freedom Scientific. Trekker was the first stand-alone accessible GPS product. StreetTalk™ adapted the Destinator™ 3 GPS application for Pocket PCs to run on the PacMate line of PDAs. Both products were discontinued after limited popularity in the marketplace. In 2008, HumanWare released another version of a stand-alone GPS product, called the Trekker Breeze. The Trekker Breeze has a simple user interface utilizing nine buttons to execute the navigation commands.

After over a decade of experience, Sendero expanded from the BrailleNote to three other platforms with its Software Development Kit (SDK). Code Factory, which makes a screen reader for mobile phones and Windows PDAs, worked with Sendero to create Mobile Geo, released in September 2008. HIMS from Korea adopted this SDK for their Braille Sense and Voice Sense PDAs with a product called Sense Navigation. Freedom Scientific adopted this SDK to create a product called StreetTalk VIP GPS, thereby reviving an accessible GPS solution for the PAC Mate.

In 2010, Sendero expanded again with the addition of Sendero Maps for the PC as well as Sendero GPS LookAround for iPhone and Android devices.

Finally, there is a point-of-interest-only product for mobile phones called Loadstone. It has no street maps, only points of interest created by users or public domain points. The great thing for blind people is that there are options to fit a variety of needs and way-finding situations.

Accessible GPS Market Trends

Accessible GPS has been on the market since 2000, beginning with a laptop version that state agencies would not fund. As of the writing of this chapter, there are seven accessible GPS options and approximately 10–20% of government agencies now fund these products. The increasing prevalence of accessible GPS products can be attributed to convincing funding agencies that these products are an essential tool in independent way-finding. We estimate that 10% of people who are blind and own some adaptive technology also have a fully accessible GPS product, in the range of 15,000–25,000 users worldwide.

Accessible GPS Systems

In the previous section, there was a brief description of some of the current accessible GPS systems and how they fit into the timeline of accessible GPS development. The aim of this section is to paint a more detailed picture of all the currently available accessible GPS systems.

Accessible GPS Systems on Personal Data Assistants

As evidenced from the history of accessible GPS systems, the demand for a full-featured GPS system on a portable unit was high. The main reason for the accessible GPS explosion on various PDAs is that many blind and visually impaired individuals already own and extensively use these devices. These devices offer a choice of Braille or QWERTY keyboards and option of speech and Braille output. Preference between these devices is fundamentally a personal choice. However, the devices that are the most portable and have the easiest user interfaces are the most popular.

All of the following are essentially running the same GPS software due to the fact that they are developed using the same SDK. The difference is in the hardware platform.

Sendero GPS for the BrailleNote Apex, PK, and mPower

The BrailleNote products run a proprietary software called KeySoft which includes fully accessible applications, such as a word processor, book reader, Web browser, email, memo recorder, media player, calculator, streaming audio, and instant messaging chat (Figures 5.1 and 5.2). The accessible GPS, Sendero GPS, is just another application added to the above list.

Sense Navigation for the Voice Sense and Braille Sense

The Braille Sense, Braille Sense OnHand, Braille Sense U2, and Voice Sense PDAs, from HIMS Inc., offer similar applications to the BrailleNote, but in addition also offer a DAISY player, Twitter, and FM radio (Figures 5.3 through 5.5). The Sense line of products, like the previously mentioned BrailleNote line, operates on a proprietary user interface, but it is very similar to Windows. The Braille Sense OnHand and the Voice Sense QWERTY have built-in GPS receivers ensuring that one is never without their GPS receiver.

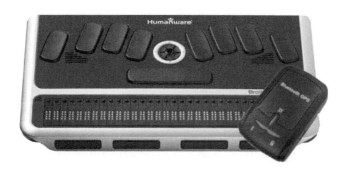

FIGURE 5.1
BrailleNote Apex with GPS receiver.

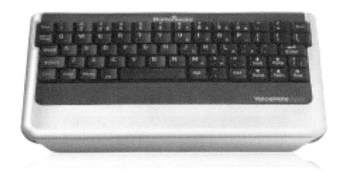

FIGURE 5.2
VoiceNote Apex QWERTY.

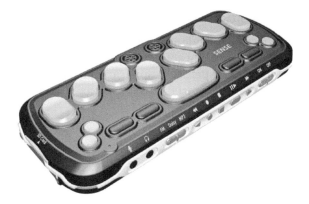

FIGURE 5.3
Voice Sense.

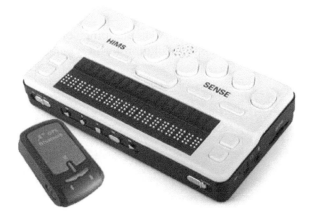

FIGURE 5.4
Braille Sense OnHand with GPS receiver.

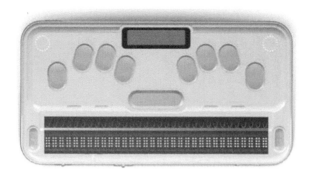

FIGURE 5.5
Braille Sense.

StreetTalk VIP for PAC Mate Omni

The PAC Mate Omni, from Freedom Scientific, provides an accessible version using their JAWS screen-reading software for Windows Mobile (Figure 5.6). It provides the standard Microsoft applications including Word, Excel, Calendar, Outlook, Inbox, Contacts, Internet Explorer, and Windows Media Player.

Future Platforms

As of this writing, the GPS system currently being called Nearby Explorer is being developed by American Printing House for the Blind (APH) to run on an Android PDA, called Braille Plus from APH and Orion from LevelStar.

Accessible GPS for PCs

Sendero Maps for the PC

Not forgotten from the days of the Atlas mapping software on the PC, the demand for an accessible mapping solution for PCs persisted. The strength

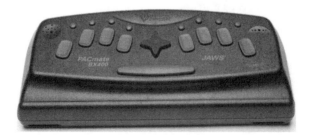

FIGURE 5.6
PAC Mate Omni.

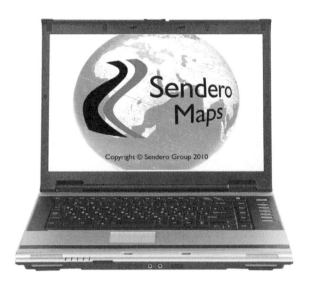

FIGURE 5.7
Laptop running Sendero Maps program.

of a PC solution is that most of the portable solutions, as powerful as they are, still cannot compete with the speed of a PC (Figure 5.7). Long routes can be created and point-of-interest searches spanning hundreds of miles can be completed in mere seconds.

Accessible GPS for Mobile Phones, Smartphones

This group of accessible GPS systems results from a high demand for portability. In this increasingly mobile world, with close to 5.3 billion mobile subscribers worldwide (International Telecommunication Union 2010), it goes without saying that many people would want access to maps and GPS on a device that they are already carrying around with them.

Mobile Geo for Windows Mobile Devices

Mobile Geo was the first accessible GPS solution for a mainstream mobile device (Figure 5.8). Compatible devices included Windows Mobile-based smartphones and Pocket PCs, and with an accessible screen reader called Mobile Speak, all the functions of the phone were accessible to the user. The input method, differing from all the previous devices, was either phone keypad or a mini-QWERTY keyboard.

Sendero GPS LookAround for the iPhone and Android

To keep up with all the mobile GPS apps for sighted individuals, a version of accessible GPS was developed for the most popular platforms, iPhone and

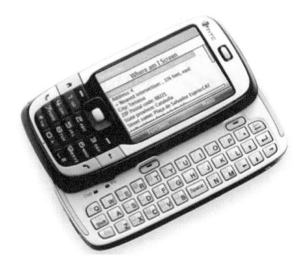

FIGURE 5.8
Windows Mobile phone running Mobile Geo.

Android, in 2010 and 2011 (Figure 5.9). This GPS provides basic environmental information, such as nearby points of interest, cross street, and current location of the user. Currently, these apps do not have the capability to create routes and no maps are stored on the phone, so, if the user does not have an active connection with the cell tower, there will be no maps available.

Stand-Alone Accessible GPS Systems

Trekker Breeze Stand-Alone by HumanWare

The Trekker Breeze was developed in 2008 to provide a simple stand-alone GPS solution that is preferred by those who do not have much technology experience (Figure 5.10). Trekker Breeze can be controlled by one hand and has nine buttons for input. It verbally announces names of streets, intersections, and landmarks as you walk. The most recent model provides routing to addresses and commercial points of interest.

Kapten Plus

Kapten Plus is a mainstream GPS product which offers voice control, utilizing the automatic speech recognition technology from Nuance. The most recent model has been improved to make its features accessible. Kapten Plus can announce the user's location and any surrounding point of interest. It can create routes as well as save locations the user has visited. Like the Breeze, Kapten uses the SIRF 3 GPS chipset. Because of its small size, it has a small patch antenna, which may have some difficulty in

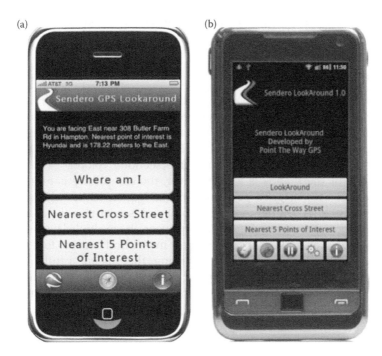

FIGURE 5.9
(a) iPhone and (b) Android phone running Sendero GPS LookAround software.

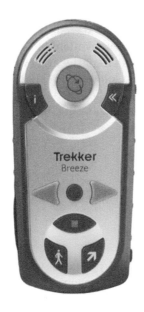

FIGURE 5.10
Trekker Breeze.

receiving satellites among tall buildings. It also functions as an MP3 player and FM radio.

Semiaccessible GPS Systems

With the advent of the iPhone and Android devices with screen readers, a number of GPS applications are anywhere from not at all accessible to semi-accessible. Some of the iPhone semiaccessible GPS apps are TomTom, GPS by TeleNav, MotionX GPS Drive, and NAVIGON. Some of the Android semiaccessible GPS apps are WalkyTalky and Intersection Explorer.

The cost for these apps is low; however, the complexity is high because these devices are designed primarily for navigation while driving and for visual feedback. When new versions come out, sometimes the accessibility becomes worse, sometimes better. In any event, the multiple layers of menus and visual display make it challenging for most blind users to find the functions in a timely manner. As of this writing, there is not a fully accessible turn-by-turn application on any type of smartphone other than Mobile Geo for Windows Mobile phones, and the Windows operating system for that product has been discontinued.

Comparing Accessible GPS Systems

Since, as the saying goes, "Not one size fits all," it is good that there are various accessible GPS systems now available to blind and visually impaired people. Every product has its strengths and weaknesses. Every user has a different set of needs. It is no longer a question of *if* a blind person should have GPS but a question of *which* GPS to have.

Primary considerations when choosing a GPS system are

1. User interface
2. Multifunctionality
3. Portability
4. Price

User Interface

A primary consideration is the type of user interface, for both input and output. In using an information-rich system like accessible GPS, it is important that the user can quickly access the necessary information to be able to travel successfully. If one is struggling with typing in an address or cannot hear the announcement, then the system has not made life easier for anyone.

The first question regarding the hardware of an accessible GPS system is what is the preferred method of input. Depending on how much the user plans on inputting addresses, custom points of interest, searching for points of interest, and so on, the choice of input will be a factor on which GPS system is chosen. The four types of input available are Braille keyboard, QWERTY keyboard, mobile phone keypad, and voice control technology.

The QWERTY options are VoiceNote mPower QT, BrailleNote Apex QT, Braille Sense QWERTY, and Voice Sense QWERTY. The Braille keyboard options are Voice Sense, Braille Sense, Braille Sense OnHand, VoiceNote mPower BT, BrailleNote Apex BT, and BrailleNote PK. The mobile phone keypad options are Mobile Geo, iPhone, and Android. The voice control options are Mobile Geo with limited voice control and Kapten Plus with full control.

While voice control can add convenience, it is one of those technologies which is always promising perfection in the future, not necessarily being a technology that works consistently in all situations. It is common in noisy outdoor environments for voice recognition to be very frustrating. There are also privacy issues. Not everyone wants the other bus passengers to know what destination you are trying to select. It is troublesome when you are talking to your device and someone speaks to you at the same time. Voice control is not nearly as accurate or private as keyboard control.

The second hardware consideration is the output, meaning how to get the information from the device. All the units have speech output and some can also have a Braille display. A Braille display can be an invaluable asset for those who extensively use them, as well as provide spelling confirmations on street names and locations, but it also increases the price.

The options for a PDA with Braille display are BrailleNote PK, Apex (BT or QT), Braille Sense OnHand, Braille Sense QT or BT, and Pac Mate with BT or QT. Although an outboard display can be added to a mobile phone or Voice Sense, this defeats the purpose of a small portable all-in-one device.

Beyond the hardware aspects of the GPS device, it is also important to consider the software aspects when determining potential productivity. The more features a product has to offer, the steeper the learning curve. However, many users invest the necessary time to learn how to use their GPS to suit their navigational needs. Different situations require different GPS functionality. Are you just walking around and want to know what streets are nearby versus researching a trip or planning a route? Are you on city streets or in the woods? Depending on the individual's intended use, it is important to choose the appropriate GPS system that will maximize productivity.

Multifunctionality

In our fast-paced world, it is not uncommon to see people checking their emails or editing a report on the way to work. It is also not unusual for a person to carry more than one electronic device. When it comes to accessible GPS, it is important to consider minimizing all the devices one has to carry. If a person already has an accessible PDA that they use for browsing the Internet, sending emails and editing documents, why not just add GPS to that device rather than add another device to the mix? Three brands of accessible PDAs have accessible GPS add-on software. If, on the other hand, a person does not need to carry a device for email, Internet or word processing, why would they carry a fully featured device when all they would use is the GPS?

Portability

Portability is very important with accessible GPS. One would think that this consideration would be straightforward, meaning the most portable device would be the most popular. However, it is not always that simple. Depending on the user, it might not be the best choice to have the most portable unit because of trade-offs with the user interface, physical layout of the device, or location information content. The ultimate goal of the multifunctional accessible GPS units was to add the GPS capability to accessible PDAs and phones that people were already carrying around with them, making portability a nonissue.

The user interface consideration was discussed in a previous section, but it resurfaces here as well. In this case, it would not matter how portable an accessible GPS system is if the user just cannot figure out how to search for an address, cannot understand the directions, or has to completely learn to use a new hardware device. Additionally, the unreliability of voice input may outweigh the benefits of a small device.

The physical layout of the device is important to a person with larger hands or poor sensitivity in their fingers. They would probably prefer to have a GPS device that weighs the least or that could easily fit in their pocket, but it would not be possible for them to use. Alternatively, a person might choose one of the relatively heavier PDAs because they already carry it to and from work, so adding GPS to that will not make a difference in portability to that person.

The location information content is another aspect that will influence a person's choice regarding portability. If the device they want weighs less, but does not have a comprehensive point-of-interest database or an unreliable GPS receiver, they will likely choose the device that can deliver more information. Another aspect that arises is the weight of the Braille display on the accessible PDAs. If the user wants to have access to the spellings of streets and points of interest or prefers to mute the speech for privacy, the weight of the Braille display would be overlooked.

The bottom line with portability is that the smaller the better as long as you do not sacrifice features and accessibility.

Price

Last but not least is the price consideration. First of all, one needs to weigh the importance of the previously mentioned aspects and determine what it is worth to have the optimal accessible GPS solution for their individual needs.

TABLE 5.1

Comparison of Accessible GPS Systems

Hardware Platform	Input Type	Output Type	Multi-Functional?	Price ($)	Portability Weight
BrailleNote, VoiceNote	Braille or QWERTY	Speech and/or Braille	Yes	1388	1.35–1.8 lbs; 612–812 g
Braille Sense, Voice Sense	Braille or QWERTY	Speech and/or Braille	Yes	1388	0.58–2 lbs; 266–914 g
PAC Mate	Braille or QWERTY	Speech and/or Braille	Yes	1499–1799	1.8–4.2 lbs; 812–1905 g
Windows Mobile-based smartphones and pocket PCs	Mobile phone keypad	Speech	Yes	788–998	0.3–0.5 lbs; 140–250 g
iPhone and Android	Touchscreen or mobile phone keypad	Speech	Yes	5	0.3 lbs; 133 g
Trekker Breeze	Few buttons	Speech	No	929	1.1 lbs; 499 g
Kapten Plus	Voice control technology	Speech	No	399	0.13 lbs; 60 g

One can pay thousands of dollars for a GPS system that can provide all imaginable location information, but if this tool is never used, the investment does not make sense. On the other hand, one can try to save some money on a GPS system just to find out that the system is not reliable or cannot do what is needed.

Next, one needs to determine available resources. Some questions to answer would be: Do they already have or can benefit from an accessible PDA like the BrailleNote or Braille Sense products? Do they qualify for outside funding sources such as grants and state rehabilitation funds?

Comparison Chart

Table 5.1 presents all the currently available accessible GPS systems summarizing the previously mentioned considerations.

User Experiences with Accessible GPS

With accessible GPS systems permeating the market, blind travelers now can access their world as never before. The blind traveler can now be actively involved in every aspect of where they are going and how they are getting there. He or she can become a navigator on a road trip, determine a bypass route when stuck in traffic, keep tabs on the taxi driver's route, learn about the sites and businesses being passed, and ride the bus without needing anyone to announce the stops. Students can also chart custom routes across the campus or hikers can do the same in the woods. There are four main benefits to having accessible GPS:

1. Access to location information
2. Teaching orientation and mobility concepts
3. Problem-solving skills/safety
4. Increased opportunities

Access to Location Information

Basic access to location information is something that can be easily taken for granted. To someone who is blind or visually impaired, it carries a greater significance because the user can learn about their surroundings and have unprecedented access to "signage," or all the visual cues that help a person navigate. Everyone has received the directions such as, go past the third gigantic tree and my house is the one on the left. If those trees were taken out, or in the case of a visually impaired person, you could not see them, and it would make finding a location much more difficult.

In addition to having access to signage, accessible GPS can also identify a point of interest or a street name that is something new, making the user exclaim, "I didn't know that was there!" During an accessible GPS demonstration, the system was announcing a restaurant that no one, including the sighted individuals, knew was there. The participants were so adamant about the restaurant not being there as they believed they would have known about it. Upon further exploration, we did indeed find the door to that restaurant. The main point being that with accessible GPS you can explore with a whole new set of eyeballs.

Another aspect of accessible GPS is the virtual exploration or the ability to "look around" to gather information about the travel environment, including street names, intersections, points of interest, city, and so on. This feature helps with mental mapping skills, so that a person can fully understand the environment, how the streets intersect, what businesses they will pass on their route, and so on, before they even travel outside.

Teaching Orientation and Mobility Concepts

Accessible GPS has proven very valuable in introducing important orientation and mobility concepts, such as left and right, cardinal directions, and clock face directions. Without adequate repetition, these concepts can be quite challenging to an individual learning orientation and mobility techniques. The beauty of accessible GPS systems is that you will hear destinations using these concepts. Travelers can also learn environmental concepts such as shapes of intersections, direction of travel, sidewalks, and types of streets.

Additionally, when accessible GPS is incorporated into the teaching curriculum, it can be applied to geography and social studies core curriculum concepts. A student can, for example, go to a place on the map and learn about it, what restaurants it has, major tourist spots, and so on.

Problem-Solving Skills/Safety

Not arguably, the most important benefit of accessible GPS is increased safety. An individual can use GPS to determine distance and direction to a destination, confirm their place in space and direction of travel, and obtain immediate access to addresses and phone numbers in case they are lost or need to call for help. At any point in a route, the user can confirm that they are where they are supposed to be; otherwise, they can determine what they need to do to fix it and if they are overwhelmed can call for help. Over the years, accessible GPS users have shared a range of all of these situations.

With Flexibility Come Increased Opportunities

Beyond the obvious orientation and mobility benefits of GPS, having access to information that provides flexibility is directly related to increasing opportunities. The better a person independently navigates, the better he or she will be prepared for obtaining a job, maintaining that job, and advancing a career. Flexibility is having the ability to navigate on the fly. This can be accomplished through a combination of tools like mobility instruction and GPS navigation. Like sighted folks, blind people need to get around effectively and GPS provides the equivalent of print signs as well as voice or Braille navigation assistance.

User Stories

Since the inception of accessible GPS, Sendero has closely followed its users and even organized events to ensure that we receive constant feedback from our users. For various years, Sendero organized a "WayFun" trip where 20 or so users would get together and explore a new city using their accessible GPS. Travelers would submit their personal stories of what they learned over the course of the trip. Additionally, users share their GPS trace files, recorded points of interest, photos, audio files, and testimonials when they embark on a solo-trip. One user recorded his trip to Yosemite, California, and submitted his route files, points of interest, and audio files, and shared all of this with all accessible GPS users (Figure 5.11).

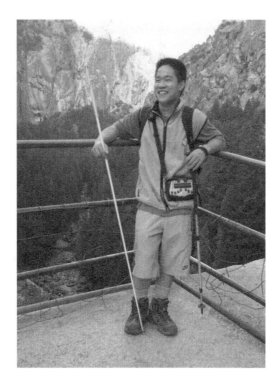

FIGURE 5.11
Accessible GPS user navigating independently in Yosemite, California.

For over 10 years, Sendero has been collecting stories from GPS users. The stories are from new users, users who have discovered another feature or have found it particularly useful on a trip, and even from veteran users.

The stories from new users are typically that of enthusiasm for their new technology. Their world is opening up to them in a way they never imagined.

> Once I really grasp the informational possibilities, I'm going to be traveliciously invincible!!
>
> **–CH**

> I'm loving my new Sendero product running on the Apex. Whether in virtual or GPS mode, the software makes it a pleasure to use. I love the information that is available at my fingertips (literally) whenever I am out walking or traveling. The occasional announcements of passing POIs and the change of street announcements makes it easy for me to walk around.
>
> **–MM**

I'm just getting started with the GPS, and already, the others who regularly ride my bus, even the driver, are interested when I tell them what we are passing. It is great to learn about places you didn't know you were passing every day.

–CC

The stories from experienced users who just discovered a new feature are similar in tone to the new user ones, since they are the people who thought they knew everything that GPS had to offer, but were surprised once again.

Today, I got on a bus without auto announce. Although I asked, the driver failed to call my stop and we passed it. When I got off the bus, I immediately turned on the Sendero Look Around application and quickly figured out where I was.

–DH

I took the GPS on the coach and was able to follow where we were going and get a lot of information about the towns we passed through. It is surprising how many places have English names which are quite different from the name they have in German. The driver was quite amused when I accused her of speeding—well over 100 Km/h is speeding in my book.

–SB

Finally, the stories from veteran users reflect on their GPS use over the years (Figure 5.12).

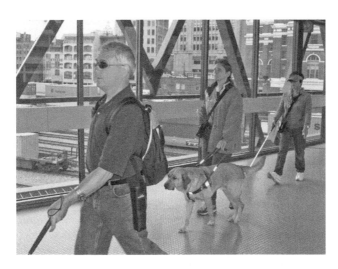

FIGURE 5.12
Group of accessible GPS users exploring a new city.

For many years after I moved to Los Angeles in 1984, I had very little knowledge of street names, the types of businesses on those streets, whether particular streets ran East/West or North/South, and so on. After traveling with GPS since 2000, and, in essence, watching what I was passing, I have a good understanding of where things are, even when I don't have my GPS with me. And, since I use GPS with a braille display, I automatically know the spellings of street names and of names for businesses. GPS does not replace the need for good mobility and orientation skills. But knowing where I am and what is around me greatly enhances my ability to travel independently whether I am on foot, on a bus, or in a taxi or private automobile.

When walking with my guide dog, AJ, I generally use Sendero GPS to tell where I am. With one-handed commands that don't interfere with my dog, I can quickly determine the name of the street I am on, the next intersection, my direction of travel, and whether I am getting closer to my destination. This removes the necessity of counting streets, and allows me to focus more on traffic sounds and the people around me.

When traveling on a bus, I set my destination to my final address. I can then tell when I am getting close to my destination. Also, I don't need to worry if the driver forgets to call my stop, or simply turns off the automatic stop announcements.

When traveling in a taxi, or with my wife or sons in a private automobile, I use Sendero GPS to quickly locate restaurants and businesses of interest, and then compute routes to those destinations. This makes me totally aware of where we are going and how we can get there. It makes me an active and helpful navigator when traveling instead of a passive passenger who is not giving any input. Having someone tell you, as a driver, which streets are coming up before you can see them can be very helpful; especially at night.

When it comes to locating things, Sendero GPS also functions as geographically-based electronic yellow pages. There are over 15,000,000 public and personal businesses included in the database for the United States and Canada. I look up items of interest either where I am, or virtually in remote locations. Since telephone numbers are included I can, for example, call in advance to see if a particular business is open, its hours of operation, and whether they have a product that I am looking for.

–RS

I remember the first time I had my Sendero GPS working with my Braille Note. I was like a child in a candy store. Why! It was for the first time that I didn't have to ask an Access driver "Where are we?" It gave me so much information that I was craving for and really didn't know what I was missing not having a GPS on the Braille Note. The most ironic thing is when I give precise directions to drivers who don't know where they are driving or I turn off speech and know when I'm being taken for a joy ride and need to correct the driver.

–MEE

References

Bacon, F. 1597. *Religious Meditations, Of Heresies.*

Bentzen, B. L. 1997. *Environmental Accessibility.* In Blasch, Weiner and Welsh (Eds.), *Foundations of Orientation and Mobility*, 2nd Edition. New York: American Foundation for the Blind.

Brusnighan, D. A., Strauss, M. G., Floyd, J. M., and Wheeler, B. C. 1989. Orientation aid implementing the global positioning system. In S. Buus (Ed.), *Proceedings of the Fifteenth Annual Northeast Bioengineering Conference*, pp. 33–34. Boston: IEEE.

Collins, C. C. 1985. On mobility aids for the blind. In D. H. Warren and E. R. Strelow (Eds.), *Electronic Spatial Sensing for the Blind*, pp. 35–64. Dordrecht: Martinus Nijhoff.

Crawford, D. W. and Godbey, G. 1987. Reconceptualizing barriers to family leisure. *Leisure Sciences*, 9(2):119–128.

Golledge, R., Marston, J., Loomis, J., and Klatzky, R. 2004. Stated preferences for components of a personal guidance system for nonvisual navigation. *Journal of Visual Impairment & Blindness*, 98(3):135–147.

International Telecommunication Union. 2010. Key Global Telecom Indicators for the World Telecommunication Service Sector. Available at http://www.itu.int/ITU-D/ict/statistics/at_glance/KeyTelecom.html.

Loomis, J. M. 1985. Digital map and navigation system for the visually impaired. Unpublished manuscript, Department of Psychology, University of California, Santa Barbara.

Ponchillia, P. E., MacKenzie, N., Long, R. L., Denton-Smith, P., Hicks, T., and Miley, P. 2007a. Finding a target with an accessible GPS. *Journal of Visual Impairment and Blindness*, 101(8): 479–488.

Ponchillia, P. E., Rak, E. C., Freeland, A. L., and LaGrow, S. J. 2007b. Accessible GPS: Reorientation and target location among users with visual impairments. *Journal of Visual Impairment and Blindness*, 101(7): 389–401.

Trimble. 2011. GPS Tutorial. Available at http://www.trimble.com/gps/index.shtml.

Weaver-Wyant, R. 2010. Moving blindly through a visually oriented world. Accessible at http://www.senderogroup.com/docs/Moving_Blindly_Through_a_Visually_Oriented_World.doc.

6

Development, Evaluation, and Lessons Learned: A Case Study of Talking Signs® Remote Infrared Audible Signage

Bill Crandall and James Marston

CONTENTS

Introduction

This chapter is a "case study" formulated in the hope of satisfying the interests of and in benefit to rehabilitation engineers and those interested in developing/manufacturing access technology, as well as orientation and mobility professionals who might have wondered about the process of bringing access technology "to the street." It describes the origin of the idea, and the twists and turns of the perennially promising wayfinding access technology, Talking Signs® remote infrared audible signage (RIAS).

The chapter begins with a physical description of the system and the demographics of those whom the technology is designed to serve. It describes, in a general way, the early laboratory experiments that specified the hardware—designs which can, in many cases, be seen in the evolved, modern implementation. Most important, however, are descriptions of the later field experiments designed to explore the breadth of wayfinding applications (intersections, identification of bus stops/buses, emergency egress, navigation in facilities); this research being primarily based upon objective measures of time, errors, restarts, and subjective measures including surveys, open-ended questions, and focus groups. Other field experiments concentrated more on how travel might be affected by factors such as cognitive awareness, mental maps, affective values, and so on. It has been the long history of positive research results that has attracted manufacturers to develop a range of impressive variants to this original wayfinding technology.

The ride has been bumpy and in order to highlight issues that others might hopefully steer around, the chapter ends with a short section on "Lessons Learned." In retrospect, most of these same pitfalls can and do confront all such endeavors.

RIAS Concepts

RIAS labels the environment so that people who cannot see or otherwise read print signs have access to that information. Using a hand-held receiver (shown on the right, Figure 6.1), a person scans the area to pick up messages from the infrared transmitters (shown on the left, Figure 6.1) labeling what is around them, such as bus stops, train platforms, ticket machines, information windows, and elevators or stairs. In addition, this system has been shown to be particularly effective in providing dynamic/real-time indications of wait time for the next bus to arrive (via text-to-speech); on-board vehicle location (next stop) recorded or via text-to-speech; vehicle and route identification (destination) recorded or via text-to-speech; and pedestrian crossing information (at intersections: walk/wait and direction/location).

In order to enhance wayfinding, the beam width of the transmitter can be adjusted to be as narrow as 6° or as wide as 360°. As you walk closer to the sign the message gets clearer and louder. Because the infrared transmitters use a communications technology called frequency modulation (FM), only the strongest of the messages are picked up (think FM car radio), only the message your receiver is pointed toward is heard. Most RIAS messages are unique and short, simple and straightforward.

If technologies are difficult to learn and hard to use, chances are that potential users will not choose to use them. This is especially true for systems meant to be used in real time—when actually traveling. RIAS is robust in this regard. Training and use are simple: the location of the Talking Sign is where the message is loudest and clearest. There is nothing the user must remember or adjust in order to use the system. The message is a label. If users walk toward the direction they are pointing the receiver at when they hear the message clearly, they are going toward the sign.

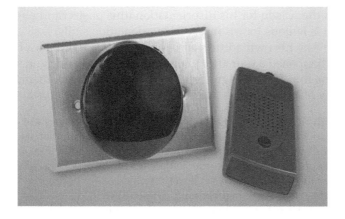

FIGURE 6.1
Remote infrared audible signage (RIAS) transmitter (left) and receiver (right).

Demographics

The U.S. Census Bureau's 2005 Household Economic Studies found that "nearly 7.8 million people age 15 and older had difficulty seeing words or letters in ordinary newspaper print, including 1.8 million being completely unable to see [such words or letters]" when using their corrected vision (Brault, 2008).

With a population rapidly shifting to larger proportions of people in older age groups, the number of people who have difficulty reading, for example, visual emergency egress signs can be expected to increase rapidly as well. Most people with severe visual impairments are 65 or over, a group growing twice as fast as the overall population. There is a per-decade increase of 1–2 million persons in the United States over 65 with functional limitations in seeing (Schmeidler and Halfmann, 1997) defined as difficulty seeing ordinary newsprint with their best-corrected vision. These seniors are still potentially very mobile, but impaired vision is very likely to restrict their confidence and ability to travel independently.

Formation of the Technology: The "Idea"

Anything that has been around a while will develop apocryphal stories, and the one around the idea for Talking Signs has been one of those. Just so, "Necessity is the Mother of Invention" stories that are hard to displace—largely because knowing the protagonist gives it such a truthful ring. Accordingly, the legend goes: One evening Bill Gerrey, Smith-Kettlewell (S-K) electronics engineer, became disoriented while walking home after a late evening bout of drinking. Because Bill is blind, he patiently waited on the street until he could hail someone to point him in the direction toward home. An add-on to this story has Bill losing his cane to a sidewalk construction hole as the reason for his disorientation (this postscript being required because Bill is famous for his impeccable orientation skills).

The truth—by his own admission—is much more mundane. The story is real, only it happened a year after a convergence of tinkering and serendipity produced the first Talking Signs prototype. From Bill's documentation of the early history of Talking Signs (Gerrey, 1991):

> At Smith-Kettlewell, events happened so fast that everyone is still debating as to who thought of which part first. I can tell you that, as far as I know, Pete Neiberg and I were the first to modulate the Z-axis of an oscilloscope with a tape recorder and detect the beam with a cadmium-sulfide cell into a Radio Shack pocket amplifier. Not to be forgotten is the main character, Bill Loughborough. These experiments went on in his laboratory. He recognized the inevitability of this system before the rest of us admitted to it. It was his work with infrared beacons and games that led us down the infrared path.

Loughborough was keen to create a running game where relatively sedentary children would be motivated to stretch themselves, both physically and emotionally. He wanted a beep-beep infrared beacon to aid nonsighted runners in traversing a clear path. On the other hand, Bill Gerrey wanted an aid to navigation and therefore the idea of replacing the beeps with speech messages came quickly to him, followed immediately by these talking beacons being used as signs that talked (for the first few years the devices being called "Talking Lights"). All these ideas and what was to follow occurred in several hours of conversation over drinks at the corner's "Don't Call It Frisco."

Surprisingly, the issue of whether this development should be radio frequency or infrared never came up because it was so obvious to these engineers that the directionality of the infrared light signal can be precisely controlled whereas the radio frequency signal tends to be omni-directional; an infrared exit sign and an infrared entrance sign could be installed back-to-back without one interfering with or being mistaken for the other. The decision whether the technology should be amplitude modulation (AM) or FM was settled once a prototype revealed the crosstalk interference existing between AM transmitters. As previously noted, FM receivers select only one signal at a time, based upon signal strength at the receiver end. This fixes the crosstalk problem. The second issue was interference by bright lights. Imagine these little LEDs on a pole with the blazing sun lined up behind them: David and Goliath! Another one of these S-K boys, Jules Madey, created a "front end" for the receiver that is the hallmark of RIAS design: one that is practically immune to this immense volume of superfluous, interfering sunlight pouring into the RIAS receiver, thereby allowing the system to function uniformly indoors as well as out of doors. Technically, the RIAS world revolved around Jules for he hand-assembled the receivers and transmitters and programmed the voice messages for the early RIAS experiments and installations. He then designed a receiver front end which retained the solar background suppression of the original units but was more suitable for mass production.

The first blooming of installations occurred due to passage of a supportive 1990 resolution by the San Francisco Board of Supervisors, and with strong advocacy from the City's Department of Public Works, Talking Signs had arrived!

Ward Bond/Talking Signs, Inc.

In the early 1990s, C. Ward Bond visited several disabilities conferences seeking potentially useful applications for his new product—the Infogrip chording keyboard. At one of these conferences, Ward ran into Loughborough and based upon the ensuing relationship, in 1993 Ward, along with Loughborough, John Hilburn, and Bill Crandall, created Talking Signs, Inc. (TSI) to manufacture and deploy products based on prototypes developed by the S-K's Rehabilitation Engineering Research Center (RERC) in San Francisco.

TSI engaged founding member Hilburn's Baton Rouge electronics company, Microcomputer Systems, to bring the hardware into line with modern communications technology. Prototypes and patent applications resulting from the venture include infrared location and communications in passenger conveyance vehicles and facilities; automated transactions machines; automatic variable output control of LEDs; transmitter array cover; emergency egress system; and multilanguage/multichannel system.

Things began to move quickly. By 1994, systems were being installed in the New Main Library in San Francisco and the Lighthouse International in Manhattan. Under Department of Transportation (DOT) funding, a comprehensive demonstration project was developed in the Powell Street Station for the Bay Area Rapid Transit (BART) and a demonstration was set up throughout the L' Enfant Plaza Metro Station in Washington, DC. Other San Francisco projects included Talking Signs at intersection crosswalks in the Civic Center, the Caltrain station, throughout Yerba Buena Gardens, transit platforms for Muni, the Main Library, the Ferry Landing, the Courthouse, Moscone Center West, and were installed throughout City Hall as part of its earthquake renovation. All in all, 2012 units had been installed in San Francisco as of 2011.

Elsewhere, as a result of the recommendation by the American Foundation for the Blind, the Mashantucket Pequot Tribe installed 300 Talking Signs in the cultural museum on their reservation in Connecticut. In the late 1990s, Talking Signs, Inc. developed a strategy to install Talking Signs in airports. Bona fide interest was developed at O'Hare, Reagan National, Los Angeles, Ottawa, and from the Port Authority of New York and New Jersey. On the morning of September 10, 2001 representatives of the Airport Division of the Port Authority and Kennedy, LaGuardia and Newark Airports met with Ward Bond on the 64th floor of the World Trade Center and agreed to begin a pilot project at LaGuardia Airport. Of course, everything changed a day later; perhaps it is time to restart such an initiative.

American National Standards Institute

An American National Standards Institute (ANSI) standard for RIAS was published in 2003. This important American standard harmonizes with the nomenclature of the ADA Accessibility Guideline (ADAAG). This is also an important prelude to the International Standards Organization (ISO). We wait.

Evolution of Experiments from Lab Tests to "Real World"

Every so often engineers will visit the S-K Eye Research Institute to discuss their idea of yet-another-ultrasonic-cane. When we disclose to them the history of such unutilized endeavors (see discussion in Chapters 3 and 8), the general reaction is that these other guys must have been doing something wrong because their idea is such a good one! Perhaps because Talking Signs started out in an institution focused on solutions for people who cannot see (or cannot see well) by people who either were themselves blind or who worked closely with people who were, each step of development was a sure-footed one. The early experiments were explicitly designed to evaluate the efficacy of the fundamental concept.

SK Exp 1

The first Talking Signs research centered on laboratory-based engineering and basic human factors. John and Lesley Brabyn (Brabyn and Brabyn, 1982) studied intelligibility of Talking Signs messages from the receiver versus high-fidelity recorded speech. Given the primitive state of speech encoding into the TS transmitter in those early days, it is surprising that after 60 trials for each of the 18 participants there were no (well… 2.9%) differences in accuracy scores between conditions, and with participants reporting "a high level of confidence and a low level of uncertainty in their correct answers."

SK Exp 2

The Brabyns' second study (Brabyn and Brabyn, 1983) was to compare time of travel for locating specific doorways in an unfamiliar building using TS versus Raised Print. TS condition mean travel time 64.4 s versus 86.2 s for the Raised Print condition.

> Participants had no prior experience with electronic navigation systems and received minimal training during the experiment with the device being tested however, 86% of the participants expressed considerable previous familiarity with raised-print labeling. Thus, we feel that the performance test used in this experiment was conservative.

SK Exp 3

In 1985, Shenkman (1986) on sabbatical to S-K from Sweden studied the receiver's best angle of light opening to maximize efficiency in detecting the presence of a Talking Sign. The result was that the wider the opening—(the greater the receptive angle)—the more likely the detection will occur. Performance did not increase after a receiver angle reached 24°. Shenkman acknowledged the common sense notion that there is a trade-off between ease of detecting the presence of a TS and the accuracy of locating one, but he did not attempt to quantify this by performing the experiment. Taking this angle-accuracy trade-off into consideration, later laboratory experiments at S-K established the standard for *receiver angle of acceptance*.

Field Experiments and Selected Findings

After the positive results of S-K in-house lab tests, multiple experiments by various researchers, investigating a wide range of locations, problems, and populations, were conducted.

ACB Convention

The first evaluation of TS "outside" of those conducted by S-K took place at the American Council of the Blind (ACB) convention in San Francisco in July 1993 (Bentzen and Mitchell, 1995). The "bake-off" was between Verbal Landmarks® (VL) induction loop (very localized, nondirectional radio) way-finding system and Talking Signs directional infrared messaging. "...the "real-world" setting of a busy convention site in a major hotel provides unquestionable face validity to the study and undoubtedly helped to high-light strengths and weakness of the technologies that might have been less apparent in the laboratory" (Bentzen and Mitchell, 1995). Both systems employed a personal receiver, but the similarities diverged from there. The VL receiver began picking up walking instructions only when users were within 5 feet of the transmitting inductive loop. Therefore, users were required to go to a particular "start" location in order to pick up the instruc-tions. In contrast to verbal directions *to the destination*, the TS receiver began picking up verbal labels *at the destination* from between 10 and 100 feet away (depending on adjustment of the transmitter). Therefore, users could pick up messages regardless of their start location.

Participants using TS reached the destination 45–70% sooner and with less distance traveled than those using VL. They were also less likely to require assistance and less likely to "give up." The results of the ACB study show that in this paradigm, TS has a clear performance advantages in both travel time and travel distance over a system that lists travel directions. In subjective ratings from the questions and survey, TS showed significantly better scores than VL for such items as (1) ease of use, (2) ease of compre-hension of message, and (3) desirability in both familiar and unfamiliar areas.

Quickly following these strong results was a series of other studies, con-ducted in order to determine applicability of the RIAS technology to other print-reading disabilities and to various other travel situations, such as public rights-of-way and public transportation, shown by surveys to be high on the list of people's information needs. Because Crandall was (and is) part of the Talking Signs business, his function after being motivator for funding the projects has been to be the gofer for the experiments, handing over responsibilities for design, running subjects, data analysis, and so on to outside consultants.

SK Exp 4

Results from testing the ability of 16 blind participants to navigate 6 indoor and outdoor routes (6 on each of two visits or a total of 12 trials) on the campus of San Francisco State University (Crandall et al., 1994) indicates that, in addition to other positive outcomes, significantly more routes were successfully completed with the use of Talking Signs (with minimal verbal travel instructions) than without Talking Signs (but with longer verbal travel instructions).

SK Exp 5

Eighteen blind participants used TS in locating (1) a bus poles or bus shelters and (2) one of three San Francisco Municipal Railway (Muni) buses parked at a curb. The bus pole was located in the midst of newspaper racks and was therefore especially difficult for the participants to locate by touch (Crandall et al., 1996). In addition, dog guides are trained to guide owners away from obstacles; therefore, bus poles seem to fall into that category of things to be avoided. Thus raised print labeling on bus poles was shown to be ineffective; none of the 18 participants located a bus pole using their conventional techniques while 15 of the 18 did so when using Talking Signs.

Participants were statistically more successful in locating the shelter which was near the curb using the Talking Signs system than using tactile signs, whereas they were essentially equally successful when using either system for locating and identifying the shelter which was along the building line. Perhaps this was due to the participants' tendency to follow ("shoreline") the building line where there would be a greater chance of physically encountering the shelter.

In addition to the more objective results on travel performance, the study also gave us an opportunity to ask auxiliary questions; not only were these participants already experts in blindness but now they had become experts in how they wanted to use the TS technology. Participants were asked to vote— in rank order—their preferences for "Destination" messaging. Here is what they wanted: route number, bus destination, and name of operator (company), but not name of bus routes, or direction of travel. And here is what they wanted to see as messaging at bus stops and shelters: number of bus route, destination of bus, transit operator, but not names of bus route or schedule. "In order to allow generalization of results, the environment was completely free of obstacles and the 'bus driver' (the experimenter) was always available to immediately identify the bus once the door to the bus was reached."

"I wish we could do it over" finding: You may not get too far into a study when the performance of the participants indicates what you'd not thought of when designing the experiment. But, when the experiment starts, the show must go on! So, it's better to plan from every angle, carefully piloting with participants that represent the target population, otherwise you may end up evaluating the experimental *design* and not the experimental *treatment*! This experiment was a case in point; the pedestrian path to the buses was clear, allowing participants to shoreline the curb directly to the bus. Participants themselves volunteered that under more typically challenging conditions, the Talking Signs system would make identifying and locating buses much easier. As a result, we lay victim to the "Ceiling Effect" where all the data piles up at one end of the scale—either because the task is too easy or because it is too difficult. In this case, all participants—regardless of treatment—arrived at the bus at nearly the same time. True, in the *No Talking Signs* condition participants could have been delayed in identifying the bus because, as often happens, the bus driver is on break. But what started out as a feature of our design (generalizability of results) ended up being a bug.

SK Exp 6

Previous research indicates that Talking Signs users independently learn many characteristics of the system that we did not specifically teach them in the short training preceding test trials. Ease of use, learning to scan, ease of picking up messages, and following the sign to the destination are thought to be related to the level of training and indicate a need to evaluate training requirements for effective and safe use of the system. A very detailed manual of instruction based upon the protocol followed in this experiment was produced for use by future Trainers (Bentzen et al., 1995). The study therefore focused on the question: "What is the minimum amount of training required for a person to effectively and safely use the Talking Signs?" To answer this question, we evaluated the travel characteristics of 36 visually impaired people who used the system as an aid to navigation through a complex subway station in downtown San Francisco (Powell Station) for the Bay Area Rapid Transit (BART) and the San Francisco Municipal Railway (Muni) (Crandall et al., 1995a,b). Ninety-six TS transmitters were installed in the Project ACTION/US Department of Transportation-funded demonstration/ evaluation. The broad cross section of participants was divided into three groups, each group being matched for varying levels of mobility skills, degree of residual vision (self-reported), method of travel (guide dog or cane), presence of hearing impairment, and self-reported level of spatial thinking. Testing involved the participants navigating a multiplicity of travel routes classified as "easy," "medium," or "hard." Each of 3 groups of 12 participants was given a different level of training in the proper use of the wayfinding system. The type of training varied, depending upon the group, from a hands-on one-hour training session given by our instructor, to hands-on training for 15 min, and to a self-directed "home study" session by the participant. During the one-hour testing period, participants traveled as many of the total number of routes as possible.

It is important to know where the misfit between the user and the technology lays so that either the technology or the training procedures (or both) can be altered to make the system more efficient and reliable for the user. Participants were scored on the reasons for failing to complete routes. These included: ineffective scanning, failure to monitor messages, no concept of pointing, misinterpretation of message, poor grip, ineffective exploration, problems with reflections, and apparent poor spatial reasoning.

We found that participants in all groups were readily able to learn to use the infrared signage system in order to acquire the necessary wayfinding information and travel through the transit station without assistance, although, in general, participants with less training traveled fewer routes successfully. Within the limits of the one-hour test period, 35 of the 36 participants successfully completed at least two easy routes utilizing TS as their only aid; 23 successfully completed at least two additional medium routes, and 17 successfully completed at least two additional hard routes. During the course of the experimental testing, the TS transmitters were used by participants a total of 500 times. The lesson here is that had TS not been available, the participants would have had to get some form of information or assistance, or to make their travel decisions on less definitive information 500 times.

SK Exp 7

The problem of providing emergency information in buildings to individuals who are visually impaired is complex because emergency procedures vary according to the type of emergency, extent of emergency, size of building (single floor or high-rise), occupancy (i.e., hotel or office building), and type of building construction (i.e., fire and smoke-secure guest rooms) (Crandall et al., 2000). There is little research that compares the use by persons with visual impairments of different formats for obtaining wayfinding information, especially in this context of emergency situations.

In order to model the effectiveness of communicating emergency information in a number of accessible formats, a paradigm was established where participants read or listened to instructions for going to an exit stairway and then traveled to that stairway. Specifically, communication effectiveness was determined by objective and subjective measures for each of the following five accessible formats: Braille; raised print; tactile maps; push-button audible signs; RIAS.

Among other findings, the major conclusions are that both RIAS and push-button route directions enable blind users who are not severely hearing impaired to access emergency egress information in an efficient manner. Auditory information is preferred above tactile information, but it is not accessible for persons who are severely hearing impaired. Braille results in more efficient access to egress information than raised print and tactile maps and is the preferred tactile format.

After seeing how well TS helped the visually impaired community, we were curious if it was useful for other groups with special needs.

Other Disabilities

SK Exp 8 and 9

Two studies involved persons with developmental disabilities in a transit facility, one in the SEPTA system in Philadelphia (Bentzen and Crandall, 1995) and one in San Francisco's BART. In collaboration with The Arc (Association of Retarded Citizens) of San Francisco, a human factors evaluation, involving 15 developmentally delayed clients, was performed to determine the effectiveness of TS use for this group (Crandall et al., 1999a,b). Discussions with our colleagues at The Arc indicated that many of their clients might be able to travel more independently, with better orientation, greater safety, and increased confidence in complex environments, with the assistance that TS could provide.

These discussions also allowed us to explore the special adaptations to the technology (location and messaging) appropriate to the needs of this population and provided the opportunity for us to learn the training requirements specific to this population.

Developmentally delayed people who are unable to understand print signs were able to auditorily identify and go to destinations with the help of Talking Signs messages. The repeating messages also gave people who were cognitively impaired the opportunity to listen to messages repeatedly, to help them pick up and understand the information. In the broadest sense, RIAS comprises a menu of choices and reminders for the traveler—signs confront them with the options available at any given point in their travels and remind them where to go next. Talking Signs are directional, so that the traveler can "look around." Once the appropriate destination is recognized, the traveler can move in that direction.

The Talking Signs system is an excellent aid to travel for persons with developmental disabilities. In our study, it enabled them to independently confirm the location and identity of key features in a transit station such as the correct fare gate, the correct side of a platform, or the correct exit from a platform or station to a street or to a connecting bus or train. Given only 30 min of training in use of the technology, all participants successfully used TS messages to make travel decisions such as identifying a particular exit, entrance, or side of a transit platform.

Would these participants use the system in their daily life? Throughout the experiment, all participants continued to need verbal reminders and occasional physical assistance in holding the receiver correctly. The most common problems were forgetting to use the receiver or forgetting to move it around to get a clear message. Perhaps training and practice could aid in independent use of the RIAS system.

Congressional Project: RIAS

The Federal Transit Administration of the U.S. Department of Transportation (DOT) managed the remote infrared audible signage model accessibility project (RIAS MAP), providing 309 Talking Signs in six Seattle Sound Transit rail/bus stations in the Puget Sound Region. The key objective of the demonstration was to assess the benefits of RIAS for people who are visually impaired, or cognitively or learning disabled. A major study of this program was carried out by The Volpe National Transportation Systems Center (Petrella et al., 2009) examining the impact accessible transit has on the lives of people with vision loss in terms of education, work, and general quality of life.

On the basis of the findings from the evaluation, RIAS technology enhanced multimodal accessibility for nearly all study participants. In general, RIAS technology enabled users to navigate the transit system more efficiently and with greater confidence and independence, though users felt that the coverage and placement of transmitters was better at some stations than at others. Respondents indicated that the most important information provided by RIAS was the location of the bus bays and train platforms, with accompanying information on the bus numbers, directions, and destination. The installation of signs at bathrooms and drinking fountains was useful, but was deemed less of a priority.

UCSB Experiments

A widely different approach of investigation into the needs of blind travelers and technological solutions was started at the University of California Santa Barbara (UCSB). Two geographers whose research interests were transportation, spatial cognition, mental map development, and behavioral geography (how humans interact with the environment) developed a survey for 55 visually impaired persons designed to determine attitudes toward, and use of, transit, and to determine why this population exhibited a paucity of transit participation. The main finding that Dr. Reginald Golledge and his then graduate research assistant James Marston (who were themselves visually impaired) found was that the lack of information about transit and travel services and how to efficiently find and use the vehicles and systems, were the most important factors influencing their low usage rate (Golledge et al., 1995, 1996b, 1997; Marston et al., 1997).

The survey led to research to find technologies that could increase the amount and quality of information that this population had indicated they needed. The UCSB research interest was not just in the technology's efficacy, but in how it could affect travel behavior and access to opportunities; in short, how it might lead to increased access impacting a person's quality of life.

In 1996, Golledge and Marston attended a demonstration of Talking Signs, newly installed at the San Francisco Public Library. Marston had been looking for "real-world" research projects that could aid the blind and increase access to opportunities, and was very impressed with the labeling and directional information provided by this technology.

UCSB Exp 1

Their first experiment at UCSB using the devices was a simple geometric installation of four stanchions, placed in a square or rectangular pattern on an open field. Twenty participants (ten blind and ten blindfolded) were asked to find and travel to each of the four posts, both with and without the Talking Signs transmitters. Participants were asked to identify the shape they had just traveled, and also to try to bisect the shape (i.e., walk from home base to first and second base, and then walk directly to home plate). Rating questions were asked to determine user satisfaction.

UCSB Exp 2

Once the efficacy of the system was established (corroborating the previous studies by others), the UCSB group wanted to determine if some real-world usage could be established that could lead to changes in travel behavior and mode choice, and extend activities for this population. They designed an experiment at a circular bus loading area on the campus, with an installation of three TS that led the 20 participants (10 blind and 10 blindfolded) from one side of the circle to the other side, where buses were boarding. Many different bus routes served the campus; a TS transmitter was installed on the front window of one of the buses. When the specific bus came into the bus circle, participates identified it, walked around the circle, and tried to find the bus before it departed. Often, there were three or so buses at the boarding area. A major problem in blind transit use is identifying the proper vehicle to board, so identification of the bus and location of the door is a very important item of information to make transit use safe and more efficient (Golledge et al., 1998a,b). Various ratings and travel ease questions were answered after the experiment.

Results showed statistically significant improvement in time and errors to walk to and locate the boarding area and find the proper bus for boarding. With TS, participants were able to walk to the proper bus without searching for each bus and arrived before the bus left the area. Without TS, many buses left the area before the participants were able to identify the correct bus among the many at the boarding area.

UCSB Exp 3

Building on the feedback from users and the promising results of the field tests, a much larger, "real-world" experiment was conducted. Twenty-nine visually impaired participants walked from the local Braille Institute, crossed a street, and found a mid-block bus stop equipped with a transmitter. They then identified a bus that was equipped with a transmitter, which announced the bus number, direction, and destination. They boarded the appropriate bus and traveled to the transit center terminal where there were 10 transmitters installed. Participants identified and traveled to all signed locations, learning the interior environment, and then found a labeled bus in the crowded bus terminal boarding area for the return trip. Many more ratings and discussion questions were asked to determine how this added information affected transit tasks and spatial knowledge, in addition to data on walk and search times, errors, and other performance measures (Golledge and Marston, 1999).

This population learned the layout of transit amenities such as ticket windows, doorways, change machines, public phones, bathrooms, and so on much faster and with fewer errors when using the TS device. The study showed that all participants were able to find a mid-block bus stop using the TS receiver. It also showed statistically significant improvement in finding the proper bus for boarding at a crowded bus terminal boarding area.

UCSB Exp 4

Results in the previous experiments were quite positive and led to many more as yet unanswered research questions. A major experiment was designed to take advantage of a new installation that was a high-traffic use, multimodal train station in an urban environment. No researcher interference was used to control traffic flow and other environmental conditions, thus this was a true "real-world" experiment. Thirty volunteers with a range of vision impairment, but mostly with no useful vision, participated. Data included: error and walking times to find various labeled amenities in the environment, with five simulated transfers from one form of transit to another, stopping to find a total of 20 amenities on the way. In addition to the objective methods to collect those times and errors, the investigators collected a multitude of subjective data. These included getting a good baseline of trip-making frequency, transit mode use, and other historic data from each subject before starting the experiment. After the test, many of these same questions were asked for direct comparisons to pretest histories. The investigators also looked at how spatial orientation and learning was affected by the condition being presented. They asked question pre- and posttest about actual and perceived transit mode use, transfer behavior, and so on. Of particular interest were a series of five open-ended questions that allowed participants to tell us in their own words how the technology usage affected their travel patterns and states of mind (Marston, 2002; Marston and Golledge, 2000, 2003; Marston and Church, 2005).

In this experiment, 51 locations were labeled in and around a multimodel terminal. The ability to find and travel to many different locations using the RIAS signage was statistically significant, when compared to the participants' regular method of travel. Participants were significantly faster finding the bus shelter with the device than when using their regular method. In fact, many people could not find the shelter in the allotted time without the device. It is notable that when there were no other people around to ask, there were no usable cues to find a bus shelter.

Spatial Cognition

Once the efficacy of a navigation device has been evaluated, the true utility of the information delivered to the user can be shown by the impact it has on learning an environment through increased spatial cognition. A mental map of an environment is a valued step beyond simply being able to follow step-by-step route instructions. The UCSB investigators first evaluated spatial cognition previously developed in their *UCSB Exp1* where users walked a route and identified the shape of two paths; one was a square and the other a rectangle. Those using TS were much better in this simple task. The ability to make shortcuts is very important to this population and a second phase in that experiment was to see if participants could bisect the shape and travel directly from "second base" to "home plate." The results also showed that TS had a positive effect on this ability.

In *UCSB Exp 3*, participants using TS were able to learn the location of labeled landmarks much better when using the system. Those two small successes led to an experiment designed to more fully test the accumulation of spatial knowledge with the use of a wayfinding device.

In *UCSB Exp 4*, participants walked five simulated transit transfer routes (e.g., from train gate to subway fare machine) visiting a total of 20 locations during the five transit transfer routes. After several routes had been completed, participants were starting to get some knowledge of possible routes, doorways, and other locations. For two of the 20 locations they were asked to walk to and locate, there were shorter routes "shortcuts" they could use if they understood the location of doorways that they had not used before. They might, for example, have learned of the door's location by hearing it being used or through their understanding of traffic flows. A typical blind traveler will stick to known and previously used routes. And so, the ability to make a shortcut using an unfamiliar route would demonstrate that spatial information had been acquired and processed. Using the TS system while walking previous routes, some users picked up on the existence of other amenities, destinations, and new doorways. Of the two paths where a shortcut was possible, 89% and 100%, respectively, of the totally blind participants were able to make the shortcuts. When not using TS, but their regular method of travel, 18% and 27%, respectively, of the totally blind participants made the shortcuts. After the experiment was completed, 20 spatial relationship questions were asked to both TS users and non-TS users. 88% of the TS users, and 44% of those using their regular methods, had correct answers.

Intersections

So far, we have summarized how RIAS solves everyday problems in many different travel contexts. Below, we offer an example of one very serious and challenging problem faced by people who cannot see (or cannot see well) and how TS experiments demonstrated the efficacy of the RIAS solution.

Crossing points are the places in any journey where the traveler is most vulnerable to danger in the form of collisions with passing vehicles that can result in serious injury or death. At signalized intersections in busy urban areas, many confusing cues are presented to the blind traveler who must rely primarily on traffic sounds to determine the geometry of intersections, the nature of traffic control, and when it is safe to cross. In addition to knowing the state of the pedestrian signals, it is important to also have the correct alignment to the destination in order to travel safely in the confines of the crosswalk area. Walking at the wrong time, or not being aligned properly, can be deadly. It is not surprising that anecdotal evidence abounds that stressful street crossings cause many trips not to be made.

Taking these needs together, S-K developed a unique Audible Pedestrian Signal solution for evaluation. Each RIAS transmitter unit (mounted atop the conventional visual pedestrian display—see Figure 6.2) has transmission in two directions with a separate message on each. The front message is a narrow beam aimed across the street at pedestrians waiting to cross. This

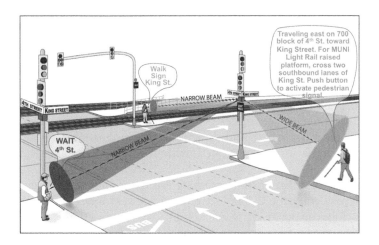

FIGURE 6.2
Separate messages come from the front and rear of the Talking Signs accessible pedestrian signal (APS) unit; the (rear) "orientation message" tells the users where they are and what direction they are traveling while, at the same time, the (front) "pedestrian crosswalk indicator message" tells users the condition of the pedestrian signal.

message is linked to the pedestrian signal and says, for example, either "Walk Sign 4th Street" or "Wait 4th Street." The rear message is a wide beam aimed down the sidewalk toward pedestrians as they approach the intersection. This message gives intersection specific information. For example: "Traveling East on the 700 block of 4th Street toward King Street. For Muni Light Rail raised platform, cross two Southbound lanes of King Street. Push button to activate pedestrian signal."

SK Exp 10

Twenty subjects, most who consider themselves to be good to excellent travelers, all negotiated four intersections of various configurations with a total of 80 crossings with TS and 80 without (Crandall et al., 1998, 2001). For each of the 160 street crossings, the following types of objective performance data were collected for each subject: safety, precision, independence, and knowledge of each crossing maneuver. TS provided a clear advantage in each measure.

Following each crossing, participants were asked about: information they used for alignment; how they knew when it was safe to cross; shape the intersection; type of traffic control; and other information they found to be useful. Other subjective data were obtained from participants regarding their evaluation of the usefulness of different features of the system.

Data showed that TS at intersections significantly improved safety, precision, and independence in street crossing, as well as knowledge of intersections, for good, frequent, independent blind travelers, using a long cane or dog guide, including those with hearing loss. Talking Signs also resulted in improved street crossing for persons who considered themselves relatively poor travelers, and who did not normally travel in unfamiliar areas (Bentzen et al., 1999).

UCSB Exp 4

When provided with definitive information about the onset of the walk interval, users can be confident they have the right of way at a street crossing. Attention can then be fully placed on other acoustic information for crossing, such as the location, speed, and direction of turning vehicles. Both the fear of injury and the stress associated with the need to get assistance are decreased.

As the stress and fear of street crossing can reduce many people's ability to travel independently, the UCSB researchers were very interested to see if TS at street crossings can positively affect mobility. Two intersections were equipped with TS. One was a four-lane street (one way but for a bus lane in the other direction), with slow and congested traffic. The other was only a two-lane street, but with very high speeds, leading to an expressway on-ramp.

Participants crossed these intersections both with and without the RIAS receiver. Times to cross the streets were much faster when using the system. In the more difficult crossing, the high-speed two-lane street, 3 of the 15 participants that used their regular method of travel could not/would not cross the street in the 4 min that were allotted when using their regular methods. In addition, there was a very significant difference in the alignment both at the beginning of crossing, and at arrival at the other curb cut. All people using the device were properly aligned at both ends, while those using their regular methods often deviated from the crosswalk (Marston, 2002).

These "Intersection" experiments resulted in development by two manufacturers of an enhanced RIAS-based system, one strictly RIAS, and the other a hybrid speak-out/RIAS.

Partnerships

Over the years, TSI attracted several important strategic partnerships that have resulted in major technological advances and enhancements to the list of international projects in Japan, Norway, Italy, and Canada. Close communication between human factors researchers and hardware development partners has raised the level of the technology while at the same time increased true functionality to users.

Mitsubishi Precision

In 1998, Mitsubishi precision (MPC) chose to license Talking Signs system for further development for several reasons: RIAS already had a certainty position in this field in the United States and Europe; for users it was determined to be of superior utility compared to other available wayfinding systems; and additional support for future international standardization would be needed to secure wide international build-out of the system.

MPC's engineers did a terrific job of listening to their constituents and then thinking outside the box in producing RIAS devices that had very advanced capabilities. Their "Personal" system—a portable RIAS transmitter—remains asleep until awakened by a trigger sent from the hand-held receiver, thereby conserving batteries; a "hands-free" receiver is users' most often requested addition. MPC's solution is a unit that clips onto the glasses frame, having an infrared detector on the front and on the rear, and an "air tube" that carries the sound to the ear without obstructing the ear. For use in museums where delivering wayfinding as well as artifact-specific narrative is desirable, in addition to speech messages, the "Museum System" (a kind of "random access" speech player) uses a code unique to each RIAS sign to index into and activates the receiver's on-board flash memory containing extended speech narration specific to that sign. RIAS research has also taken place in Japan (Tajima et al., 2001, 2002; Kurachi et al., 2005).

MPC has installed Talking Signs in over 50 cities in Japan including 300 intersections (for the Japanese National Police Agency), museums, department stores, recreation centers, town halls, railway stations (for Japan National Railway West), hospitals, and a university. Outside of Japan, Mitsubishi has installed TS in Norway at the town center of Krinstiansand, and in Oslo at the Headquarters of the Norway Association for the Blind as well as the new Oslo Opera House.

MPC's participation in development of a new Japanese Industry Standard (JIS) for wayfinding devices includes the American National Standards Institute (ANSI) specification of RIAS. The Japanese government is currently in the process of establishing an International Standards Organization (ISO) standard based on these ANSI and JIS standards.

Luminator, Next Bus, and Polara Engineering

On the basis of the research at S-K (Crandall et al., 1996), Luminator developed and manufactured a mature product for buses under license from TSI. NextBus, Inc. collaborated with S-K to embed RIAS using text-to-speech conversion into approximately 800 bus shelter signs in San Francisco. Polara Engineering, Inc. has made several important improvements on the RIAS prototype evaluated by Crandall et al. (1998).

Solari di Udine

Under license from TSI, Solari di Udine (Italy) developed and deployed a state-of-the-art TCP/IP Ethernet/IEEE 488-based system that allows

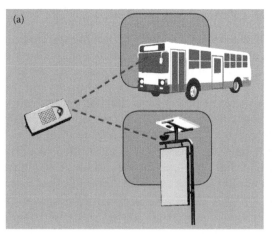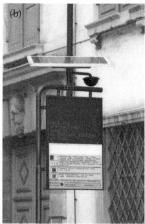

FIGURE 6.3
The RIAS receiver identifies the oncoming bus from up to 150 feet away and also bus stops, giving real-time information such as bus destination and next bus arrival times (a). Detail of photovoltaic, wireless bus pole (b).

real-time updating of messages (wirelessly) and—like the Luminator system—transmits bus destination information to awaiting riders when an approaching bus is 150 feet away. When the bus leaves a stop, an internal system immediately begins transmitting the name of the next stop, allowing riders to hear, at will, the upcoming stop through their receiver.

In addition, this development incorporates various options (GSM/GPRS/WiFi) for communicating wirelessly with a server and operating independent of the mains by virtue of incorporating photovoltaic cells into their bus pole RIAS device. These were rather easy design and manufacturing steps for Solari to take because they had already deployed a large number of stand-alone parking payment systems that employ these same wireless/photovoltaic technologies (Figure 6.3).

Future Directions

Many attempts have been made to address and resolve the wayfinding needs of blind, visually impaired, and other disabled travelers. Although various degrees of technical success have been realized, these efforts have, for the most part, been failures in the "functional" sense. These failures have generally fallen into the following categories: (1) the technologies have been too expensive for consumers to purchase and maintain; (2) usage has required learning a complex and nonintuitive interface, which in turn required training and practice; and (3) the technologies have not been accurate or reliable. Finally, the costs to install and maintain these technologies have been perceived as being excessive, and therefore from a marketing standpoint, rendered economically unfeasible.

The research and development program at S-K aims at employing recently developed methods and technologies in order to improve the prospects for enhanced functionality and deployment by collaborating with others in creating a unified wayfinding and information platform that is popular with users because it is ubiquitous and enhances user experience; is popular with regulators and owners/operators because of low production, installation and maintenance cost; and is popular with manufacturers because it serves the large market of diverse disabilities (Crandall, 2011).

However, success in deployment of accessible wayfinding systems involves a great deal more than the technology; the legal mandate (as a civil right) has to be acknowledged and then converted into meaningful requirements. Only then can enforceable regulation bring about a fertile-enough climate in which these technologies could flourish. Even after these steps are complete, support is required to turn systems that *could* flourish into ones that *can* flourish. These dynamically interconnected components are aggressive grassroot support from users; bold action by standards setters and enforcers; support from facilities owners and/or operators; and the perception of a market adequate enough in size to promote commercialization.

Barriers to Deployment

If the system we have just looked at is really all that useful, then why do we not see more Talking Signs being made available and used by people who can benefit from enhanced access to information as they travel? Developing wayfinding systems is not enough. No matter how good they might be in helping to solve the problem of independent travel, unless they are deployed, they might as well not exist. Systems are solutions only when adequately supported. This points directly to the need for regulation, funding for implementation, education, support from access consultants, and strong efforts by members of the disabled communities themselves to promote the requirement and deployment of these systems.

Civil Rights versus Guidelines, Standards, and Regulations

Accessibility guidelines, standards, and regulations include minimal wayfinding information—labeling on "Exit" doors, for example, that is accessible to travelers who are blind or who have low vision—chiefly in the form of signage that is sufficiently large, high in contrast, and with highly readable, well-spaced fonts to be used by people with low vision, as well as numbers for permanent rooms and spaces in Braille and raised print for those with no usable vision. This does not mean, however, that people who are blind or who have low vision do not have a civil right under the ADA to wayfinding information such as directional signs, informational signage, and maps, or to wayfinding information based on technologies such as RIAS and GPS that is sufficiently accurate and includes information in outdoor settings of particular relevance to them, such as slope, texture, acoustic cues, exact locations of bus stops, and traffic control information as well as amenities located inside of buildings such as elevators, restrooms, boarding platforms, and information desks. However, because accessible wayfinding information is not specifically covered by ADA Accessibility Guidelines* or ADA Standards for Transportation Facilities, it is seldom seen as a priority in transit or public accommodations, and its provision is enforceable only through negotiation with the U.S. Department of

---

* But see *ADAAG 2.2, Nov. 1996–Equivalent Facilitation* which "permits the use of alternative designs and technologies that provide substantially equivalent or superior access to and usability of a facility. Such innovative approaches may also be useful in providing access to facility types for which no specific standards have been written."

Transportation, the U.S. Department of Justice, or through judicial action. A variety of accessible wayfinding technologies exists, many of which have the potential to enhance wayfinding not only for people who are visually impaired, but also for those who have cognitive or mobility impairments. Until there are guidelines and standards that mandate it, it is unlikely that there will be widespread availability of accessible wayfinding technologies, particularly those that require installation and maintenance. Meanwhile, people with print-reading disabilities remain without reasonable accommodation to the information they need to safely and efficiently navigate in the public arena.

Consumer Demand and Demand by Consumers

Good solutions come and go for lack of a market. On the one side, the limited economics of market pressure within the transit industry itself do not provide the incentive necessary for agencies to support accessible wayfinding technologies. On the other side, consumers with impaired vision who could benefit from these systems heretofore have not been unified in their advocacy for accessible wayfinding to pressure regulators, jurisdictions, and properties (i.e., public accommodations as well as public rights-of-way) into providing what is needed for their safe and independent travel. Disagreement about the proper role of assistive wayfinding technology paralyzes regulators, manufacturers, and institutions. We reap what we sow.

Support from access consultants is critical, for they are the most direct link between wayfinding systems and facilities.

Outreach and education create the environment where these systems are integrated into the daily life of travelers. But are conventional programs such as those provided by orientation and mobility specialists up to the task of training their students in the use of these technologies? Perhaps organizations such as Project ACTION—which adopt specialized curricula on an as-needed basis—could set in motion a broad program of outreach and training.

The Waiting Game

Waiting for faster, cheaper, and easier solutions results only in endless discussions around the theme "new technologies." These are distractions from applying the very adequate solutions already in existence. While playing the "Waiting Game," a whole segment of our population continues being deprived of equitable environmental access—as if the benefits of these products and services to date were irrelevant. In addition, if developers and manufacturers lack confidence that their efforts will result in a meaningful deployment, why would they bother? And investors will surely stay away.

Interacting Forces

Just as a chain of *individual* activities must successfully be completed in order for travelers to reach physical destinations, so must a number of powerful, interacting forces (cultural, educational, historical, economic, political, and social) come into play in support of these technologies. The powers of these *societal* and *economic* forces dwarf the remarkable *technical* solutions that so far have been dramatically underutilized. Direct support from these powerful domains is required for technological systems to be developed, deployed, and ultimately used by the people who heretofore have lacked efficient and sufficient access to signage information. If these societal and economic activities were aligned in support of the needs of the public, the synergies produced would lead to a significant gain in freedom and independence in travel. Like the synergies present in the technologies we presently have, all of these social and economic factors are necessarily interconnected—each component strongly influencing and being influenced by the many other components.

Lessons Learned

Every endeavor has its unique and constantly changing set of challenges and pitfalls and, as a "case history," this chapter represents only one such endeavor. The list of "Lessons Learned" presented below highlights a small sample of what became obvious to us—but only after the fact. It is hoped that by presenting these points here and now, some grief will be spared those in our field who are just now setting off in a similar pursuit.

1. Strike while the iron is hot—promotions and retirements of partners and potential clients can immediately halt further development of prospective projects; they are off with a whole new set of "challenges."

2. The patent process is very expensive relative to the assets of a small or start-up company. Seriously evaluate the cost/benefit for each patent application and have a good rationale for making the investment. Like so much in business, "you never know." Be willing to cut loose; patents are expensive to get (in dollars, but also time) and expensive to maintain. In the United States, you start paying at the time of filing.

3. Remain on guard to protect the result of the hard won and costly investments made to develop intellectual property. At minimum, create an official "paper trail" to document any attempts to breach the fence around this valuable asset.

4. Never commit in writing without consulting a lawyer (or two!).

5. Maintain control over product, pricing, and installation.

6. Be realistic about your expectations; separate out bona fide interest of partners and potential clients from their natural tendency to want to "say yes" to supporting the needs of people with disabilities.

7. Buy-in from your end users is critical; otherwise it is "all dressed up and no place to go."

8. Bring prospective users into all phases of development.

9. Ensure that outreach and training are given as much attention as the hardware. Training, such as that provided by orientation and mobility specialists (see Chapter 3), must include training in use of wayfinding technologies.

10. In the Talking Signs case, personal receivers are part of the transmitter/receiver *system*. In similar cases where multiple components are required for use, funds for all components need to be included in the budget.

11. Stay in contact well after the work is completed so the facility owner/manager knows that support is readily available.

References

Bentzen, B., and W. Crandall. 1995. Optimal Characteristics for Signage Systems in Transit Stations for Persons with Visual or Cognitive Disabilities. Report of research conducted under contract to KRW.

Bentzen, B., W. Crandall, and L. Myers. 1999. Wayfinding system for transportation services. Remote infrared audible signage for transit stations, surface transit, and intersections. *Transportation Research Record*, 1671: 19–26.

Bentzen, B., and P. Mitchell. 1995. Audible signage as a way finding aid: Comparison of Verbal Landmarks® and Talking Signs®. *Journal of Visual Impairment and Blindness*, 89: 494–505.

Bentzen, B., L. Myers, and W. Crandall. 1995. Talking Signs® System: Guide for Trainers. Final Report, National Easter Seal Research Program. Project ACTION.

Brabyn, J., and L. Brabyn. 1982. Speech intelligibility of Talking Signs. *Journal of Visual Impairment and Blindness*, 76: 77–78.

Brabyn, L., and J. Brabyn. 1983. An evaluation of "Talking Signs" for the blind. *Human Factors*, 25(1): 49–53.

Brault, M. 2008. Americans with Disabilities: 2005. Current Population Reports, P70–117, U.S. Census Bureau, Washington, DC. http://www.census.gov/prod/2008pubs/p70–117.pdf.

Crandall, W. 2001. Getting there when you are blind: Talking Signs. *Scope: National Academy of Ophthalmology*, 5(1): 8–10.

Crandall, W., B. Bentzen, L. Myers, and P. Mitchell. 1995a. Transit Accessibility Improvement through Talking Signs® Infrared Remote Signage: A Demonstration and Evaluation. Final Report, National Easter Seal Research Program. Project ACTION.

Crandall, W., B. Bentzen, S. Rosen, and P. Mitchell. 1994. Infrared Remote Signage for the Blind and Print Handicapped: An Orientation and Mobility Study. Final Report, National Easter Seal Research Program.

Crandall, W., B. Bentzen, L. Myers, and D. Steed. 1995b. Talking Signs® Remote Infrared Signage: A Guide for Transit System Managers. Final Report, National Easter Seal Research Program. Project ACTION.

Crandall, W., B. Bentzen, and L. Myers. 1996. Talking Signs® Remote Infrared Signage for People Who Are Blind or Print Disabled: A Surface Transit Accessibility Study. Final Report, National Easter Seal Research Program. Project ACTION.

Crandall, W., B. Bentzen, and L. Myers. 1998. Remote Signage Development to Address Current and Emerging Access Problems for Blind Individuals. Part I. Smith-Kettlewell Research on the Use of Talking Signs® at Light Controlled Street Crossings. NIDRR #H133G60076. The Smith-Kettlewell Eye Research Institute.

Crandall, W., B. Bentzen, and L. Myers. 1999a. Remote Signage Development to Address Current and Emerging Access Problems for Blind Individuals. Part II. Smith-Kettlewell Research on the Use of Talking Signs® for Use by People with Developmental Disabilities. NIDRR #H133G60076. The Smith-Kettlewell Eye Research Institute.

Crandall, W., J. Brabyn, B. Bentzen, and L. Myers. 1999b. Remote infrared signage evaluation for transit stations and intersections. *Journal Rehab. Research & Development*, 36(4): 341–355.

Crandall, W., B. Bentzen, and L. Myers. 2000. Remote Signage Development to Address Current and Emerging Access Problems for Blind Individuals. Part III. Emergency Information for People with Visual Impairments: Evaluation of Five Accessible Formats. NIDRR #H133G60076. The Smith-Kettlewell Eye Research Institute.

Crandall, W., B. Bentzen, L. Myers, and J. Brabyn. 2001. New orientation and accessibility option for persons with visual impairments: Transportation applications for remote infrared signage. *Clinical and Experimental Optometry*, 84(3): 120–131.

Gerrey, W.A. 1991. Introduction to Talking Signs®. *Smith-Kettlewell Technical file*, 12(4).

Golledge, R., C. Costanzo, and J. Marston. 1995. The Mass Transit Needs of a Non-Driving Disabled Population. Institute of Transportation Studies, Research Reports, Working Papers, *Proceedings 102965*, Institute of Transportation Studies. UC Berkeley.

Golledge, R., M. Costanzo, and J. Marston. 1996b. Public transit use by non-driving disabled persons: The case of the blind and vision impaired. (California PATH Working Paper UCB-ITS-PWP-96–1): Partners for Advanced Transit and Highways (PATH).

Golledge, R., J. Marston, and C. Costanzo. 1997. Attitudes of visually impaired persons toward the use of public transportation. *Journal of Visual Impairment and Blindness*, 91(5): 446–459.

Golledge, R., J. Marston, and C. Costanzo. 1998a. Assistive Devices and Services for the Disabled: Auditory Signage and the Accessible City for Blind and Vision

Impaired Traveler. California PATH Working Paper, UCB-ITS-PWP-98-18, Report for MOU 276.

Golledge, R., J. Marston, and C. Costanzo. 1998b. Assistive Devices and Services for the Disabled. Final Report. University of California Achievement Field Station PATH Division Grant #MOU 276.

Golledge, R. G., and Marston, J. R. 1999. Towards an accessible city: Removing functional barriers to independent travel for blind and vision impaired residents and visitors (California PATH Research Report No. UCB-ITS-PPR-99-33 for PATH project MOU 343): California PATH Program, Institute of Transportation Studies, University of California, Berkeley.

Kurachi K., S. Kitakaze, Y. Fujishima, N. Watanabe, and M. Kamata. 2005. Integrated pedestrian guidance system using mobile device. In *Proceeding on 12th World Congress on ITS*. San Francisco.

Marston, J. 2002. *Towards an Accessible City: Empirical Measurement and Modeling of Access to Urban Opportunities for those with Vision Impairments, Using Remote Infrared Audible Signage*. Unpublished dissertation. Santa Barbara, California.

Marston, J.R., and Church, R.L. 2005. A relative access measure to identify barriers to efficient transit use by persons with visual impairments. *Disability and Rehabilitation*, 27(13): 769–779.

Marston, J., and R. Golledge. 2000. Towards an Accessible City: Removing Functional Barriers to Independent travel for Blind and Vision Impaired: A Case for Auditory Signs. Final Report, University of California Berkeley: University of California Transportation Center, Grant # UCTC 65V430.

Marston, J., and R. Golledge. 2003. The hidden demand for activity participation and travel by people with vision impairment or blindness. *Journal of Visual Impairment and Blindness*, 97(8):475–488.

Marston, J., R. Golledge, and C. Costanzo. 1997. Investigating travel behavior of non-driving blind and vision impaired people: The role of public transit. *The Professional Geographer*, 49(2): 235–245.

Petrella, M., L. Rainville, and D. Spiller. 2009. Remote Infrared Audible Signage Pilot Program Evaluation Report Prepared by: The Volpe National Transportation Systems Center Economic and Industry Analysis Division 55 Broadway Cambridge, MA 02142. Report Number: FTA-MA-26-7117-2009.01.

Shenkman, B. 1986. The effect of receiver beamwidth on the detection time of a message from Talking Signs, an auditory orientation aid for the blind. *International Journal of Rehabilitation*, 9(3): 239–246.

Schmeidler, E., and D. Halfmann.1997. Statistics on visual impairment in older persons, disability in children, and lie expectancy. *Journal of Visual Impairment and Blindness*, 91:602–606.

Tajima, T., T. Aotani, K. Kurachi, and H. Ohkubo. 2002. Evaluation of pedestrian information and communication systems-a for visually impaired persons. In *Proceedings of the California State University Northridge Conference on Technology and Disability*. Los Angeles, CA.

Tajima, T., K. Yachi, T. Aotan, K. Kurachi, and H. Ohkubo. 2001. Pedestrian information and communication systems for visually impaired persons. In *Proceedings of the California State University Northridge Conference on Technology and Disability*. Los Angeles, CA.

7

Evaluating the Effectiveness of Assistive Travel and Wayfinding Devices for Persons Who Are Blind or Visually Impaired

James Marston and Billie Louise (Beezy) Bentzen

CONTENTS

Introduction

Technological advances and increased computing power have led to many new assistive devices in recent years, for people who are blind or who have low

vision. Unfortunately, many of those designed to help travelers who are visually impaired navigate and travel safely have not been widely adopted. This
chapter addresses the evaluation of assistive devices for travel and wayfinding, with the hope that concrete examples of good experimental procedures
and a better understanding of the target audience, can assist in the development of devices that are user-friendly to a wide range of travelers who are
visually impaired, and which provide positive benefits to independent travel.

A grant to the Smith-Kettlewell Eye Research Institute, "Fundamental
Issues in Wayfinding Technology" (the Wayfinding Project) was awarded in
response to a request from the National Institute of Disability and
Rehabilitation Research to provide guidance for the evaluation of wayfind-
ing technologies for people who are blind or visually impaired. This project
included two activities that directly provide information for this chapter.
Human factors research to validate a research protocol was conducted by
Alan C. Scott, Billie Louise Bentzen, Linda Myers, Janet M. Barlow, and James
R. Marston. A survey of the wayfinding needs of travelers with visual
impairments was conducted by Joshua A. Miele and James R. Marston.
Summaries of both of these activities can be found online.*

Numerous systems or devices intended to help visually impaired people
plan and travel routes independently have been developed in recent years,
but few have met with much success (Ross, 2001; Loomis et al., 2007; Giudice
and Legge, 2008). Lack of success has sometimes resulted because the developers did not understand the needs of visually impaired travelers and the
great diversity of this population, and developed products for which there
was no interest. Sometimes it was because the devices were too expensive for
visually impaired individuals, and sometimes it was because the technology
required expensive changes to the built environment such as the addition of
hardware to buildings, costly or time-sensitive updates to databases, or monitoring by others. Sometimes it was because the devices were hard to use,
were cumbersome, or were not cosmetically appealing.

Effective evaluation of travel and wayfinding devices throughout the
developmental process can lead to more useful and more widely accepted
end products. Good evaluation can guide developers in refining devices to
be acceptable and attractive to end users, it can guide funding agencies in
determining the likelihood that money invested in development is likely to
result in a commercially viable product, and it can guide purchasers. Effective
evaluation answers the following questions.

- Does the technology enable people who are visually impaired to do
  what it is designed to do?
- Does the technology increase users' confidence that they will get to
  destinations safely, without getting lost, and with reduced stress?
- Does the technology perform technically, as it is intended to do?

---

* http://www.ski.org/Rehab/wayfinding.html

- Is the technology user-friendly for a wide range of people who are visually impaired, including the majority of legally blind people who are over the age of 65, have some usable vision, and are likely to have age-related hearing loss?
- Is the user interface acceptable to end users?

This chapter looks at measures of success and efficacy that have been developed in previous projects by us and others. We review different types of measures and point out benefits and problems of using each one to assess the value of various devices and technologies.

Know the Target Population

To a large extent, development has been technology-driven. Attempts have been made to answer the question: "How can this technology be adapted to users who are blind?" rather than: "What information is needed by travelers who are visually impaired, and how can it best be presented to them?" All too often, technologies are developed that show a lack of understanding of the complex and heterogeneous nature of those who make up the visually impaired community. There is a wide range in skills, abilities, and level of independence. The range of usable vision differs widely between individuals, and often within each individual by lighting conditions, complexity of the environment, time of day, fatigue, and other factors. In addition, wayfinding by visually impaired travelers is influenced by age, age of onset of vision loss, degree of training, and concomitant disabilities, including hearing loss. Interviews or familiarization with a small group of people with low vision or total blindness is not sufficient for drawing any conclusions about wayfinding by people who are visually impaired. Developers need to make it a point to get to know and understand the wide range of characteristics of people who are blind or who have low vision before beginning to conceive of assistive technologies. They must also listen carefully to the feedback from people who use the technology. In the experience of the second author of this chapter, a person who was totally blind was asked by a technology developer to travel a simple, indoor route with a technically sophisticated but cumbersome prototype that attempted to provide step-by-step route directions at appropriate times. It also provided information about landmarks along the way. After arriving at his destination, the participant said "All I need is the directions." The developer considered this comment to be irrelevant, instead of realizing that the complexity of the user interface and the additional information it provided might have been interfering with this participant's sense of satisfaction in travel, and that this could be the case for many other potential end users.

TABLE 7.1

Results of the Survey Administered to Visually Impaired People as Part of the Wayfinding Project

The Six Criteria Offered to Participants	Percent of Participants Choosing Each Criterion among Their Top Three (%)
Getting where you want to go	86
Feeling safe while traveling	79
Low stress while traveling	55
Not getting lost along the way	42
Getting there quickly	23
Not needing to ask for directions or information	11

In deciding how to evaluate wayfinding technologies, it is helpful to know what criteria visually impaired travelers think are most important in evaluating successful travel. A survey was administered to people who were visually impaired as part of the Wayfinding Project. The survey asked 466 visually impaired respondents to select the top three out of six stated criteria that might be used to define a successful independent trip. The major results are summarized in Table 7.1.

Clearly, the respondents thought successful completion of trips and feelings of safety and low stress were the most important criteria. Time advantages were not rated highly, and having to ask people for help was not a problem with this group. Most successful blind travelers realize that sometimes asking for help is the best way to recover from disorientation, or to learn new routes or environments.

To learn whether a technology facilitates travel and wayfinding by people who are blind or visually impaired, whether the technology performs technically as it is intended to do, and whether people who are blind or who have low vision are able to use the user interface, human factors experiments in which participants use the technology to perform tasks for which it was intended are the most informative. To learn whether people who are blind or who have low vision find that the technology provides wayfinding information they want, whether they find it easy to use, and whether they find it comfortable or convenient to use, subjective methods such as surveys or interviews are the most informative.

Performance Measures

Performance measures, also called objective measures, record observable human behavior, such as whether a participant deviates from the intended path of travel or reaches a destination independently. Performance measures are the only means to establish that an improvement in performance of way-finding tasks is probably attributable to the use of a technology.

Reaching the Destination

Participants reaching a destination without need for assistance is the primary performance measure for evaluation of technologies intended to facilitate travel from a start point to a destination. If there is a statistically significant difference in the number of participants, or in the number of trials in which participants reached the destination without assistance, as compared to a baseline or another technology, this indicates that it is likely that the difference can be attributed to the technology. (See Bentzen et al., 1999 for an example of the use of this measure.)

Number of Deviations from Intended Route (Path Confusions)

The number of deviations from a route is sometimes used as an indication of goodness of wayfinding on the route. However, what an observer with unimpaired vision may consider deviations from a route may be deliberate deviations from straight line travel in order to pick up additional cues, such as grass or building lines, or landmarks that may confirm that travelers are exactly where they think they are, so number of deviations is not always a perfect reflection of wayfinding.

Recovery from Route Deviations

Independent recovery from route deviation is a very meaningful performance measure of the effect of a wayfinding technology. Some technologies may be very good at helping travelers who are off-route or confused to get back on track. Others may be very good at providing information about the precise location of the traveler, but not be designed to provide information to help users get back on track. (See Crandall et al., 1999 for an example of the measure of recovery from disorientation.)

Time to Reach a Destination

Time to perform a task has long been used in psychology, human factors research, and other cognitive science fields to measure individuals' ability to understand and react to various inputs. An apparent assumption in much research on wayfinding technologies is that a reduction in the time to reach a destination represents a worthwhile improvement in the experience of independent travel. However, as previously mentioned, visually impaired people did not consider getting to a destination quickly to be as important as other criteria for a successful trip, and the measure has potential problems. Participants need to reach the destination on each trial, or there may be so much missing data that statistical analysis is not possible. If participants need assistance to recover from deviations from the intended route, the time required for them to obtain assistance may be impracticable, and it may be necessary to establish an arbitrary time limit for recovering from disorientation or for getting assistance.

A common finding when having participants travel using relatively unfamiliar technology is that using the technology (holding it properly, pushing the correct buttons or keys, entering a query in the correct format, and so on) may take a good deal of time. This may result in participants taking longer to reach the destination than under a baseline condition, even though for experienced users of the technology, the destination might have been reached more quickly using the information provided by the technology. For these and other reasons, time to complete a task is not recommended as a main variable for measuring efficacy of a device compared to a "no device" condition. However, in some situations, time is a very informative measure (Loomis et al., 1998, 2005; Klatzky et al., 2006; Marston et al., 2006, 2007). These experiments were comparing the efficacy of different interface designs for guidance and the use of time-to-destination for all these experiments made it easy to compare results. Some experiments measure the walking speed per foot or meter and compare this to participants' normal walking speed. Most experiments, however, compare completion of the task to some other type of baseline.

Distance Measures

Distance can also be used as a measure of walking efficacy (Church and Marston, 2003). This measurement is difficult to collect in some experiments, but if one is testing GPS, virtual reality, or other trackable devices it is quite simple to collect these data. Sometimes there is a direct correlation to time measurements; however, sometimes distance reveals something about the technology being studied. For example, a study of different personal guidance system interfaces (Loomis et al., 1998) found that although virtual sound always produced the shortest travel times, the distance traveled was quite similar across treatments. This indicated that all the device interfaces had equivalent accuracy, but that the shorter time must have been because acquiring and facing the correct heading was faster and easier with the virtual sound. Since the distances were similar, the time differential must have occurred when searching for a new heading direction at waypoints, and when adjusting heading on the route. All participants in this experiment were able to finish all routes, adding validity to the recorded times. In experiments where all subjects or all conditions cannot achieve completion, recorded time loses its robustness.

Evaluating Spatial Learning

Some wayfinding technologies may be particularly effective for enabling users to form good cognitive maps of the area in which they use the technology.

Blind travelers who have formed good cognitive maps may be able to take shortcuts in areas where they have previously used the technology (see Chapter 6); and/or decrease their need for use of the technology, or need for assistance on subsequent trips in the area.

Spatial cognition theory points to a progression in how people understand space and acquire spatial knowledge. People normally learn the location of landmarks, and then learn the routes between them. Routes are at first a series of "walk straight," "find a cue or landmark," "turn left or right," until arrival at a destination. Over time, most people, whether or not visually impaired, start to integrate these landmarks and routes into an overall spatial concept of the space, a type of "bird's eye view," survey view, or cognitive or mental map (Strelow, 1985; Sholl, 1996; Montello, 1998). Once a mental image of space is developed, people can use their knowledge to try novel routes to various destinations, make shortcuts, understand what to do when a desired and known path is blocked, or when they need to make some kind of detour. Instead of simply following known routes (A to B, B to C), they are able to integrate their location with desired destinations, and make direct progress to their goal (directly from A to C). Some techniques and devices for the blind have the possibility not only to help users accomplish a goal (cross a street, discover and find locations indoors, or follow outdoor routes with GPS) but also to help the user understand spatial relationships in the environment.

There are a number of ways to measure the effect of a wayfinding technology on spatial learning. Pointing accuracy can be measured: after participants have traveled a route, have them stand in one location and point to where they started, or to other locations they have located along the route. The ability to make spontaneous shortcuts can be used as a measure of spatial understanding. The need for additional information from the technology can be measured by recording the number of times the device was used to get spatial information. The accuracy of participants' maps or models of the area traveled can be measured, as can the accuracy of responses to spatial questions regarding the area traveled (Jacobson et al., 2001; Blades et al., 2002; Marston, 2002).

Special Measures for Evaluating Devices for Safety and Wayfinding at Street Crossings

Measures of street crossing are often broken down into a number of tasks, each of which can be objectively measured: identify the end of a block; locate the crosswalk; locate and push the correct pushbutton, if any; align to cross; determine when to start crossing; and maintain correct heading while crossing. The most common way for researchers to measure the ability of pedestrians who are visually impaired to identify the end of a block is to have participants stop when they think their next step will be on the street (Bentzen and Barlow, 1995; Hauger et al., 1996).

While it is important that pedestrians cross within the crosswalk, there is legally no significance to whether they cross in the middle of a crosswalk or not. Many pedestrians who are visually impaired prefer to begin crossing from a position close to the curb ramp, on the side farthest from the center of the intersection, rather than begin crossing from the curb ramp, itself. The most ecologically valid measure of locating the crosswalk is therefore simply whether the pedestrian begins to cross from within the crosswalk—anywhere within the crosswalk. See Bentzen et al. (1999) for the first example of the use of this frequently used measure.

If it is necessary to actuate a pushbutton in order to get a pedestrian timing at a signalized intersection, pedestrians need to locate and press the correct pushbutton. There are often two pushbuttons on a corner, one for crossing in each direction. A number of measures are used for pushbutton actuation: participant located and pushed the correct button on first attempt; participant located and pushed incorrect button; and participant located the incorrect button first, rejected that button, and then located and pushed the correct pushbutton (Scott et al., 2008).

Aligning to cross, or establishing a heading toward the opposite end of the crosswalk, prepares pedestrians who are visually impaired to begin crossing in the correct direction, that is, in the direction indicated by the crosswalk. Alignment clues typically used by pedestrians who are visually impaired include traffic on the street parallel to the intended crossing and traffic idling at the stop line of the street to be crossed. Traffic is not always present at an intersection, however. Also, at intersections having complex geometry, traffic on the parallel street may not be parallel to the crosswalk, and stop lines may not be perpendicular to the crosswalk, so these clues are unreliable. There are a number of challenges in measuring alignment.

The perception of straight-ahead (or aligned) by people with visual impairments is not necessarily consistent with the facing direction of the head, torso, or feet, all of which may face a slightly different direction. Therefore, an experimenter cannot be certain what part of the anatomy of a participant represents the participant's intended direction, nor the direction the participants will take when they begin to cross. Any static measurement of alignment is therefore subject to considerable error. Measurement tools are also challenging. While compass devices have sometimes been used to measure alignment, they are very sensitive to variations in mounting position that are necessitated by individual anatomy, and they are subject to fluctuations caused by metal in the vicinity. (Bentzen and colleagues have found that variability in compass readings may be caused by poles, keys, or a cell phone in the pocket of the participant or experimenter, a belt buckle, or a watch on either the participant or the experimenter.)

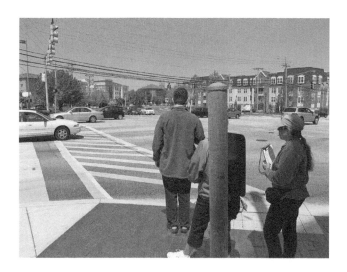

FIGURE 7.1

It is easy to see that if this blind research participant crosses this street in Towson, Maryland, he will end up walking into the middle of the intersection. His alignment was recorded as "outside the crosswalk" and "toward the center of the intersection," very crude measures, but accurate enough to reveal differences attributable to APS with prototype wayfinding features, and very meaningful to pedestrians who are blind as well as to traffic engineers who are major consumers of this research.

In a series of evaluations of the effects of Accessible Pedestrian Signals (APS) on street crossing, measures of the alignment of participants who were blind were made by observation, in a way that was both ecologically valid for blind pedestrians, and meaningful to traffic engineers.

Participants made crossings at four unfamiliar, complex, signalized inter-sections in various cities (Bentzen et al., 1999, 2004, 2006; Barlow et al., 2005, 2009; Scott et al., 2008). Researchers stood behind participants and judged whether, if participants traveled in the direction they appeared to be facing immediately prior to beginning to cross, they would complete their cross-ings within the marked crosswalk lines (see Figure 7.1). Results of some experiments showed significant differences in alignment accuracy attribut-able to APS conditions.

The measure is crude because participants' apparent facing direction is not always the direction toward which they will begin crossing. It is also crude because crosswalk widths vary, and because a slight difference in the posi-tion of the experimenter observing the accuracy of alignment can make par-ticipants appear to be aligned within or outside the crosswalk width. However, the measure is valid because it does not require that participants stand still until a measurement is made, or that where they begin crossing is controlled or precisely known. It is a meaningful measure for traffic engi-neers, because it is whether a pedestrian is in or outside a crosswalk that determines whether he or she is making a legal crossing (see Figure 7.2).

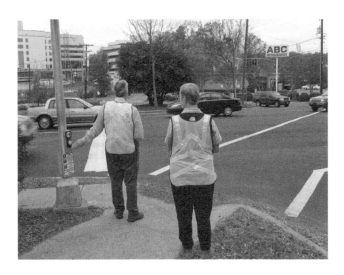

FIGURE 7.2
This blind research participant in Charlotte, North Carolina, has pushed an APS pushbutton and is aligning to cross. He is keeping his hand on the arrow that will vibrate when it is time to cross because the traffic is very loud and he is not sure he will be able to hear the audible walk indication. He has used traffic idling at the stop line, as well as traffic on the cross street, to help him to align. However, the crosswalk is not parallel to the stop line or perpendicular to the traffic on the cross street. When he crossed the street, he walked parallel to the stop line, entirely outside the crosswalk.

A more precise measure of alignment at crossings has recently been used by Bentzen and colleagues to measure the effects of six different cues on alignment. Participants walked down plywood ramps having cues that could be rotated to face in different intended crossing directions relative to the slope of the ramp, located the cues and used them to align, and then continued down the ramp and onto a parking lot for a distance of 10 ft. Participants' headings over the first 10 ft (3 m) of walking were measured and these trajectories were compared with the intended trajectories (Scott et al., 2011a).

Pedestrians who are blind need to maintain an accurate heading in the direction of the crosswalk while crossing. All pedestrians who are blind veer to some extent, especially in very wide crossings. Technologies that assist pedestrians who are visually impaired in maintaining a heading across the street can help them avoid the dangers of veering into an intersection where there is moving traffic, or of becoming disoriented if they do not finish their crossings where they expect to. Typical cues for maintaining one's heading while crossing are: maintaining a direction of travel parallel to and at a consistent distance from parallel traffic; traveling in front of cars stopped at a stop line; following the crowning of a street, which typically slopes down toward corners to facilitate drainage; and following other pedestrians.

As for measuring alignment, there are major challenges in measuring the ability of pedestrians who are blind to maintain a heading while crossing a street. Where people who are visually impaired walk as they cross a street is highly unpredictable. In addition to any wayfinding technology, where they travel in relation to a crosswalk is influenced by where they start. They may start from where they intersect the curbline, to maintain their proprioceptive sense of straight ahead; they may start near the pushbutton, which is rarely near the centerline of a crosswalk; they may prefer to start from a curb ramp, which is often not in the center of a crosswalk; or they may prefer to start from a defined curb, perhaps on the side of the curbramp farthest from the center of the intersection. Where visually impaired pedestrians travel in relation to a crosswalk is also influenced by which cues they use to maintain a heading while crossing. In addition, they may attempt to travel directly toward the sound of an APS, which is seldom located in the center of the crosswalk. Where they travel may also be influenced by a common preference for traveling farther from versus closer to the center of the intersection.

Measuring participants' positions as simply "inside" or "outside" the crosswalk, either at the completion of the crossing, or also at various distances along the crossing, allows participants to travel in a natural way, can capture differences in maintaining a heading that are meaningful to engineering and enforcement personnel, and makes it easy to obtain data by direct observation (Scott et al., 2008; Barlow et al., 2009). However, this is a relatively coarse measure that may not capture small but significant differences in maintaining heading that may be attributable to a technology. Increasing the number of distances at which maintaining heading with regard to the crosswalk is measured makes it more likely that small changes in heading that are attributable to hearing and responding to an APS beacon will be picked up. In ongoing research, Bentzen and colleagues are measuring accuracy at three distances in addition to the end of the crossing, and also recording where participants are within the width of the crosswalk and how far outside the crosswalk they sometimes are.

Participants' positions in relation to the centerline of the crosswalk can also be measured. This is a fairly precise measure that is likely to capture small, but statistically significant differences. However, it may require interrupting the natural flow of participants' travel to position them in a precise location for starting to cross and it requires actual or virtual marking of the crosswalk. (See Wall et al., 2004; Scott et al., 2011a,b for examples.)

The time at which pedestrians who are visually impaired begin to cross the streets has important implications for their safety. At signalized intersections, beginning to cross at the wrong time in the signal cycle, or beginning to cross too long after the onset of the walk signal can result in pedestrians being in the crosswalk in the presence of conflicting perpendicular vehicular movement. Measures of the time at which pedestrians begin to cross include: whether they do or do not begin their crossing during the walk interval (the interval during which pedestrians are intended to initiate crossings, as indicated by a walking person or the indication WALK), and the interval during which they begin crossing (WALK, flashing DON'T WALK—during which they should be completing crossings, or steady DON'T WALK—during which they should not be in the crosswalk). The interval during which participants completed their crossings is also often recorded. Delay in beginning to cross after the onset of the walk interval, or, in the absence of a pedestrian signal, the onset of parallel traffic, are also sometimes measured. In general, in comparison to crossings at complex, unfamiliar, signalized intersections with no APS, APS have resulted in a greater likelihood that participants who had little or no vision would start crossing during the walk interval and complete their crossing before the onset of perpendicular through vehicular traffic. APS have also significantly reduced the delay in starting to cross (Scott et al., 2008; Barlow et al., 2009).

Choosing an Appropriate Baseline Measure

In evaluating wayfinding technologies or other assistive devices for people who are blind or who have low vision, the choice of a baseline against which to judge whether the technology did or did not result in improved wayfinding or performance is essential. The authors have read or reviewed numerous evaluations of assistive technologies for travel and wayfinding that simply report measures of travel with a technology but do not compare it with any baseline, so no valid conclusions can be drawn about the effect of the technology.

It is often not feasible to obtain a number of sufficiently similar potential users to divide them into two or more groups who travel with and without the technology—a between-groups design. It is much more common that evaluation of technologies will use a within-subjects design, in which the same participants use the technology and travel the same or similar routes with and without the technology. For traveling relatively simple routes, it is sometimes successful to have participants obtain wayfinding information in the same ways they normally would as they travel in unfamiliar environments—chiefly by asking for assistance and directions. This is the most ecologically valid comparison. However, a baseline of travel using customary sources of wayfinding information, with no constraints, may be so impractical that an experiment cannot be conducted because of time and distance constraints, or the data may be impossible to analyze because it has so many variables. Here are some typical things that happen when travelers who are visually impaired ask other travelers for wayfinding information:

- Other travelers provide wrong information, either because they do not know where the destination is, or because they mix up left and right.

- Information is not understandable because it is not conveyed in useful ways, for example, people often point to the direction the blind person should travel, rather than expressing the direction in words.
- Other travelers do not speak the same language, so the question is not understood.
- Other travelers engage in off-topic conversations with the visually impaired traveler.
- Other travelers insist on guiding the visually impaired traveler to the destination or next landmark.

Any of these occurrences may make measures of time to travel, rate of travel and/or distance, and off-course deviations useless, or at least hard to interpret. In the Wayfinding Project, participants traveled both indoor and outdoor routes, each using information provided by one of two wayfinding technologies, and traveled similar routes using verbal directions prepared by an Orientation and Mobility (O&M) Specialist. Wayfinding information for the indoor route was provided by remote infrared audible signage (Talking Signs, see Chapter 6), and wayfinding information for the outdoor route was provided by accessible GPS (see Chapter 5).

Finding the right baseline to use, especially when testing a single technology, is quite important and sometimes it is revealing to use more than one baseline calculation. For example, in an experiment testing Talking Signs at a multimodal train station in San Francisco, visually impaired participants performed five simulated transit transfer tasks, locating 20 objects during the experiment (Marston, 2002; Marston and Church, 2005). One group of 15 participants used the technology while another group of 15 used their regular method of travel; this allowed for between-subject comparisons. The 20 location tasks varied in difficulty and interlocation distance and thus did the required time and effort to reach these locations. To compare results to the optimal walking time for each location task in the experiment, a sighted user who was familiar with the area was used to establish a baseline time. As expected, none of the visually impaired people with or without the technology completed the tasks as fast as the sighted and familiar user. The sighted user who was familiar with the area made of course no errors, and had no need to ask for assistance. However, a sighted person who had never been to the area was also asked to complete the routes and find the 20 locations. This unfamiliar first-time user made several errors in searching for locations and once had to ask for assistance to find a certain location. Two interesting findings came about by using those two different baselines.

Several people with mild vision loss were able to perform all 20 tasks in the same time or a bit faster than the unfamiliar first-time user. The types of travel tasks for the visually impaired participants had a wide range of difficulty, and the real purpose of having the familiar sighted baseline was to determine the "time penalty" of locating various places without the use of vision. For example, walking to the street corner was a simple task, when using O&M skills and listening for the traffic. However, finding a bus shelter for a specific bus, with no accessible information, or finding a poorly placed fare machine, was much harder without vision, and without the device.

Two different baselines were also used in an experiment on a city street and on a path in a park, testing guidance from two different interfaces for a personal guidance system (PGS) (Marston et al., 2006). The travel times for the two devices were quite similar, but it would have been almost impossible to compare those two treatments to walking times with no treatment, as the routes and environment were very complicated. As the PGS had some lag time before it delivered the instructions, it was decided to test three sighted people who walked the route with vision, but did not make any movements until the system gave instructions. Therefore, they experienced the same waiting times at waypoints; the users also had to carry and use the equipment, which put them on par with the blind participants. Using those times as a baseline revealed that one of the totally blind participants was only about 10% slower than the average of the three sighted participants. That remarkable showing by a blind person validated the efficacy of the system being tested. The two researchers running the experiment, who were quite familiar with the routes, having walked with the participants and observed potential obstacles repeatedly, decided to blindfold themselves after the experiment and see how quickly they could complete the route. Their dismal results showed the importance of using only SKILLED blind travelers. Blindfolded sighted people, with great knowledge of the route and obstacles, were no match for the orientation and navigation skills the blind learn over time.

In research on street crossings cited earlier, Bentzen and colleagues have compared baseline crossings without APS to crossings with APS (Scott et al., 2008), compared baseline crossings with standard APS to crossings with prototype beaconing APS (Barlow et al., 2009), or compared baseline crossings with standard APS to crossings with tactile guidestrips.

An appropriate baseline that enables conclusions to be drawn about cost/benefit of a wayfinding technology is to have the participants learn routes from an O&M instructor with repeated trials until they can perform the task at an optimum level, recording the instructional time needed. This baseline can then be compared to the amount of time it takes trained users of the technology to travel similar routes on the basis of information from the technology.

Designing Unbiased Evaluations

Choosing the proper environment to test products is important as the choice of the environment may bias the results. It is a good idea to have some visually impaired people or trained O&M specialists investigate the planned environment and offer suggestions and comment on problems that might not be otherwise apparent to the researcher. It is especially important to make sure that any baseline test (such as comparison to no treatment) be ecologically valid. For example, if a location-based device is tested to find a doorway to a specific room and there is no Braille room number that can be used in a baseline condition with no device, there is no ecological validity because participants would have no way to determine that they were at the correct room without any identification.

The choice of environment is very important when testing navigation devices like accessible GPS. Accessible GPS should not be evaluated in urban canyons where there is not good availability of at least three positioning satellites for accurate triangulation of location. Some areas, such as city sidewalks, are "bounded", with streets on one side and buildings on the other (Gaunet and Briffault, 2005; Gaunet, 2006). Skilled travelers who are visually impaired can easily follow routes along city streets and thus a no-treatment baseline might be justified. However, if the route is not well defined or bounded, such as sporadic gravel paths in a park (Marston et al., 2006), there is no validity when testing in a no-treatment condition.

Assuring correct installation of technologies as well as their correct functioning is important to the conduct of unbiased evaluations, especially when two technologies are being compared. In research by the second author that compared two technologies involving transmitters and receivers, Talking Signs and Verbal Landmark (Bentzen and Mitchell, 1995), in order to control for possible bias of researchers, each company was asked to install its transmitters along routes in a hotel in the manner in which they were intended to function to enable people to get from the beginning to the end of each route. However, one company installed many more transmitters than the other, which may have biased the outcome of the comparison. Each company was also asked to provide technical support throughout the evaluation but one company did not provide support and their technology did not function consistently well. Thus statistically significant differences in the ability of participants to reach destinations could have been attributable to differences in number of transmitters, and/or differences in consistently correct functioning of equipment, as well as to the differences in the way in which information was provided by each technology. No statistical test of interaction between these factors was possible because they were completely overlapping. On the basis of both objective performance (getting to the destination) and subjective questions following route travel, researchers concluded that there were significant differences in the ability of people who were visually impaired to successfully use the information provided by the two technologies. However, subjective data were needed along with performance measures to help interpret the results of this biased evaluation.

Caution should be used in any design in which performance is to be compared on similar routes or tasks with and without a technology, or with two different technologies. No two routes or street crossings are identical; subtle differences in ambient sound, slope, building lines, or vehicular and pedestrian traffic may result in differences in the ease and accuracy of travel. When different technologies, or technology versus no technology, are being used to travel different routes, the best design is to have a portion of the participants travel one route under one condition, and the other route under the other condition, and then have a comparable portion of the participants travel the routes with the reverse assignment of wayfinding conditions.

Selecting Participants

Selection of participants for research evaluating travel and wayfinding technologies requires careful consideration. People who are visually impaired differ in many ways, which can affect their ability to benefit from technologies. Yet, the preponderance of research on travel and wayfinding by people who are visually impaired has been limited to participants who have little or no vision (no light perception, or no more vision than light perception). This means that they can see no forms, edges, or shadows. Samples are frequently limited to participants between the ages of approximately 20–60. However, the large majority of people who are visually impaired have some object perception that they are likely to use for orientation, obstacle avoidance, and detection of landmarks, and the large majority of people who are visually impaired are also over the age of 65, by which age they normally are experiencing some degree of age-related hearing loss.

There are a number of reasons for the common limitation of evaluation of wayfinding and travel technologies to such a small group. When evaluating technologies with participants who have low vision, it is difficult or impossible to determine whether differences in performance are attributable to the technology or are attributable to the amount and type of low vision. When evaluating technologies with elderly people, hearing loss and cognitive factors may reduce the likelihood that observed differences will be found, and it may not be possible to determine whether it is age, hearing loss, or cognitive limitations that are interfering with the usefulness of the technology. The presence of some degree of hearing loss may result in difficulty and inability to benefit from technologies with audible output, particularly when they are intended to be used in travel situations with high ambient noise. Remaining peripheral vision permits some people who are elderly to retain high wayfinding skills, though they may have difficulty with such tasks as face recognition or reading. They may not appear to benefit from a wayfinding technology. Thus, either hearing loss in older people who are visually impaired, or the presence of good peripheral vision may result in statistical outcomes showing no benefit of the technology.

However, research conducted under the Wayfinding Project with a varied sample of 41 participants suggests that using a restricted sample (i.e., adults less than 60 years old, with little or no vision and unimpaired hearing) is likely to reflect differences that would be found with visually impaired populations with low vision and with hearing loss, although some care ought to be taken in generalizing for people with concurrent visual and hearing impairments. A similar result was found in research in which participants had to judge whether it was the street in front of them or the street beside them that was being signaled by an APS. Performance of participants with low vision was in the same direction as performance of participants who had little or no vision, although differences in performance by participants with low vision were not significant (Scott et al., 2006). Interestingly, performance by groups of participants with three different types of cognitive disabilities, who were not visually impaired, was also in the same direction, though differences were not significant.

Research participants with low vision may experience less improvement in wayfinding tasks when using wayfinding devices than participants who are totally blind because their wayfinding may be quite good without the technology. People who have reduced acuity but full visual fields generally have less difficulty with wayfinding than people who have limited visual fields, but whose acuity may still be quite good. People who are totally blind generally have more difficulty with complex wayfinding tasks than people who have some vision; therefore they are more likely to demonstrate significantly improved wayfinding when using a technology.

If a technology does not appear to benefit elderly people who are visually impaired, characteristics of aging that frequently accompany visual impairment may make it hard to determine whether it is the technology *per se* that is not beneficial, or whether other individual characteristics may be contributing to the appearance of no benefit. Common characteristics of aging include: hearing loss; decrease in attentional field; reduced information-processing ability; increased time to learn new tasks or information; poor night vision; increased sensitivity to glare; reduced stamina; and limited experience with technology. If a technology does not appear to benefit older participants (especially), the problem may be with the user interface. If use of a keyboard seems to have interfered with success in using a technology, interactive speech might be a more successful interface. The problem may also be that the physical and attentional demands of the wayfinding task selected for evaluation are too demanding. Improvement in wayfinding might have been seen if, for example, an experimental route had been shorter.

Blindfolded participants who have no visual impairment should not be used in the evaluation of travel and wayfinding technologies. They are not used to wayfinding without full visual information; this can result in appearance of no benefit because they may not perform the task/s well either with or without the technology. On the other hand, they are likely to have quite good wayfinding concepts and spatial reasoning, as the presence of full vision is a chief contributor to the development of spatial skills and rea-soning in children. This can result in appearance of no benefit because per-formance without the aid is already quite good, or result in the appearance of benefit because a small amount of additional spatial information may be more readily understood and incorporated into wayfinding when underly-ing spatial skills are good. Blindfolded sighted participants should also not be used because their subjective experiences of performing wayfinding tasks are limited to the experience of performing the tasks without visual input; this is a very small part of what it means to be blind or visually impaired. It is only the experience of living with visual impairment that enables partici-pants to make judgments about such issues as comfort or convenience of a technology, or whether the technology solves real problems in useful ways.

An ideal participant group would contain all the relevant characteristics of people who are blind or visually impaired and are potential users of the technology, in the same proportion as they exist in the total population of potential users. Selecting a random sample of people who are visually impaired in which each person has an equal chance of participating in the research would be a way to achieve this ideal group. However, visual impair-ment is a low incidence disability; therefore it is difficult to get a significant random sample within a feasible distance from the experimental site. Participants must actually use the technology, and they will typically need to use the technology in the same location. Therefore, selection of partici-pants from various geographic regions is not usually possible.

For reasons of cost, time, and availability of prospective participants, it is usually impossible to have samples larger than 20–40 participants. Many evaluations have fewer than 10 participants. However, evaluations using 10–20 participants have commonly revealed significant effects of travel and wayfinding technologies.

Convenience sampling is often the only feasible choice for evaluation of travel and wayfinding technologies. Typically, a sample is drawn from peo-ple in a small geographic area, who are readily available to the researcher, and who fit the most important criteria for the purpose of the research. However, with convenience sampling, great care is needed in interpreting results. Conclusions cannot be generalized with any certainty to a larger population, who may differ in a variety of characteristics that can affect travel and wayfinding. Convenience sampling is improved when attention is paid to balancing or limiting some characteristics.

If the technology is very new, and the goal is simply to demonstrate that a technology having certain characteristics is useful to at least some people who are visually impaired, it may be appropriate to limit the participants to a small group of 8–12 people who are most likely to be able to use and to benefit from the technology (such as people with little or no vision) who are good travelers, and who are familiar with travel and wayfinding technolo-gies. Positive results of an evaluation of this kind with such a limited group will not be generalizable to the larger group of more varied people with visual impairments, but may be a sufficient basis on which to decide whether further development of the technology should be pursued.

If a technology is well developed, perhaps commercially available and in use for travel or wayfinding by people with visual impairments, it is more appropriate to include a larger group of participants with a wider selection of characteristics. However, results will still not be generalizable to particular groups of people with visual impairments, such as elderly people or people with hearing or cognitive disabilities, or to people with low vision. The most common plan is to use one relatively large group, usually including at least 15–20 participants, having the characteristics determined to be essential for the purposes of the evaluation, and excluding those characteristics that would make it most difficult to interpret the results of the research.

Distractions and Cognitive Demands While Traveling

Safety must be a major concern when designing products to assist visually impaired travelers. Distractions from the device and cognitive demands placed on the user can interfere with safe travel. Several commercial products for blind travelers, GPS-based and Talking Signs, advise against using the device while walking to enhance safety and avoid liability concerns. If the proposed device requires attention from the traveler while in motion, questions about interference with normal mental processing and decisions should be addressed in the experiment. As device development matures, it might be advisable to see if various interface modifications or user-selection options can reduce the demand on processing channels. This can be done by research methods known as interference tasks. For examples of interference tasks using an N-back test to determine the relative cognitive demands of devices having different user interfaces, see Giudice et al. (2008); Klatzky et al. (2006, 2008).

Subjective Measures: Efficacy and Performance Evaluated by Participants

All too often the ultimate user of technology or new techniques is ignored in the planning and testing stages of development of assistive devices for persons with visual impairments. Sometimes the research team shows little understanding of the needs and of the wide range of abilities of this population. There seem to be too many research products that, while designed and developed with the best of intentions, and with exciting and innovative technology, do not meet the needs of users. Items can be prohibitively expensive, be bulky, or draw unwanted attention to the user; they may use cognitive channels that are needed for other activities or for environmental monitoring for travel cues or safety concerns. Some devices work well only after long and arduous amounts of training and adaptation to using new sensory modalities. Others might require so much attention and reliance on the device that other skills are not used, leading to an almost robot-like usage, and attention to safety may be compromised.

Whether because a developer's aim is to keep development and manufacturing cost low, or because he or she does not understand the wide range of potential users, many devices do not offer options to fit the needs of the highly diverse population of potential visually impaired users. Some devices and techniques seem to be designed for the totally blind person who has no other functional or sensory problems. The vast majority of people with visual impairments, however, has some sight, are often elderly, and might have many other issues, such as loss of hearing, problems using complicated devices, arthritis, and other disabilities that make carrying and using a device much more difficult than for younger users. For example, when evaluating what users with vision impairments wanted in a GPS device, whether in surveys or post-test evaluations, it has been found that users would like many types of options (Golledge et al., 2004; Marston et al., 2006, 2007).

Users should be able to offer their opinions. They should be allowed to give input on how well they thought a device worked, whether it had any effect on their perceived safety, whether it had any effect on their emotional state, such as stress or fear, how hard it was to learn to use, whether there were any negative effects, whether they would actually want to use or carry/wear the system, and specifically, if the device makes the tasks it was designed for easier to perform. This kind of information is not obtainable through objective performance criteria.

People with disabilities often report that they feel that the biases and attitudes of researchers lead to experiments and products that do not reflect the needs or situations of their special population, and that the results obtained lack validity for them. Good research must consider the attitudes and needs of the target population and involve them in planning and seek their input as part of the evaluation (Kitchin, 2000, 2001). Who better to ask to evaluate products and techniques then those who are intimately involved every day with vision loss? Who best to know if a product or technique is valuable, easy to use, makes tasks easier, does not affect (or maybe increases) safety, and leads to a feeling of increased quality of life?

The following kinds of information may be obtained from users by means of surveys, rating scales, or focus groups:

- Did participants think the technology gave them useful information?
- Could participants understand the information?

- Was this the type of information that participants wanted to have?
- Would having this information make it easier for participants to travel independently?
- Would having this information make participants more likely to travel independently?
- Would participants be likely to use the technology if it was available to them?
- Did the technology increase the participants' confidence that they would not get lost?
- Did the technology increase the participants' confidence that they would be safe as they traveled?
- Did participants feel comfortable and graceful as they used the technology?
- Did participants feel unduly conspicuous as they used the technology?
- Did participants think the technology was easy to use?
- Did participants think the technology was easy to learn to use?
- Did participants think the technology was comfortable?
- Did participants think the technology was convenient?
- Was the user interface of an appropriate weight or configuration, for example, mounted on the long cane, hand-held, or head-mounted?
- Was the appearance of the user interface acceptable?
- Was the volume adequate in the situations in which the technology might be used?
- Were vibrotactile signals sufficiently noticeable?
- Were switches easy to identify?
- Were switches easy to operate?

Often a survey, rating scale, or focus group is used in conjunction with performance measures.

Evaluation through Questions and Rating Scales

Evaluation sometimes uses closed questions that restrict responses to options such as yes/no or agree/disagree, or may use ratings. Using closed questions has the advantage that they place relatively low cognitive demand on participants, they make it easy to record data, they make it easy to analyze data to obtain quantifiable results, and they are amenable to automatic recording and summarizing of data. Disadvantages are that they may not capture actual opinions, and that they do not give participants the opportunity to make helpful suggestions that developers may not have thought of, or that may help developers focus improvements on what is most important to users. Likert scale questions are sometimes used to get around some of the problems in obtaining meaningful answers to yes/no questions. In Likert scale questions, respondents are asked to indicate the strength of their agreement with statements about a particular issue using a scale usually of 1–5 or 1–7, with one end of the number scale representing "strongly disagree," and the other end, representing "strongly agree." An issue might be stated as follows: "When using the technology, I felt confident that I would not get lost."

It is a good idea to have users rate the difficulty, stress, anxiety, and other problems with various tasks before participants complete the tasks with new devices or techniques. Comparing these responses to those made after the experiment can reveal the amount of improvement that the users feel they received. Often, those rating differences are quite large and offer insight into the needs of this group, and to the efficacy of devices (Golledge et al., 1998; Golledge and Marston, 1999; Marston, 2001, 2002; Marston and Golledge, 2003, 2004). There is more validity in asking pre- and postexperiment questions about the same attributes and feelings, than in asking a set of questions after the experiment that require participants to consider how they would have felt when doing the task without the device.

Evaluation Using Open-Ended Questions

The first author has noticed that participants who were visually impaired appreciated that they were allowed to answer open-ended questions and give suggestions and opinions. These can take a lot of time to collect and are more difficult to score and analyze, needing some kind of parsing and qualitative analysis, but they have been invaluable as a way to truly understand how the end user feels about the product and potential problems in daily living and travel. By releasing the user from the strict confines (and possible biases) of researcher-defined criteria, open-ended questions are valuable as they can inform the experimenter of new directions for future research. The first author uses them in all experiments because they have led him in directions he had not thought of; sometimes they even reveal research questions that have never been covered in the literature. For example, when asking the participants how the use of auditory signs in transit tasks differed from their regular methods, there was a very large emphasis on being independent and not having to ask for help. By asking participants where they would like to use certain devices, new ideas about uses and locations were often offered. Affective states, like stress, anxiety, feelings of safety, and well-being can be discovered without having to specifically ask those questions.

If possible, open-ended questions should be asked before any discussion or rating questions have been asked, in order to not influence the participant.

It is a good idea to specifically ask participants whether they had any negative opinions, as some people do not want to hurt the researcher's feelings or belittle the research.

Evaluation Using Focus Groups

Focus groups are a form of subjective research in which a group of people are asked about their perceptions, opinions, beliefs, and attitudes toward a product, service, concept, or idea. Questions are asked in an interactive group setting where participants are free to talk with other group members.

There are many advantages to using focus groups. Focus groups:

- Can offer insight into statistical findings—especially if unexpected outcomes occur;
- Can provide a more fully nuanced understanding of participants' opinions;
- Can encourage participants to interact with each other, sharing their opinions and questioning the assumptions and opinions of others;
- Can stimulate more thought on questions than is typical for surveys;
- May lead to changes of opinion throughout the discussion, and to a more definitive conclusion;
- Offer opportunities for validation of individual opinions, when similar opinions are expressed by others.

There are also disadvantages to using focus groups. Participant selection, the questions asked, how they are phrased, how they are posed, in what setting and by whom, affects the answers obtained from participants.

- Results are inevitably influenced by the moderator or researcher who is conducting the focus group, even if that moderator does not have any vested interest in the technology.
- Participants may provide responses they feel the moderator wants to hear.
- Lack of anonymity or confidentiality can inhibit truthful response.
- Researcher has less control over a group than a one-on-one interview.
- Data is hard to analyze because opinions and insights may shift in the course of conversation.
- Requires highly skilled moderator.

- Requires getting the group to agree to a time and place, and to show up.
- The number of participants is too small to be a representative sample of even a small population.

Focus groups are only meaningful in the evaluation of a technology after participants have traveled using that technology for relevant tasks. If participants have not actually used the technology, there is no way to know whether what participants are imagining and providing opinions about is much like the actual technology.

Evaluating Performance of the Technology

Technologies are not ready for systematic and quantifiable evaluation unless they have been demonstrated to function flawlessly, on repeated consecutive trials. It has been a rather common experience of both authors that developers are not sufficiently rigorous in laboratory testing of devices prior to scheduling human factors evaluations. When technologies do not consistently perform as they are intended to do, it is difficult to interpret the results of human factors testing.

During human factors testing, it is useful to include measures of the technical functioning of the device. The following list suggests some possibilities.

- Does the technology provide information when it is supposed to do so?
- Does the technology provide accurate information?
- Does the technology correctly and accurately indicate to users when they are off-route?
- Does the technology respond with the correct type of information in response to key strokes or voice commands?

In the validation research for the Wayfinding Project, the data sheet had provision for recording whether GPS technology provided information that it should have automatically provided at the five waypoints on the route. The automatic information messages occurred 69.1% of the time, with only 7 of 41 participants receiving all five messages such as the name of the street ahead or an instruction to turn. The data sheet also had provision for recording whether GPS technology provided accurate information. The automatic information messages were accurate 86.5% of the time, but 20 of 41 participants received at least one inaccurate message. The automatic turn prompts were presented at an appropriate time 79.0% of the time, but 15 participants received at least one inaccurate turn prompt or failed to receive a turn prompt that should have been provided. Finally, 9 of 41 participants received at least one inaccurate off-route message during their GPS wayfinding trial. In these instances, participants were informed by the GPS system that they were off route, when in fact they were not. It is clear that GPS technologies are still quite inaccurate in many urban settings and still sometimes give completely wrong information. (The Wayfinding Project research was conducted in an urban area, but surrounding buildings were all relatively low; it was not in an urban canyon.) However, accessible GPS users who are skilled at interpreting the information are able to accept the inaccuracies and learn to reject wrong information, and may find much satisfaction in the use of the technology despite its technical inadequacies (La Grow et al., 2009).

Summary

There are many important considerations in evaluating the effectiveness of assistive devices for travel and wayfinding. In any evaluation, the following questions need to be answered.

1. Does the device solve a problem or fill a need that is experienced by people with visual impairments?
2. Can the device be demonstrated through performance measures to improve travel and/or wayfinding for a substantial proportion of travelers who are visually impaired?
   a. Is the research design unbiased?
   b. Is there an appropriate baseline?
   c. Is the participant group appropriate for the stage of development of the technology?
   d. Is the route or task appropriate to the technology?
3. Does subjective research demonstrate that people who use the technology experience benefits that they consider meaningful?
4. Is the technical performance of the device robust?

When the answers to all of these questions are positive, it is appropriate to conclude that the time, effort, and expense of developing the technology have been well spent, and that there is a reasonable likelihood that commercialization of the device will be worthwhile.

References

Barlow, J. M., Bentzen, B. L., and Bond, T. 2005. Blind pedestrians and the changing technology and geometry of signalized intersections: Safety, orientation, and independence. *Journal of Visual Impairment and Blindness.* 99, 587–598.

Barlow, J. M., Scott, A. C., and Bentzen, B. L., 2009. Audible beaconing with accessible pedestrian signals. *AER Journal: Research and Practice in Visual Impairment and Blindness*, 2(4), 149–158.

Bentzen, B. L., and Barlow, J. M. 1995. Impact of curb ramps on safety of persons who are blind. *Journal of Visual Impairment and Blindness*. 89, 319–328.

Bentzen, B. L., Barlow, J. M., and Bond, T. 2004. Challenges of unfamiliar signalized intersections for pedestrians who are blind: Research on safety. *Transportation Research Record: Journal of the Transportation Research Board* (1878), 51–57.

Bentzen, B. L., Crandall, W. F., and Myers, L. 1999. Wayfinding system for transportation services: Remote infrared audible signage for transit stations, surface transit, and intersections. *Transportation Research Record: Journal of the Transportation Research Board* (1671), 19–26.

Bentzen, B. L., Scott, A. C., and Barlow, J. M. 2006. Accessible pedestrian signals: effect of device features. *Transportation Research Record: Journal of the Transportation Research Board* (1982), 30–37.

Blades, M., Lippa, Y., Golledge, R. G., Jacobson, R. D., and Kitchin, R. M. 2002. Wayfinding by people with visual impairments: The effect of spatial tasks on the ability to learn a novel route. *Journal of Visual Impairment and Blindness*, 96, 407–419.

Church, R. L., and Marston, J. R. 2003. Measuring accessibility for people with a physical disability. *Geographical Analysis*, 35(1), 83–96.

Crandall, W., Brabyn, J., Bentzen, B., and Myers, L. 1999. Remote infrared signage evaluation for transit stations and intersections. *Journal of Rehabilitation Research and Development*, 36, 341–355.

Gaunet, F. 2006. Verbal guidance rules for a localized wayfinding aid intended for blind pedestrians in urban areas. *Universal Access in the Information Society*, 4(4), 338–353.

Gaunet, F., and Briffault, X. 2005. Exploring the functional specifications of a localized wayfinding verbal aid for blind pedestrians: Simple and structured urban areas. *Human Computer Interaction*, 20(3), 267–314.

Giudice, N.A., and Legge, G.E. 2008. Blind navigation and the role of technology. In A. Helal, M. Mokhtari, and B. Abdulrazak (Eds.), *Engineering Handbook of Smart Technology for Aging, Disability, and Independence*, pp. 479–500, John Wiley & Sons.

Giudice, N. A., Marston, J. R., Klatzky, R. L., Loomis, J. M., and Golledge, R. G. 2008. *Environmental learning without vision: effects of cognitive load on interface design.* Paper presented at the 9th International Conference on Low Vision, Montreal, Quebec, Canada.

Golledge, R. G., and Marston, J. R. 1999. Towards an accessible city: Removing functional barriers to independent travel for blind and vision impaired residents and visitors (California PATH Research Report No. UCB-ITS-PPR-99–33 for PATH project MOU 343): California PATH Program, Institute of Transportation Studies, University of California, Berkeley.

Golledge, R. G., Marston, J. R., and Costanzo, C. M. 1998. Assistive devices and services for the disabled: Auditory signage and the accessible city for blind or vision impaired travelers (California PATH Working Paper No. UCB-ITS-PWP-98-18): University of California, Berkeley California PATH Program, Institute of Transportation Studies.

Golledge, R. G., Marston, J. R., Loomis, J. M., and Klatzky, R. L. 2004. Stated preferences for components of a personal guidance system for non-visual navigation.
Journal of Visual Impairment and Blindness, 98(3), 135–147.

Hauger, J. S., Rigby, J. C., Safewright, M. P., and McAuley, W. J. 1996. Detectable warnings at curb ramps. *Journal of Visual Impairment and Blindness*, 90, 512–525.

Jacobson, R. D., Lippa, Y., Golledge, R. G., Kitchin, R. M., and Blades, M. 2001. Rapid
development of cognitive maps in people with visual impairments when
exploring novel geographic spaces. *IAPS Bulletin of People-Environment Studies
(Special Issue on Environmental Cognition)*, 18, 3–6.

Kitchin, R. M. 2000. The researched opinions on research: Disabled people and disability research. *Disability and Society*, 15(1), 25–48.

Kitchin, R. M. 2001. Participatory action research approaches in geographical studies
of disability: Some reflections. *Disability Studies Quarterly, Fall*, 21(4, Symposium
on Disability Geography: Commonalities in a World of Differences), 61–69.

Klatzky, R. L., Giudice, N. A., Marston, J. R., Tietz, J., Golledge, R. G., and Loomis, J. M.
2008. An N-back task using vibrotactile stimulation with comparison to an
audiotyr analogue. *Behavior Research Methods*, 40(1), 367–372.

Klatzky, R. L., Marston, J. R., Giudice, N. A., Golledge, R. G., and Loomis, J. M. 2006.
Cognitive load of navigating without vision when guided by virtual sound versus spatial language. *Journal of Experimental Psychology: Applied*, 12(4), 223–232.

La Grow, S. J., Ihrke, E., Ponchillia, P. E., Sullins, C. D., Owiti, S. A., and Lewis, L. 2009.
User perceptions of accessible GPS as a wayfinding tool. *AER Journal: Research
and Practice in Visual Impairment and Blindness*, 2(3), 111–120.

Loomis, J. M., Golledge, R. G., and Klatzky, R. L. 1998. Navigation system for the
blind: Auditory display modes and guidance. *Presence: Teleoperators and Virtual
Environments*, 7(2), 193–203.

Loomis, J. M., Golledge, R. G., Klatzky, R. L., and Marston, J. R. 2007. Assisting way-
finding in visually impaired travelers. In G. L. Allen (Ed.), *Applied Spatial
Cognition: From Research to Cognitive Technology* (pp. 179–203). Mahwah, N.J.:
Lawrence Erlbaum Associates.

Loomis, J. M., Marston, J. R., Golledge, R. G., and Klatzky, R. L. 2005. Personal guidance system for people with visual impairment: Comparison of spatial displays
for route guidance. *Journal of Visual Impairment and Blindness*, 99(4), 219–232.

Marston, J. R. 2001. Empirical measurement of barriers to public transit for the vision-
impaired and the use of remote infrared auditory signage for mitigation.
*Proceedings of the California State University Northridge Conference on Technology
and Disability*.

Marston, J. R. 2002. Towards an Accessible City: Empirical Measurement and
Modeling of Access to Urban Opportunities for those with Vision Impairments,
Using Remote Infrared Audible Signage. Unpublished Dissertation, University
of California, Santa Barbara.

Marston, J. R., and Church, R. L. 2005. A relative access measure to identify barriers to
efficient transit use by persons with visual impairments. *Disability and
Rehabilitation*, 27(13), 769–779.

Marston, J. R., and Golledge, R. G. 2003. The hidden demand for activity participation
and travel by persons who are visually impaired or blind. *Journal of Visual
Impairment and Blindness*, 97(8), 475–488.

Marston, J. R., and Golledge, R. G. 2004. Quantitative and qualitative analysis of barriers to travel by persons with visual impairments and its mitigation through accessible signage. Paper presented at the TRANSED 2004, 10th International Conference on Mobility and Transport for Elderly and Disabled People, Hamamatsu, Japan.

Marston, J. R., Loomis, J. M., Klatzky, R. L., and Golledge, R. G. 2007. Nonvisual route following with guidance from a simple haptic or auditory display. *Journal of Visual Impairment & Blindness*, 101(4), 203–211.

Marston, J. R., Loomis, J. M., Klatzky, R. L., Golledge, R. G., and Smith, E. L. 2006. Evaluation of spatial displays for navigation without sight. *ACM Transactions on Applied Perception*, 3(2), 110–124.

Montello, D. R. 1998. A new framework for understanding the acquisition of spatial knowledge in large-scale environments. In M. J. Egenhofer and R. G. Golledge (Eds.), *Spatial and Temporal Reasoning in Geographic Information Systems* (pp. 143–154). New York: Oxford University Press.

Ross, D. A., 2001. Implementing assistive technology on wearable computers. *IEEE Intelligent Systems*, 16, 47–53.

Scott, A. C., Barlow, J. M., Bentzen, B. L., Bond, T. L. Y., and Gubbe, D. 2008. Accessible pedestrian signals at complex intersections: Effects on blind pedestrians. *Research Record: Journal of the Transportation Research Board* (2073), 94–103.

Scott, A., Barlow, J, Guth, D., Bentzen, B. L., Cunningham, C., and Long, R. 2011a. Nonvisual cues for aligning to cross streets. *Journal of Visual Impairment and Blindness*, 105, 648–661.

Scott, A., Barlow, J, Guth, D., Bentzen, B.L., Cunningham, C., and Long, R. 2011b. Walking between the lines: Nonvisual cues for maintaining heading during street crossing. *Journal of Visual Impairment and Blindness*, 105, 662–674.

Scott, A. C., Myers, L., Barlow, J. M., and Bentzen, B. L. 2006. Accessible pedestrian signals: The effect of pushbutton location and audible WALK indications on pedestrian behavior. *Transportation Research Record: Journal of the Transportation Research Board* (1939), 69–76.

Sholl, M. J. 1996. From visual information to cognitive maps. In J. Portugali (Ed.), *The Construction of Cognitive Maps*. Dordrecht: Kluwer Academic Publishers.

Strelow, E. R. 1985. What is needed for a theory of mobility: Direct perception and cognitive maps-lessons from the blind. *Psychological Review*, 92(2), 226–248.

Wall, R. S., Ashmead, D. H., Bentzen, B. L., and Barlow, J. 2004. Directional guidance of audible pedestrian signals for street crossing. *Ergonomics*, 47(12), 1318–1338.

8

Sensory Substitution of Vision: Importance of Perceptual and Cognitive Processing

Jack M. Loomis, Roberta L. Klatzky, and Nicholas A. Giudice

CONTENTS

Introduction

For most activities of daily life, vision is the preeminent sense for humans. Over one million optic nerve fibers of each eye transfer vast amounts of information to the brain every second, and a large fraction of the cortex is involved in the processing of this information. The most obvious effect of losing vision is a significant decrement in performance of actions that rely on the spatial resolution and wide field of view that vision provides, particularly under tight temporal constraints (see Chapters 2 and 4). Returning a tennis serve or driving in city traffic are examples. Nonetheless, the ability of many blind people to perform tasks that we generally think of as visually guided, like steering a bicycle around obstacles (using echolocation), is testimony to the potential of other sources of information to substitute for visual input. This form of sensory substitution, allowing one or more of the remaining spatial senses to take the place of vision, is possible because hearing and touch are also informative about the environment. Expanding these natural sensory substitutions with compensatory strategies and theoretically motivated technologies would no doubt enhance the capabilities of blind and low-vision individuals.

Over the past two centuries, inventions have come into use that augment the natural substitution of one sense by another. Braille provides access to text, and the long cane supplements spatial hearing in the sensing of obstacles, borders between surfaces underfoot, and so on. Over the last five decades, electronic devices, many based on computers, have emerged as more effective ways of promoting vision substitution (see the edited volume by Warren and Strelow, 1985 for a good introduction, and Giudice and Legge, 2008 and Levesque, 2009 for recent reviews). Access to text has greatly expanded with electronic Braille displays and synthetic speech. For obstacle avoidance and sensing of the local environment, a number of ultrasonic sensors have been developed that use either auditory or tactile displays (Brabyn, 1985; Collins, 1985; Kay, 1985; see also Chapter 3). For navigation through the larger-scale environment, assistive technologies now include GPS-based navigation systems (Chapter 5) and remote infrared audible signage (Chapter 6).

In the remainder of this chapter, we examine the potential for new technologies to assist blind people by substituting for information that is otherwise visually encoded. We do so through the lens of cognitive science and neuroscience, which leads to an understanding of the information processing capabilities of individuals with and without sight. Our overarching message is that while great potential for sensory substitution exists, there are clear constraints on the utility of new technologies that stem from perceptual and cognitive processing. Unfortunately, these constraints have neither been widely recognized nor their implications understood by researchers in the field. Besides discussing these constraints, we will offer examples of effective assistive technology and suggest guidelines for the development of future devices. The organization of the chapter is as follows: In the first section of the chapter, we begin with a distinction between general-purpose and special-purpose sensory substitution, which obviously differ in the range of activities they are intended to support. To aid in evaluating these approaches, we present a general theoretical framework for sensory substitution that relies on knowledge about perceptual and cognitive information processing. We then consider different bases for sensory substitution, ranging from functional equivalence and brain plasticity to artificial intelligence. After a brief section on the implications of differences between blind and sighted people for sensory substitution, we end with some recommendations for the design process.

General-Purpose and Special-Purpose Sensory Substitution

An approach that has been tried in the past is general-purpose substitution of vision by touch. This is perhaps best exemplified by the pioneering work of Paul Bach-y-Rita and Carter Collins (Bach-y-Rita, 1967, 1972; Collins, 1970), who used a video camera to drive a tactile display of vibrotactile or electrotactile stimulators. Each 2-D visual image is represented by an isomorphic tactile image on some surface of the body, such as the back or abdomen. The premise behind such an approach is that with sufficient practice, people will eventually be able to interpret the tactile stimulation well enough to perform many activities that would otherwise be extremely challenging, if not impossible. The early research offered tantalizing evidence of success with simple tasks (Bach-y-Rita, 1972). In addition, the early research (e.g., White, 1970; White et al., 1970) provided fascinating results that led to a great deal of subsequent interest by scientists and philosophers in what has been termed "distal attribution" (e.g., Auvray et al., 2005; Auvray and Myin, 2009b; Epstein et al., 1986; Loomis, 1992; O'Regan and Noë, 2001; Siegle and Warren, 2010). Distal attribution (or externalization) refers to experiencing tactile stimulation on the skin surface as objects external to the user. This occurs when the user is allowed to manipulate the video camera and observe the contingencies between motor activity and the resulting changes in tactile stimulation. Importantly, distal attribution can be obtained with just a single tactile stimulator (Siegle and Warren, 2010). Besides the research on distal attribution, investigation of performance on spatial tasks has continued to be done by Bach-y-Rita and his colleagues as well as by others (e.g., Bach-y-Rita, 2004; Bach-y-Rita and Kercel, 2003; Chebat et al., 2011; Sampaio et al., 2001; Segond et al., 2005). Despite the many years of research, no general-purpose vision-to-touch translator has emerged that is sufficiently robust and reliable for use in everyday life. The same can be said for projects pursuing the goal of general sensory substitution of vision using audition (e.g., Auvray et al., 2009a; Capelle et al., 1998; Meijer, 1992; Veraart, 1989).

In light of the failure of general-purpose vision substitution for use in everyday life, efforts today are more commonly directed toward the creation of special-purpose devices that enable specific activities such as pattern identification, perception of spatial layout, control of locomotion with respect to the near environment (mobility), and navigation through the large-scale environment (orientation and wayfinding). Small-scale successes have been demonstrated for some simple tasks like walking around obstacles (e.g., Auvray et al., 2009a; Chebat et al., 2011; Collins, 1985; Jansson, 1983; Segond et al., 2005). Unfortunately, too many researchers developing sensory substitution devices, while touting the fascinating work on distal attribution and encouraged by good performance on simple tasks, have neglected the basic science on perceptual and cognitive processing in the design and evaluation of their devices. In the following section, we indicate how the ultimate success of any device for substitution across perceptual channels fundamentally depends on how the required information is matched to the capabilities of the human perceptual-cognitive system.

Theoretical Framework for Special-Purpose Sensory Substitution

Any effort to compensate for the absence of vision by substituting another information channel comes down to the use of touch or hearing, the other spatially informative senses. Extending earlier theoretical work (Collins, 1985; Kaczmarek, 2000; Loomis, 2003; Loomis and Klatzky, 2007; Veraart, 1989; Veraart and Wanet, 1985), we propose that a principled approach to using touch or hearing as a substitute for vision in connection with a particular function comprises two essential steps. The first is to identify the optical, acoustic, or other type of information (e.g., ultrasound) that is most effective in enabling that function. The second step is to determine how to display this information to the remaining spatial senses of touch and hearing. Besides the use of direct spatial cues, display methods include using spatial language that is presented, for example, through synthetic speech or electronic Braille.

Step 1: Identifying Informational Requirements for a Task

The first step, then, requires research to identify what information is necessary to perform the function. As an example, consider obstacle avoidance while walking. Usually, a person walking through a cluttered environment with adequate lighting is able to use vision to avoid collision with obstacles. Precisely what information sensed using vision, ultrasound, radar, laser range finding, or some combination thereof, best affords obstacle avoidance? One way to address this question is purely experimental—in the case of visual information alone, degrade a person's vision by limiting the field of view and spatial resolution to learn the minimum amount of visual information that affords a desired walking speed and accuracy. Cha et al. (1992) performed such an analysis using pixelized displays to determine the fewest number of points in a square matrix needed for effective travel through an environment containing obstacles. An alternative approach is strictly theoretical: given some form of reflecting energy (e.g., light, radar, or ultrasound) and a corresponding receiver, use computational modeling to determine the least information required by an ideal observer to perform the task.

Regrettably, there has been little research of either kind on the informational requirements of visually based behaviors. Without this research base, the motivation for design and development of sensory substitution devices, or assistive technology more generally, has unfortunately often been ad hoc. Even when relevant research is available, it has sometimes been overlooked in the face of attractive (read: "sexy") new technology or engineering design.

Step 2: Coupling Task Information with the Substituting Modalities

The second step in designing a sensory substitution system is to couple the critical environmental information with the substituting modality or modalities (touch and audition). This coupling involves two different factors: sensory bandwidths of the afferent pathways of the source and substituting modalities and the nature of higher-level processing. Vision, hearing, and touch each can be characterized by their sensory bandwidth, which refers to the rate at which information from the peripheral sense organs can be transmitted via the afferent pathways to the brain.

The sensory bandwidth for vision has two components, spatial bandwidth and temporal bandwidth. The spatial bandwidth is the product of (1) the total number of resolvable pixels in each eye, which in turn is determined by the total field of view and the visual acuity at each retinal position, and (2) the number of noticeably different levels of brightness and color at each pixel. The temporal bandwidth refers to the rate of information processing for each pixel. The components of sensory bandwidth for vision have been investigated extensively using psychophysics (e.g., Olzak and Thomas, 1986; Watson, 1986; Winkler, 2005). The spatial bandwidth component is closely related to the number of optic nerve fibers from each eye. Because the spatial bandwidth of vision is far greater than that of the other two senses, attempting to use some isomorphic spatial mapping from a video camera into the spatial dimensions of touch or hearing inevitably means a huge loss of information. To support this claim in connection with touch, we describe some research by the first author comparing the spatial bandwidths of vision and touch, work that was aimed at understanding why tactile sensory substitution of vision met with limited success. In a number of studies, he showed functional equivalence between tactile pattern perception and blurred vision, in which blurring (low-pass spatial filtering) was used to reduce the spatial resolution of vision (relative to pattern size) down to the level of touch. Some of the studies were done using an early version of the Tactile Vision Substitution System developed by Bach-y-Rita and Collins (Bach-y-Rita, 1967, 1972; Collins, 1970). The particular system used had a

20 × 20 array of vibrotactile stimulators placed across the back. The system included a 20 × 20 array of lamps that were illuminated when the corresponding vibrotactors were activated. In two separate studies on letter recognition (Apkarian-Stielau and Loomis, 1975; Loomis and Apkarian-Stielau, 1976), it was found to be necessary to drastically blur the visual display in order to bring letter recognition performance for vision down to that of touch; indeed, the diameter of the subjective blur circle associated with each illuminated bulb was wider than the visual display (Apkarian-Stielau and Loomis, 1975). These two experiments indicated that much of the spatial information within the tactile display was being eliminated by the intrinsic spatial filtering of the cutaneous system and thus not reaching the processing stages involved in recognition. More refined research was done later using raised characters, including letters and Braille, on the fingertips, along with low-pass spatial filtering of the corresponding visual characters

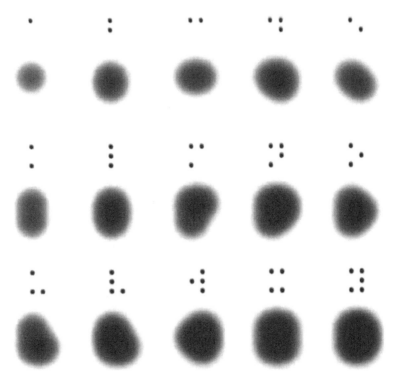

FIGURE 8.1

Depiction of how Braille characters are low-pass filtered during cutaneous processing. The visually blurred versions here are recognized with about the same level of accuracy (75%) as the alphabetic Braille characters presented to the stationary finger pad of the index finger (Loomis, 1981; see also Loomis, 1982, 1990). Much of the internal spatial detail is filtered out, but variation in shape allows good recognition performance by someone familiar with Braille. (Only a subset of the alphabetic characters is depicted. In the experiments cited, the tactile characters were slightly larger and more elevated than Braille characters used for actual reading.)

(Loomis, 1981, 1982, 1990; Loomis and Lederman, 1986). This work made it clear that much of the spatial information in patterns covering the fingertip is filtered out in cutaneous processing (see Figure 8.1).

Because of the limited spatial resolution of cutaneous processing, the number of resolvable pixels for any circumscribed region is orders of magnitude smaller than the corresponding number for vision. Here, we provide a comparison between vision and the distal pad of the index finger. The binocular field subtends $200 \times 130°$ (Harrington, 1971). Using estimates of visual resolution as a function of eccentricity out to $30°$ (Wertheim, 1894; reprinted in Westheimer, 1987) and extrapolating the best fitting curve out to $65°$, a conservative lower bound for vision is about 700,000 resolvable points for the central $65°$ of vision. In contrast, an upper bound for the distal pad of the index finger is just 330 resolvable points, assuming a spatial resolution of 1.2 mm (Legge et al., 2008). Consequently, the spatial bandwidth of the four fingertips (thumb excluded) would still be more than 500 times lower than that of vision. To convey a sense of how impoverished is the information being transmitted by the fingers, Figure 8.2b, depicts the spatial information

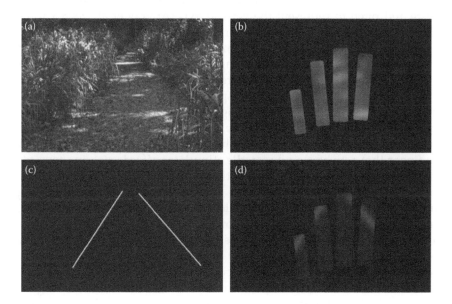

FIGURE 8.2
(a) An outdoor scene with a path. (b) Using the analogy between touch and blurred vision (Loomis, 1981, 1982), the scene is viewed through apertures representing four of the fingers with low-pass spatial filtering that is approximately that of the fingers. In reality, the fingers would scan the tactile facsimile of the path and pick up task-relevant information. Even so, at any one instant, the variations in intensity would convey little information about the path for this scene. (c) A scene limited to high contrast lines representing the edges of the path in (a). (d) The high-contrast scene viewed through apertures representing four of the fingers under the same field restriction and filtering as in (b). Now, the variations in intensity are quite informative about the edges of the path despite the same degree of field restriction and filtering.

sensed by the four fingers using the functional equivalence of touch and blurred vision (Loomis, 1981, 1982).

Much less research has been done on the spatial bandwidth of spatial hearing (see Blauert, 1997 for a review of spatial hearing in general). The parameters specifying the location of a sound source are distance, azimuth, and elevation. Most research that bears on spatial bandwidth has been done using tasks in which a sound source is successively presented in two locations. The resulting measure of discrimination is much finer than the measure of spatial resolution, which would involve spatially separating two identical sources until the two can be perceived as distinct (Loomis, 1979). Even so, measures of discrimination indicate poor precision along each of the three spatial dimensions (Ashmead et al., 1990; Blauert, 1997; Perrott and Saberi, 1990; Strybel and Perrott, 1984), making spatial hearing a poor candidate for sensory substitution based on spatial isomorphism. Accordingly, few researchers have attempted to convey information about 2-D spatial patterns using any pair of these auditory dimensions (for one who did, see Hollander, 1994). The more common approach, as will be discussed later, is to use azimuth or the passage of time to represent the horizontal axis of a figure and pitch to represent the vertical axis (Auvray et al., 2005; Cronly-Dillon et al., 1999; Kramer, 1994; Meijer, 1992).

Because the informational requirements of different tasks vary dramatically, some tasks will be possible using the spatial isomorphism of hearing or touch to substitute for vision, others not. Steering toward a point of light in a dark room requires very little spatial information; indeed, aiming a single photocell toward the point of light is sufficient. Thus, such a task is a good candidate for auditory or tactile substitution of vision. In connection with haptic touch, Lenay et al. (1997) have shown that a single photocell on the finger that activates a vibrotactile stimulator affords steering toward a point. Slightly more complex locomotion tasks, such as walking through a field of high-contrast obstacles, have also been shown to be feasible (e.g., auditory: Auvray et al., 2009a; tactile: Chebat et al., 2011; Collins, 1985; Jansson, 1983). Figure 8.2c,d shows how high-contrast information relevant to task performance can afford successful mobility in spite of the spatial bandwidth limitations of touch. At the other extreme of informational requirements is normal driving in a city environment with lots of cars and pedestrian traffic. Here, the required information is immense, ensuring that sensory substitution based on isomorphic mapping of raw visual data from a video camera onto the spatial dimensions of hearing or touch will fail (Collins, 1985).

In addition to sensory bandwidth, of which spatial bandwidth is the most limiting component, the other factor placing limits on the effectiveness of certain assistive technologies is the nature of higher-level processing for vision, hearing, and touch. For example, the fact that visual display of the acoustic speech signal (e.g., the speech spectrogram) has yet to lead to successful visual substitution of speech, despite the higher sensory bandwidth of vision, indicates that vision does not have access to specialized speech processing associated with hearing (Zue and Cole, 1979). Similarly, research suggests differences in higher-level processing of vision and touch in connection with the perception of 3-D objects and their depictions. Illustrating this is the challenge of using the sense of touch to recognize raised pictures of common objects (for review, see Wijntjes et al., 2008a). A study by Loomis et al. (1991) points to one of the reasons for the poor performance. They compared haptic recognition of raised pictures with visual recognition of the same pictures viewed on a computer display. In the haptic condition, observers felt raised pictures with one finger or two adjacent fingers, while in the visual condition, observers moved a stylus over a touch tablet to sequentially reveal portions of the picture on a stationary aperture on the display. The visual aperture was equivalent in "field of view" to the sensing surface of the one or two fingers. In addition, the computer display was optically blurred to reduce visual spatial resolution to that of touch. Recognition performance was nearly the same for vision and touch for the "one finger" condition (about 47% correct with 95 s response latency). Doubling the field of view produced a dramatic increase in performance for vision (80% correct with 60 s latency) but only a very modest increase for touch. For unrestricted field of view (no aperture), visual performance was 100% with 1.3 s latency. In another study, Klatzky et al. (1993) found that feeling raised pictures with five fingers instead of one improved performance about the same as doubling the visual field of view in the earlier study. Besides confirming the results of other studies showing poor haptic recognition of pictures of common objects, these two studies indicate that the effective haptic field of view increases more slowly with physical field of view than does the effective visual field of view (see also Craig, 1985). This means that the impoverished scene information depicted in Figure 8.2b, for visual apertures overestimates what is actually available with haptic sensing. A possible reason for this smaller effective field of view is that working memory, which is involved in the integration of sequentially presented information over space and time, has lower capacity for touch than for vision (Gallace and Spence, 2008). Another likely reason that haptic recognition of pictures falls short of visual recognition of pictures is that the figural processing associated with visual perception is less accessible by touch (Wijntjes et al., 2008b). This is almost surely the case for congenitally blind observers, who perform worse than adventitiously blind observers (Heller, 1989; Kennedy and Fox, 1977; Lederman et al., 1990).

Still another example of differences in high-level processing between touch and vision comes from research on the recognition of 3-D objects. Newell et al. (2001) had participants learn the shapes of objects either by visual or haptic exploration, during which all surfaces of the objects were perceived. The recognition phase was performed with the same or different modality, and the objects were in their original orientations or reversed orientations. The results indicated that vision preferentially encodes the front surfaces of objects during learning, whereas, touch preferentially encodes the back surfaces.

The focus so far has been on spatially isomorphic sensory substitution, but many of the successes in sensory substitution and assistive technology, as detailed in this volume, make use of technology that is not spatially isomorphic. Foremost is speech synthesis that can deliver linguistic information in the form of environmental labels, spatial descriptions of the environment, or commands to the user. GPS-based navigation systems for blind people offer the best examples (Chapter 5). In some versions, the linguistic information is supplemented by perceptual information about environmental location using virtual sound or haptics (Klatzky et al., 2006; Loomis et al., 2005). A primary reason that GPS navigation systems have been so successful is that GPS technology provides the user with access to information critical for navigation without overwhelming the user with irrelevant information. Other examples of effective assistive devices are those using ultrasonic sensors to aid in obstacle avoidance (Kay, 1985; for a recent summary see Giudice and Legge, 2008). Although these devices have not been widely adopted, a blind person learning to use such devices can reliably avoid obstacles because they provide the essential information for obstacle avoidance while excluding extraneous information that serves only to confuse.

In this section, we have presented the two essential steps in developing sensory substitution devices. The first, identifying the required information for a function, is too often ignored by researchers and developers. Even if not, relevant research may be lacking, requiring that the developer of a new system do preliminary testing. The second step, effectively coupling the required information to the user, is too often given insufficient consideration. Even if the requisite information can be translated into appropriate stimulation for the substituting modality, there are perceptual and cognitive processing limitations that might stand in the way of successful sensory substitution. With these considerations in mind, we discuss a number of bases for implementing successful sensory substitution.

Bases for Sensory Substitution

The general goal of sensory substitution is to allow functionality associated with one modality to be provided by another. The ideal would be to produce comparability of function. If inputs from two sensory channels lead to matching behavioral performance in some task, we say that at least for purposes of that task, the channels demonstrate *functional equivalence*. For some tasks, quite different representations such as object names and visual depictions can produce equivalent performance. Generally, sensory substitution falls short of this goal.

There are multiple bases by which touch, hearing, and language might singly or jointly lead to substitutability with vision. Building on what is known so far, we can identify some of these bases, which we discuss in this section. They are not exclusive of one another, and effective sensory substitution for a given activity (e.g., navigation) is likely to rely on more than one. Cattaneo and Vecchi (2011) provide an excellent review of research relating to some of these potential bases.

Functional Equivalence through Spatial Isomorphism

Spatial isomorphism between representations from two modalities ensures that parameters extracted from one will match those of the other, without systematic bias. While spatial isomorphism of representations certainly supports equivalence of function, it is not by itself sufficient. An additional key requirement is the existence of processes that can operate on the spatial parameters of the isomorphic representations so as to produce comparable performance. Under the assumption that this requirement is met, spatial isomorphism has been one of the most prevalent bases proposed for sensory substitution.

This leads to the question of whether spatial representations achieved by vision and other modalities are, to at least an approximate degree, isomorphic. We say approximate because differences in spatial bandwidth and working memory limitations must be taken into account. Consider first the sense of touch, as the greatest amount of work on spatial isomorphism has concerned touch/vision correspondence. Some studies do suggest that the visual and haptic channels, after adjusting for differences in the processing limitations of touch, produce isomorphic representations of simple 2-D and 3-D shapes (Klatzky et al., 1993; Lakatos and Marks, 1999; Loomis, 1981, 1982, 1990; Loomis et al., 1991).

Work of the present authors provides evidence for isomorphism between vision and other modalities with respect to the spatial layout of multiple objects relative to the observer. These studies demonstrate comparable performance after encoding spatial layout from different modalities, vision, hearing, or spatial language. Equivalence was found for vision and hearing, for example, in a task of spatial updating of self-position in the absence of visual feedback (Klatzky et al., 2003); importantly, the targets were matched for their encoded (as opposed to physical) locations, by placing each visual target at the perceptual distance of the corresponding auditory target. Comparable performance has also been found for judgments of relative direction (pointing to a target from the perspective of another) for maps encoded through vision or touch (Giudice et al., 2011), and across multiple spatial targets encoded by vision and spatial language (Avraamides et al., 2004).

To the extent that spatial isomorphism exists, within the constraints of differential processing limitations, touch should be able to substitute for vision in tasks that take spatial parameters such as distance and direction as inputs.

One such task is cross-modal integration, where information about the same spatial magnitude, potentially with a discrepancy, is provided to multiple senses, and a jointly determined estimate must be achieved (Ernst et al., 2000; Heller et al., 1999; Rock and Victor, 1964). In a seminal paper, Ernst and Banks (2002) tested a maximum-likelihood model for integration of information about the size of a step-edge conveyed by vision and touch. The model assumes that the two channels combine their perceptual outputs by means of a weighted average, where the weight corresponds to the reliability (inverse variability) of the channel. The results indicated that metrically appropriate spatial information was provided by both channels, but with substantially less reliability for touch than for vision. This finding is in keeping with earlier proposals that spatial processing is less "modality-appropriate" for touch than vision (Welch and Warren, 1980).

Another paradigm for assessing the consequences of spatial isomorphism is cross-modal matching, a task where an object is first sensed by touch and then identified by vision, or vice versa. A substantial literature on this topic indicates that cross-modal matching across vision and touch can be achieved with accuracy well above chance (Abravanel, 1971; Newell et al., 2001; Phillips et al., 2009). Performance in the cross-modal case does not generally exceed the level of unimodal matching achieved by the lesser modality. However, gains from using a second modality may be found when one sense guides the other to otherwise unavailable or ambiguous information (Phillips et al., 2009; Wijntjes et al., 2009). Cross-modal matching has even been demonstrated for plastic molds of real faces, a complex stimulus that may invoke specialized spatial processing mechanisms normally associated with vision (Casey and Newell, 2007; Dopjans et al., 2009; Kilgour and Lederman, 2006).

Recently, a novel test of cross-modal matching was implemented with three blind subjects who had just recovered sight, a situation that exemplifies the classic test posed by the philosopher Molyneaux (Held et al., 2011). Within 48 h after surgery, the patients succeeded at intramodal but not cross-modal matching from touch to vision. However, 5 days later, without further training, touch-to-vision matching improved significantly. While the implications of these results are not entirely clear, they cast doubt on the naïve assumption that touch provides inputs to an otherwise functional visual channel in the blind. Also disconfirmed is the idea that modality-independent representations formed by blind individuals can be automatically accessed by vision if it becomes available. Such "amodal" representations are discussed in the next section.

On the whole, our review suggests that vision can be translated into touch at a direct spatial level, albeit with considerable reduction in bandwidth. However, this translation does not guarantee a seamless transition to functionality. We next consider a related question, namely, whether visual representations achieve substitution by translation into an amodal level. This form of representation might be spatially isomorphic to the source modality, but amodality could exist without isomorphism.

Functional Equivalence through Amodal Representations

Translation from one sensory channel to another can occur between representations that preserve their modal origins, as long as modality-specific processes allow functionality. An alternative basis for functional equivalence is the convergence of multiple channels onto a common representation. The target representation has variously been called multimodal, metamodal, amodal, and unimodal. These terms convey different meanings. Metamodal designates a type of common computation that can be performed on inputs from varying modalities (Pascual-Leone and Hamilton, 2001). The term multimodal implies that the target representation is somehow differentiated or "tagged" by its modal source, but yet functions independently of that tag. This type of structure has also been called supramodal (Struiksma et al., 2009). Our preferred hypothesis is that the common representation is amodal, which implies that it is abstracted from its modal source. Gallace and Spence (2008) have suggested that an amodal spatial representation is associated with conscious information-processing, in contrast to the unconscious, modality-specific representations that feed into it.

The third term, unimodal, refers to the possibility that information from multiple sensory channels can be converted to a single, privileged channel. Presumably, when sighted people process spatial information, the privileged channel would be the visual modality. In support of the primacy of visual processing, it has been demonstrated that when sighted individuals are deprived of sight, tactile spatial processing comes to activate cortical regions otherwise associated with visual input. Blind individuals as well show activation in normally visual areas when performing spatial tasks. (See Sathian and Lacey, 2007; Sathian and Stilla, 2010, for reviews.) Sathian and Lacey (2007) pointed to the ambiguity of these results, for they may reflect recoding of tactile stimuli into visual images, or it may be that visual regions of the brain process amodal representations.

A growing body of neuroscience evidence suggests that regions traditionally considered to be sensory specific may normally be involved in multimodal, if not amodal, processing of specific stimulus dimensions. Two complementary techniques are often used. Brain imaging techniques, such as functional MRI (fMRI) and positron emission tomography (PET), allow identification of the structures that are active in specific tasks, whereas transcranial magnetic stimulation (TMS) produces temporary disruption of these brain regions during the same tasks. The first assesses correlation; the second, causality.

From such studies, it appears that some regions at least are organized around commonality of what is computed (shape, motion, face, spatial location, etc.), rather than modality per se (for further discussion, see Pascual-Leone et al., 2005). Various groups studying sensory substitution or developing these devices have pointed to studies showing that what are thought of as primary visual projection areas are activated by auditory and tactile stimulation based on camera input (de Volder and Catalan-Ahumada, 1999; Kupers et al., 2010; for other reviews, see Part 2 of Rieser et al., 2008). Occipital regions of sighted individuals known to be involved with judging visual grating orientation have been shown to be activated during discrimination of tactile grating orientation on the finger (Sathian et al., 1997), and TMS applied to these "visual" regions have led to disruption of the same tactile task (Zangaladze et al., 1999). The lateral occipital complex (LOC), an area known for visual object selectivity, has been shown to be recruited for haptic object perception in sighted individuals (Amedi et al., 2001, 2002), suggesting a general processing region for object geometry.

Further, common processing regions between blind and sighted people have been shown for various stimuli across sensory inputs. Wolbers et al. (2011a) recently reported that sighted and age-matched blind subjects showed activation in the parahippocampal place area (PPA), a region previously shown to be involved with processing of visually presented scenes, when haptically exploring Lego-block models of rooms. Functional connectivity analyses were specifically directed at the question of whether visual imagery was involved. While covariation between the PPA and occipital regions was observed for visual processing of scenes by the sighted subjects, it was absent for the haptic condition in either blind or sighted. These results implicate an amodal representation of 3-D scene geometry in the PPA, rather than convergence on a unimodal one. It has also been found that the Fusiform Face Area (FFA), a region in the fusiform gyrus that responds preferentially when viewing human faces compared to objects or other body parts (Kanwisher et al., 1997), is not exclusive to visual face processing. Category-sensitive activity has been found in the FFA for haptic face recognition in both sighted (Kilgour et al., 2004) and blind participants (Goyal et al., 2006). Finally, another specialized brain region called hMT+ in human cortical region V5, long known to be recruited for visual motion (Watson et al., 1993) has recently been shown to be involved in auditory motion detection in blindfolded sighted subjects (Poirier et al., 2005) and both auditory and tactile motion in blind participants (Poirier et al., 2006; Ricciardi et al., 2007; Wolbers et al., 2011b).

A question of practical and theoretical importance remains, however: When an empirical association between a brain area and some information-processing activity is identified, what does this mean in terms of necessity and sufficiency? With respect to necessity, when a brain area conventionally associated with one modality is activated by inputs from another, as is the case when occipital activation accompanies a tactile discrimination task, the role of the activation is unclear. While it could be essential to the task at hand, it might also reflect "downstream" transmission of activation from another area that actually performs the task. Regarding sufficiency, there is no way to guarantee whether the activation observed in the apparently cross-modal area is sufficient for the task. TMS has been used to disrupt processing and so demonstrate causality, but disrupting a single link in a complex chain could be sufficient to impair performance.

Paralleling the studies from neuroscience addressing the question of whether amodal representations exist are a number of behavioral studies, including those described earlier supporting spatial isomorphism across modalities. Another methodology is predicated on the assumption that switching between modal representations would impose costs on spatial processing, in terms of time or error. The test is then to ask whether spatial judgments that involve multiple locations encoded from different modalities are penalized, relative to their intramodal counterparts. One study supporting amodality demonstrated that judgments of relative direction could be performed across locations encoded from two different modalities, vision and touch, without significant cost relative to unimodal conditions (Giudice et al., 2009).

We view the evidence for amodal representations as a reason for optimism about at least some forms of sensory substitution. Substitutability is, of course, still limited by the detail and precision in the substituting modality, as determined by modality-specific sensory bandwidth and noise. For example, an amodal representation of spatial layout derived from audition would not be expected to achieve the precision of one derived from vision. However, within the constraints of the haptic system, behaviors that draw on an amodal representation normally encoded from vision could exploit the one encoded from touch without further transformation. This is the premise behind maps for blind people using embossed materials and electronic displays (Ungar et al., 1996; Wall and Brewster, 2006). A person who has lost vision needs no special training to understand the relation between tactual maps and visual maps. However, because close tactual facsimiles of visual maps are too complex to be readily interpretable, tactual maps usually are created with the minimum detail necessary (see Chapter 9).

Synesthesia: Exploiting Natural Correspondences

In this section, we consider whether sensory substitution could be "bootstrapped" on natural correspondences between modalities, or synesthesia. More specifically, synesthesia is the spontaneous response of one sensory channel to inputs in another (Harrison and Baron-Cohen, 1997; Martino and Marks, 2001). A channel in this sense may correspond to a sensory modality, as when a musical pitch invokes the impression of a color, or it may refer to intramodal feature correspondences such as between graphemes and colors, the most common form of synesthesia. The phenomenon has been demonstrated with objective performance measures. For example, while nonsynesthetes may have to search for a target grapheme among similar elements in a serial fashion, color/grapheme synesthetes may find that the target "pops out" by triggering a unique color response (Edquist et al., 2006).

The incidence of synesthesia in the general population has been estimated to be about 4% (Simner et al., 2006). Heritability and sex-linked patterns point to a genetic basis for the phenomenon. Bargary and Mitchell (2008) have suggested that it arises from structural anomalies in the brains of synesthetes that lead to deviant cross-activation across cortical areas.

Given its rarity and the presumed minimal role for learning, synesthesia cannot be considered a general scheme for sensory substitution. However, more generally prevalent associations across sensory modalities, which Martino and Marks (1999; 2001) call *weak* synesthesia (in comparison to the *strong* form just reviewed), might be useful. For example, Marks (1978) has shown that most people have access to systematic intermodal pairings, such as associations between color and pitch or temperature.

One particularly intriguing candidate for synesthetically based substitution involving vision is the common association between pitch height (i.e., frequency) and vertical position in the visual field. In an early study, Pratt (1930) reported a directly linear relationship between log frequency and visual height. Walker et al. (2010) found that 3–4-month-old infants who were shown a ball moving in time with a changing pitch looked for a longer time when the height of the ball was yoked to a higher pitch than with the reverse mapping. Similarly, pitch height was associated with the sharpness of points on a star.

Should we take this as evidence for innate pitch-height synesthesia? Walker et al. acknowledge that learning was possible even with such young subjects. It should also be noted that the evidence for a cross-modal correspondence in infants does not indicate its directionality. Higher pitch could have been associated with visual items being either higher or lower on the display, and the directionality could vary across subjects without this being picked up by the design. However, the fact that correspondences were exhibited at all in this age range argues at least for a developmental readiness to learn cross-modal correlations.

A cross-cultural study (Eitan and Zimmers, 2010) casts some doubt on the potential for strong synesthesia between pitch height and verticality as a basis for sensory substitution. The authors found that while this association is common in Western cultures, it is by no means ubiquitous. Moreover, the specific pitch/vertical mappings varied across subjects, and competing associations to pitch were common. If we assume that the pitch/vertical association is a form of weak synesthesia, these results raise the question of whether in general, naturally acquired associations are consistent enough to be the basis for substitution schemes.

The pitch/vertical association has been used as the basis for devices that substitute hearing for vision (e.g., Auvray et al., 2005; Capelle et al., 1998; Cronly-Dillon et al., 1999; Meijer, 1992). Pitch is used to represent the vertical position of elements in a graph, picture, or each image of a video sequence. Horizontal position is represented by time, direction (e.g., azimuth from spatial hearing), or a tonal dimension. These devices present an accessible mapping for simple patterns, and the approach has been claimed to be useful for more complex tasks. For example, pitch/vertical mapping has enabled the interpretation of monocular cues to determine depth of a target in the field

(Renier et al., 2005). Cortical changes after training on mapping visual height and brightness to sound have been measured as well, both in visual association areas (Renier et al., 2005) and in auditory cortex after extended visual deprivation (Pollok et al., 2005). Subjective impressions of vision have also been reported by users (Ward and Meijer, 2010), which Proulx (2010) termed synthetic synesthesia. However, such reports are difficult to interpret, and methods of validation are lacking.

Rote Learning

In the absence of "boot-strapping" sensory substitution on any of the bases mentioned so far, it remains possible that arbitrary associations between sensory channels could be learned. This idea is encouraged by the theory that with deliberate practice, defined by Ericsson (2004) as "engaging in practice activities with the primary goal of improving some aspect of performance" (p. S3), humans can acquire many types of skills, from complex motor behavior to conceptual mastery such as occurs in chess. A target period of practice for a complex skill is on the order of 10,000 h.

The mapping of perceptual parameters from one sensory modality to another, even if their computations are based on entirely different input data (e.g., auditory frequencies vs. visual brightness values), can be thought of as just another skill that might be learned. If skills are developed through appropriate practice over extended time periods, such mappings too may be capable of learning.

It is encouraging in this regard to note that relatively short time periods have led to measurable improvements in sensory substitution. Only 9 h of training with a spatial array stimulator for the tongue led to a doubling of measured acuity (Sampaio et al., 2001). Geldard (1957) reported a study in which a vibration-to-alphabet scheme ("vibratese") was learned in 12 h, to a level sufficient for its use in simple text.

The task is daunting, however, when we consider that if sensory substitution is to accommodate the complexity of everyday stimulation, it must involve not just the learning of associations between specific stimuli (e.g., the pitch of a 440 Hz tone = red), but the acquisition of an entirely new sensory "language." No doubt many people could learn to associate a particular visual spectrogram display with the corresponding speech, but as has been discussed, there is limited ability to interpret novel spectrograms representing arbitrary speech segments, even after extensive practice (Zue and Cole, 1979).

The literature on skill learning indicates that mastery of complex mappings across sensory channels is likely to require extensive practice—if not 10,000 h, then certainly more than a few. This gives some reason to be cautious about how far rote learning could take sensory substitution, but mappings of at least restricted complexity might be mastered with deliberate, extended practice, particularly if begun early in life. A natural question is whether there is sufficient payoff to motivate the rote learning approach, if that is what substitution is reduced to. If the information gain is not worth the time and effort needed to approach functionality, the system may be ignored.

The proposal that rote learning can be a basis for sensory substitution implicitly assumes that deliberate practice will lead to neural changes that support new capabilities. We next discuss more generally the idea that the plasticity of the brain provides a basis for substitution.

Cortical Plasticity

There is little doubt that the brain's highly adaptive nature helps explain why sensory substitution is possible to at least a limited extent. In connection with his seminal work with the Tactile Vision Substitution System, which used a video camera to drive an electrotactile display, Bach-y-Rita (1967, 1972) speculated that the functional substitution of vision by touch resulted from cortical plasticity that allowed incoming somatosensory input to be analyzed by visual areas. Though the idea was radical for its time, cross-modal brain plasticity has been confirmed by many subsequent studies.

The brain is a highly malleable organ, and there are multiple types of plasticity that arise from its ability to change in response to sensory input. For instance, the so-called use-dependent expansion refers to plastic change resulting from prolonged focal stimulation of a peripheral organ. The reading fingers of expert blind Braille readers show expanded cortical representation in somatosensory cortex (Pascual-Leone and Torres, 1993; Sterr et al., 1998), as do the finger representations for expert string players (Elbert et al., 1995).

Much of the cross-modal plasticity research has focused on long-term brain reorganization as a result of early-onset blindness. Research in this area has shown that the visual cortex of skilled blind Braille readers is activated when they are reading Braille (Büchel, 1998; Sadato et al., 1996), and TMS delivered to these same occipital regions interferes with the perception of Braille in similar subjects (Cohen et al., 1997). Brain imaging of an adult with the rare ability to read print visually with low acuity, and also to read Braille by touch, revealed complementary organization of early visual areas. Regions normally activated by the fovea were dedicated to touch, while those normally receiving projections from the periphery were activated by vision (Cheung et al., 2009). Although auditory plasticity is not our focus here, similar recruitment and disruption of occipital regions by various auditory stimuli has also been demonstrated in blind people (Kujala et al., 2005; Merabet et al., 2009; Weeks et al., 2000).

It may be tempting from such findings to conclude that plastic change is only possible with early-onset blindness and that those who lose their vision later in life will not benefit from the increased computational resources associated with neural reorganization. While it is true that plasticity tends to be greatest before adolescence (Rauschecker, 1995), a growing body of evidence has shown that this so-called critical period is neither necessary nor limited to early life. For instance, late-onset blind individuals show many of the same cross-modal involvement of occipital regions as their early blind peers for purely spatial tasks (Goldreich and Kanics, 2003; Stilla et al., 2008), suggesting that the differences often observed with occipital activation from Braille reading by early blind individuals may be practice-related or due to nonspatial linguistic factors (Sathian and Lacey, 2007). These studies suggest that the brain is able to flexibly adapt to changes in afferent input across the life span. For reviews of cross-modal plasticity in the blind, see Merabet and Pascual-Leone (2010), Sathian and Lacey (2007), and Sathian and Stilla (2010).

Remarkably, plastic change is not restricted to permanent changes in afferent inputs, as experiments with sighted people who have been blindfolded for only temporary periods have shown demonstrable effects. Behavioral changes leading to increased discrimination of tactile grating orientation have been shown to occur within 1.5 h of blindfolding (Facchini and Aglioti, 2003), and people blindfolded for 5 days showed improved Braille discrimination performance compared to sighted controls who underwent the same training (Kauffman et al., 2002). Neuroimaging results with sighted participants after 5 days of blindfolding showed that tactile stimulation activated the occipital cortex, and application of TMS disrupted tactile perception and Braille discrimination in a similar manner as has been shown in the blind (Merabet et al., 2008). Interestingly, this same study showed that the dramatic plastic changes observed with 5 days of blindfolding were completely reversed within 24 h of removing the blindfolds. Although the mechanisms supporting this short-term plasticity may differ from long-term blindness, for example, unmasking of inhibitory connections versus forging of enduring cortico-cortical connections (Pascual-Leone and Hamilton, 2001), such findings suggest that the importance of the brain's potential for change should not be underestimated.

Image Preprocessing and Artificial Intelligence

In reflecting on mobility experiments with the Tactile Vision Substitution System, one of its developers, Carter Collins, made the following comments: "However, on testing this system outdoors in the real-world sidewalk environment, it was found that there was simply too much information which overloaded the tactile system. Perhaps 90% was the wrong kind of information, that is, comprised of interfering tactile detail in the background surrounding the objects of regard, which appeared to mask the primary mobility information. The bandwidth of the skin as an information-carrying medium is limited and apparently cannot handle the vast amount of data in a raw television image as complex as a sidewalk scene" (Collins, 1985, p. 37). He went on to suggest: "For the ideal mobility system of the future, I strongly believe that we should take a more sophisticated approach, utilizing the power of artificial intelligence for processing large amounts of detailed visual information in order to substitute for the missing functions of the eye and much of the visual pre-processing performed by the brain. We should off-load the blind travelers' brain of these otherwise slow and arduous tasks which are normally performed effortlessly by the sighted visual system.... We should extract features in the scene which are essential for mobility" (Collins, 1985, p. 41). His prescient remarks point to the vital importance of not delivering information to touch and hearing that exceeds their processing capacities, as discussed earlier. Rather, one can use either simple image preprocessing or the more powerful techniques from artificial intelligence to provide information, including linguistic information, that is more suited to the processing capacities of touch and hearing. Consider, for example, the challenge of scene perception. Video data from a video camera augmented with laser range finding could be used to select the information within a narrow depth of field in front of the user and display only the information that is important for obstacle avoidance. The work of Gonzalez-Mora et al. (2006) illustrates the use of such preprocessing in connection with an auditory vision substitution system.

Going beyond simple signal processing are artificial intelligence techniques for extracting more abstract information such as object identity, features of the environment, and impending collision targets, information that can then be presented to the user by way of perceptual displays and language (Collins, 1985; Katz et al., 2010). A nice example is the Blind Driver Project by Dennis Hong and his collaborators at Virginia Tech University in response to an initiative of the National Federation of the Blind Jernigan Institute. The group has instrumented a car with video cameras, laser range finders, GPS, and other sensors and a variety of nonvisual interfaces that include auditory commands and a haptic display of airjet stimulators that the driver can feel with the hand. Blind people are able to use the display to steer a closed course and to avoid large obstacles scattered in front of the vehicle.* An important factor in the success of the project is the result of using artificial intelligence techniques to compute the edges of the road and obstacles and to present only that information on the haptic display. Removing all of the clutter that would normally appear with delivery of the raw video stream has the same benefit as starting with only high-contrast features of the environment (Figure 8.2d). It remains to be seen whether the project will have success with demands of unconstrained real city driving.

Implications of Processing Differences between Blind and Sighted People

Given that blindness is the most common target for sensory substitution, and the indications that the lack of sight profoundly changes brain function, it is important to consider whether models of spatial information processing

---

* http://www.romela.org/main/Blind_Driver_Challenge

derived from studies of sighted individuals also apply to the blind. A related question is whether the differences in sensory experience and deliberate practice of sighted and blind affect their processing. In particular, sighted or late-blind subjects are more likely to be able to use visual mediation. For example, visual experience in interpreting 3-D cues might explain why late-blind outperform early-blind in some studies of the ability to recognize tactually presented pictures (Heller, 1989).

Röder and colleagues have suggested that early blindness alters intersensory processing by reducing integration across modalities. Sighted individuals showed a greater tendency to integrate tactile and auditory taps when judging numerosity (Hötting and Röder, 2004). Blind people also showed a greater ability to filter out stimuli from a task-irrelevant modality while attending to their spatial location, as measured by event-related potentials (Hötting et al., 2004). Studies of a group who had congenital binocular cataracts early in life indicated that their audiovisual interactions, once sight was restored, were reduced relative to controls (Putzar et al., 2007).

Neural and/or processing differences between sighted and blind have important implications for the effectiveness of sensory substitution, as studies with sighted or late-blind people might not be sufficiently capable of generalization to indicate substitutability for the congenitally blind. This point is made by a study comparing blind and sighted with respect to brain areas activated during navigation aided by a tongue stimulator (Kupers et al., 2010). Consistent with the idea that blindness induces brain reorganization, the blind produced activation more like the sighted when walking under visual guidance. With the same device, congenitally blind outperformed sighted controls on obstacle detection and avoidance (Chebat et al., 2011).

Recommendations for the Design Process

A theme throughout this chapter is that while there is significant potential for sensory substitution, basic research has also pointed to clear limitations. Unfortunately, the motivation for design of sensory substitution devices, and assistive technology more generally, has often been ad hoc rather than based on sound theory or empirical findings, and evaluations tend to be limited to controlled settings. The failure to recognize the processing constraints of perception and cognition has resulted in limited utility of sensory substitution devices for supporting real-world behaviors. In addition, naïve assumptions about the end-users, rather than systematic studies with first-person reports, have ultimately reduced the enthusiasm for these devices and their adoption by the target demographic. In this final section, we highlight some key considerations in the design of assistive technology that we hope will capitalize on the basic promise and avoid some of the pitfalls demonstrated in the past.

Understanding the Information Flow from Function to Display

As we have emphasized throughout this chapter, simply having a technological solution for converting visual input into tactile or auditory output is not sufficient for successful sensory substitution. Effective devices must consider the capabilities and limitations of the human perceptual-cognitive system that underlie the function to be supported.

We postulated that a principled approach to using touch or hearing as a substitute for vision has two essential steps: (1) identify the information that is most effective in enabling the desired function, and (2) determine how best to display this information to the substituted modality. Note that more information is not necessarily better; what is needed is to provide information that is directly relevant to the task at hand. Consider the insights about the information overload delivered via the Tactile Vision Substitution System, which were lessons learned only at the late stage of real-world testing (Collins, 1985).

Any serious effort to develop sensory substitution devices and assistive technologies must be theoretically motivated and scientifically sound. We believe that principled design, based on initial due diligence with regard to the scientific base, will aid in avoiding some of the common errors that have limited the use of sensory substitution devices. Developers of new devices should also be prepared to conduct empirical research at multiple points during the design process, including not only iterative usability testing but also basic psychophysical experiments to understand underlying processes. Practically speaking, what this means is that a group that takes on the task of creating a useful sensory-based aid will have to include expertise in related theory and methods as well as technology.

Considering the End-User from the Starting Point Onward

The starting point for many assistive technologies appears to be the laudable aim of providing a solution to a practical problem. Too often, unfortunately, the problem is envisaged by the developer, and the solution is directed by the availability of engineering and technical tools. The result is the "engineering trap": A product is developed that may be interesting and even elegant, and aims to solve a real problem, but in actuality has little functional utility or even relevance for the everyday challenges of its intended users.

Given that technology exists that may be directed at an assistive problem, avoiding the engineering trap requires adhering to several practices at the starting point of a project: (1) Identify the user population who are envisioned to have the problem; (2) Assess the user needs, that is, the elements of the solution that the target population believes are necessary; (3) Determine whether the intended implementation will be functional not only technically but also in the context of human information-processing capabilities and practical constraints. The first practice is obvious for development of visual sensory substitution devices, which are almost always designed for blind/low-vision individuals. The third practice is considered a necessary step in engineering and design, although it is generally not taken far enough. It is the second step that is often overlooked entirely, and with consequences: insufficient characterization of user needs results in devices which are not accepted and have little functional utility.

Two relatively easy and inexpensive means of consulting blind individuals are survey instruments and focus groups. Surveys are easy to administer and score but they are neither interactive nor scenario driven. The results from focus groups may be harder to quantify but the clear advantage is that they provide invaluable feedback from interactive exchange and hands-on experience with prototypes. A combined approach, including iterative input from users as the project progresses, is most informative.

User input at the starting point is needed for two critical aspects of an intended assistive technology. One is the generality or specificity of the functions the technology is intended to serve. Clearly we favor special-purpose devices that support a specific function in everyday life such as navigation, rather than general-purpose devices. A second critical aspect of technology is the learning period required in order for it to be effective. Although an intuitive system is always preferable, users are more likely amenable to a steeper learning curve when the device is providing a solution to a real-world problem that is not addressed by other technologies and that has an impact on independence, quality of life, education, and/or vocation (Giudice and Legge, 2008). Developers beware: Only first-person accounts can provide an assessment of the learning/usefulness trade-off.

End-users should be consulted not only about a device's functionality but also its aesthetic appeal. Developers unfortunately often neglect this aspect of design, operating instead on the naïve assumption that access to information is more important than aesthetic considerations. To the contrary, in a study of user preferences about body-worn assistive technologies, cosmetic acceptability was often rated as more important than the potential benefit afforded by the device (Golledge et al., 2004). Where the goal is to create technology that is minimally intrusive, the reality is that sensory substitution devices that require visible hardware such as cameras, headphones, or electrotactile stimulators are not invisible. Both form and function must be considered; aesthetic impact cannot be ignored.

Concluding Remarks

In sum, the role of a sensory substitution device is to support the demands and interests of the user and to enhance capacities that are otherwise difficult or not possible from nonvisual means. A sensory substitution device should emphasize task-specific information, carefully consider the end-user's information needs and requirements, support individualized selection of desired information, and perhaps most important, should not take over functions or provide information that the user is capable of completing and receiving without the device's assistance (Jacobson et al., 2011). Learning from past blunders and following the suggestions in this chapter will provide a good starting point for designers to develop future sensory substitution devices based on theoretically motivated, user-inspired design.

Acknowledgments

The authors acknowledge the support of NIH grant 1R01EY016817 during the preparation of this chapter. Klatzky's work on this chapter was facilitated by an Alexander von Humboldt Research Award.

References

Abravanel, A. 1971. The synthesis of length within and between perceptual systems. *Attention, Perception & Psychophysics* 9: 327–328.

Amedi, A., Jacobson, G., Hendler, T. et al. 2002. Convergence of visual and tactile shape processing in the human lateral occipital complex. *Cerebral Cortex* 1211: 1202–1212.

Amedi, A., Malach, R., Hendler, T. et al. 2001. Visuo-haptic object-related activation in the ventral visual pathway. *Nature Neuroscience* 43: 324–330.

Apkarian-Stielau, P. and Loomis, J. M. 1975. A comparison of tactile and blurred visual form perception. *Attention, Perception & Psychophysics* 18: 362–368.

Ashmead, D., Davis, D. L., and Odom, R. D. 1990. Perception of the relative distances of nearby sound sources. *Attention, Perception & Psychophysics* 47: 326–331.

Auvray, M., Hanneton, S., Lenay, C. et al. 2005. There is something out there: Distal attribution in sensory substitution, twenty years later. *Journal of Integrative Neuroscience* 4: 505–521.

Auvray, M., Lenay, C., and Stewart, J. 2009a. Perceptual interactions in a minimalist environment. *New Ideas in Psychology* 27: 32–47.

Auvray, M. and Myin, E. 2009b. Perception with compensatory devices: From sensory substitution to sensorimotor extension. *Cognitive Science* 33: 1036–1058.

Avraamides, M., Loomis, J. M., Klatzky, R. L. et al. 2004. Functional equivalence of spatial representations derived from vision and language: Evidence from allocentric judgments. *Journal of Experimental Psychology: Learning, Memory, and Cognition* 30: 801–814.

Bach-y-Rita, P. 1967. Sensory plasticity: Applications to a vision substitution system. *Acta Neurologica Scandanavica* 43: 417–426.

Bach-y-Rita, P. 1972. *Brain Mechanisms in Sensory Substitution.* New York: Academic Press.

Bach-y-Rita, P. 2004. Tactile sensory substitution studies. *Annals of the New York Academy of Sciences* 1013: 83–91.

Bach-y-Rita, P. and Kercel, S. 2003. Sensory substitution and the human machine interface. *Trends in Cognitive Sciences* 7: 541–546.

Bargary, G. and Mitchell, K. J. 2008. Synaesthesia and cortical connectivity. *Trends in Neurosciences* 31: 335–342.

Blauert, J. 1997. *Spatial Hearing: The Psychophysics of Human Sound Localization.* Cambridge, MA: MIT Press.

Brabyn, J. A. 1985. A review of mobility aids and means of assessment. In *Electronic Spatial Sensing for the Blind*, ed. D. H. Warren and E. R. Strelow, pp. 13–27. Boston: Martinus Nijhoff.

Büchel, C. 1998. Functional neuroimaging studies of Braille reading: Cross-modal reorganization and its implications. *Brain* 1217: 1193–1194.

Capelle, C., Trullemans, C., Arno, P. et al. 1998. A real-time experimental prototype for enhancement of vision rehabilitation using auditory substitution. *IEEE Transaction on Biomedical Engineering* 45: 1279–1293.

Casey, S. J. and Newell, F. N. 2007. Are representations of unfamiliar faces independent of encoding modality? *Neuropsychologia* 453: 506–513.

Cattaneo, Z. and Vecchi, T. 2011. *Blind Vision: The Neuroscience of Visual Impairment.* Cambridge MA: MIT Press.

Cha, K., Horch, K. W., and Normann, R. A. 1992. Mobility performance with a pixelized vision system. *Vision Research* 3: 1367–1372.

Chebat, D. R., Schneider, F., Kupers, R. et al. 2011. Navigation with a sensory substitution device in congenitally blind individuals. *NeuroReport* 22: 342–347.

Cheung, S.-H., Fang, F., He, S., and Legge, G. 2009. Retinotopically specific reorganization of visual cortex for tactile pattern recognition. *Current Biology* 19: 596–601.

Cohen, L. G., Celnik, P., Pascual-Leone, A. et al. 1997. Functional relevance of cross-modal plasticity in blind humans. *Nature* 389: 180–183.

Collins, C. C. 1970. Tactile television: Mechanical and electrical image projection. *IEEE Transactions on Man-Machine Systems* MMS-11: 65–71.

Collins, C. C. 1985. On mobility aids for the blind. In *Electronic Spatial Sensing for the Blind*, eds. D. H. Warren and E. R. Strelow, pp. 35–64. Boston: Martinus Nijhoff.

Craig, J. C. 1985. Attending to two fingers: Two hands are better than one. *Attention, Perception & Psychophysics* 38: 496–511.

Cronly-Dillon, J., Persaud, K., and Gregory, R. P. F. 1999. The perception of visual images encoded in musical form: A study in cross modality information transfer. *Proceedings of Royal Society of London* 266: 2427–2433.

de Volder, A. G. and Catalan-Ahumadaa, M. 1999. Changes in occipital cortex activity in early blind humans using a sensory substitution device. *Brain Research* 826: 128–134.

Dopjans, L., Wallraven, C., and Bülthoff, H. H. 2009. Cross-modal transfer in visual and haptic face recognition. *IEEE Transactions on Haptics* 2: 236–240.

Edquist, J., Rich, A. N., Brinkman, C., and Mattingley, J. B. 2006. Do synaesthetic colours act as unique features in visual search? *Cortex* 422: 222–231.

Eitan, Z. and Zimmers, R. 2010. Beethoven's last piano sonata and those who follow crocodiles: Cross-domain mappings of auditory pitch in a musical context. *Cognition* 114: 405–422.

Elbert, T., Pantev, C., Wienbruch, C. et al. 1995. Increased cortical representation of the fingers of the left hand in string players. *Science* 270: 305–307.

Epstein, W., Hughes, B., Schncider, S. et al. 1986. Is there anything out there?: A study of distal attribution in response to vibrocactile stimulation. *Perception* 15: 275–284.

Ericsson, K. A. 2004. Deliberate practice and the acquisition and maintenance of expert performance in medicine and related domains. *Academic Medicine* 79: S70–S81.

Ernst, M. O. and Banks, M. S. 2002. Humans integrate visual and haptic information in a statistically optimal fashion. *Nature* 415: 429–433.

Ernst, M. O., Banks, M. S., and Bülthoff, H. H. 2000. Touch can change visual slant perception. *Nature Neuroscience* 3: 69–73.

Facchini, S. and Aglioti, S. M. 2003. Short term light deprivation increases tactile spatial acuity in humans. *Neurology* 6012: 1998–1999.

Gallace, A. and Spence, C. 2008. The cognitive and neural correlates of "tactile consciousness": A multisensory perspective. *Consciousness and Cognition* 17: 370–407.

Geldard, F. A. 1957. Adventures in tactile literacy. *American Psychologist* 12: 115–124.

Giudice, N. A., Betty, M. R., and Loomis, J. M. 2011. Functional equivalence of spatial images from touch and vision: Evidence from spatial updating in blind and sighted individuals. *Journal of Experimental Psychology: Learning, Memory, and Cognition* 37: 621–634.

Giudice, N. A., Klatzky, R. L., and Loomis, J. M. 2009. Evidence for amodal representations after bimodal learning: Integration of haptic-visual layouts into a common spatial image. *Spatial Cognition and Computation* 9: 287–304.

Giudice, N. A. and Legge, G. E. 2008. Blind navigation and the role of technology. In *Engineering Handbook of Smart Technology for Aging, Disability, and Independence*, eds. A. Helal, M. Mokhtari and B. Abdulrazak, pp. 479–500. Hoboken, NJ: John Wiley and Sons.

Goldreich, D. and Kanics, I. M. 2003. Tactile acuity is enhanced in blindness. *Journal of Neuroscience* 238: 3439–3445.

Golledge, R. G., Marston, J. R., Loomis, J. M. et al. 2004. Stated preferences for components of a Personal Guidance System for non-visual navigation. *Journal of Visual Impairment and Blindness* 98: 135–147.

Gonzalez-Mora, J. L., Rodriguez-Hernandez, A., Burunat, E. et al. 2006. Seeing the world by hearing: Virtual Acoustic Space (VAS) a new space perception system for blind people. *Information and Communication Technologies* 2006, 2nd issue: 837–842.

Goyal, M. S., Hansen, P. J., and Blakemore, C. B. 2006. Tactile perception recruits functionally related visual areas in the late-blind. *Neuroreport* 1713: 1381–1384.

Harrington, D. O. 1971. *The Visual Fields.* St Louis, MO: Mosby.

Harrison, J. and Baron-Cohen, S. 1997. Synaesthesia: An introduction. In *Synaesthesia: Classic and Contemporary Readings*, eds. S. Baron-Cohen and J. E. Harrison, pp. 3–16. Malden, MA: Blackwell.

Held, R., Ostrovsky, Y., de Gelder, B. et al. 2011. The newly blind fail to match seen with felt. *Nature Neuroscience* 14: 551–553.

Heller, M. A. 1989. Picture and pattern perception in the sighted and the blind: The advantage of the late blind. *Perception* 18: 379–389.

Heller, M. A., Calcaterra, J. A., Green, S. L. et al. 1999. Intersensory conflict between vision and touch: The response modality dominates when precise, attention-riveting judgments are required. *Attention, Perception and Psychophysics* 61:1384–1398.

Hollander, A. 1994. *An Exploration of Virtual Auditory Shape Perception.* Unpublished M. S. E Thesis, Human Interface Technology Laboratory, University of Washington. Available at http://www.hitl.washington.edu/publications/hollander/

Hötting, K. and Röder, B. 2004. Hearing cheats touch but less in the congenitally blind than in sighted individuals. *Psychological Science* 15: 60–64.

Hötting, K., Rösler, F., and Röder, B. 2004. Altered multisensory interaction in congenitally blind humans: An event-related potential study. *Experimental Brain Research* 159: 370–381.

Jacobson, K. E., Giudice, N. A., and Moratz, R. 2011. Towards a theory of spatial assistance from a phenomenological perspective: Technical and social factors for blind navigation. Paper presented at the Conference on Spatial Information Theory (COSIT 2011), Belfast, ME.

Jansson, G. 1983. Tactile guidance of movement. *International Journal of Neuroscience* 19: 37–46.

Kaczmarek, K. A. 2000. Sensory augmentation and substitution. In *CRC Handbook of Biomedical Engineering*, ed. J. D. Bronzino Ed., pp. 143.1–143.10. Boca Raton, FL: CRC Press.

Kanwisher, N., McDermott, J., and Chun, M. M. 1997. The fusiform face area: A module in human extrastriate cortex specialized for face perception. *Journal of Neuroscience* 1711: 4302–4311.

Katz, B., Truillet, P., Thorpe, S. et al. 2010. NAVIG: Navigation assisted by artificial vision and GNSS. In *Workshop on Multimodal Location Based Techniques for Extreme Navigation (Pervasive 2010)*, 1–4.

Kauffman, T., Theoret, H., and Pascual-Leone, A. 2002. Braille character discrimination in blindfolded human subjects. *Neuroreport* 135: 571–574.

Kay, L. 1985. Sensory aids to spatial perception for blind persons: Their design and evaluation. In *Electronic Spatial Sensing for the Blind*, eds. D. H. Warren and E. R. Strelow, pp. 125–140. Boston: Martinus Nijhoff.

Kennedy, J. M and Fox, N. 1977. Pictures to see and pictures to touch, In *The Arts and Cognition*, eds. D. Perkins and B. Leondar, pp. 118–135. Baltimore: Johns Hopkins University Press.

Kilgour, A. and Lederman, S. J. 2006. A haptic face-inversion effect. *Perception* 35: 921–931.

Kilgour, A. R., Servos, P., James, T. W. et al. 2004. Functional MRI of haptic face recognition. *Brain and Cognition* 542: 159–161.

Klatzky, R. L., Loomis, J. M., Lederman, S. J. et al. 1993. Haptic perception of objects and their depictions. *Attention, Perception & Psychophysics* 54: 170–178.

Klatzky, R. L., Lippa, Y., Loomis, J. M. et al. 2003. Encoding, learning, and spatial updating of multiple object locations specified by 3-D sound, spatial language, and vision. *Experimental Brain Research* 149: 48–61.

Klatzky, R. L., Marston, J. R., Giudice, N. A. et al. 2006. Cognitive load of navigating without vision when guided by virtual sound versus spatial language. *Journal of Experimental Psychology: Applied* 12: 223–232.

Kramer, G. 1994. An introduction to auditory display. In *Auditory Display: Sonification, Audification, and Auditory Interfaces*, G. Kramer, ed., pp. 1–78. Reading MA: Addison-Wesley.

Kujala, T., Palva, M. J., Salonen, O. et al. 2005. The role of blind humans' visual cortex in auditory change detection. *Neuroscience Letters* 3792: 127–131.

Kupers, R., Chebat, D. R., Madsen, K. H. et al. 2010. Neural correlates of virtual route recognition in congenital blindness. *Proceedings of the National Academy of Sciences USA* 10728: 12716–12721.

Lakatos, S. and Marks, L. E. 1999. Haptic form perception: Relative salience of local and global features. *Attention, Perception & Psychophysics* 61: 895–908.

Lederman, S. J., Klatzky, R. L., Chataway, C. et al. 1990. Visual mediation and the haptic recognition of two-dimensional pictures of common objects. *Attention, Perception & Psychophysics* 47: 54–64.

Legge, G. E., Madison, C., Vaughn, B. N. et al. 2008. Retention of high tactile acuity throughout the life span in blindness. *Attention, Perception & Psychophysics* 70: 1471–1488.

Lenay, C., Canu, S., and Villon, P. 1997. Technology and perception: The contribution of sensory substitution systems. In *Proceedings of the 2nd International Conference on Cognitive Technology*, 44–53. Aizu-Wakamatsu City, Japan.

Levesque, V. 2009. *Virtual Display of Tactile Graphics and Braille by Lateral Skin Deformation*. Unpublished manuscript, Department of Electrical and Computer Engineering, McGill University, Montreal, Canada. available online at http://vlevesque.com/papers/Levesque-PhD.pdf.

Loomis, J. M. 1979. An investigation of tactile hyperacuity. *Sensory Processes* 3: 289–302.

Loomis, J. M. 1981. On the tangibility of letters and braille. *Attention, Perception & Psychophysics* 29: 37–46.

Loomis, J. M. 1982. Analysis of tactile and visual confusion matrices. *Attention, Perception & Psychophysics* 31: 41–52.

Loomis, J. M. 1990. A model of character recognition and legibility. *Journal of Experimental Psychology: Human Perception and Performance* 16: 106–120.

Loomis, J. M. 1992. Distal attribution and presence. *Presence: Teleoperators and Virtual Environments* 1: 113–119.

Loomis, J. M. 2003. Sensory replacement and sensory substitution: Overview and prospects for the future. In *Converging Technologies for Improving Human Performance: Nanotechnology, Biotechnology, Information Technology and Cognitive Science*, eds. M. C. Roco and W. S. Bainbridge, pp. 189–198. Boston, MA: Kluwer Academic.

Loomis, J. M. and Apkarian-Stielau, P. 1976. A lateral masking effect in tactile and blurred visual letter recognition. *Attention, Perception & Psychophysics* 20: 221–226.

Loomis, J. M. and Klatzky, R. L. 2007. Functional equivalence of spatial representations from vision, touch, and hearing: Relevance for sensory substitution. In *Blindness and Brain Plasticity in Navigation and Object Perception*, eds. J. J. Rieser, D. H. Ashmead, F. F. Ebner et al., pp. 155–184. New York: Lawrence Erlbaum Associates.

Loomis, J. M., Klatzky, R. L., and Lederman, S. J. 1991. Similarity of tactual and visual picture perception with limited field of view. *Perception* 20: 167–177.

Loomis, J. M. and Lederman, S. J. 1986. Tactual perception. In *Handbook of Perception and Human Performance: Vol. 2. Cognitive Processes and Performance*, eds. K. Boff, L. Kaufman and J. Thomas, pp. 31.1–31.41. New York: Wiley.

Loomis, J. M., Marston, J. R., Golledge, R. G. et al. 2005. Personal guidance system for people with visual impairment: A comparison of spatial displays for route guidance. *Journal of Visual Impairment & Blindness* 99: 219–232.

Marks, L. 1978. *The Unity of the Senses: Interrelations Among the Modalities*. New York: Academic Press.

Martino, G. and Marks, L. E. 1999. Perceptual and linguistic interactions in speeded classification: Tests of the semantic coding hypothesis. *Perception* 28: 903–923.

Martino, G. and Marks, L. E. 2001. Synesthesia: Strong and weak. *Current Directions in Psychological Science* 10: 61–65.

Meijer, P. B. L. 1992. An experimental system for auditory image representations. *IEEE Transactions on Biomedical Engineering* 39: 112–121.

Merabet, L. B., Battelli, L., Obretenova, S. et al. 2009. Functional recruitment of visual cortex for sound encoded object identification in the blind. *Neuroreport* 202: 132–138.

Merabet, L. B., Hamilton, R., Schlaug, G. et al. 2008. Rapid and reversible recruitment of early visual cortex for touch. *PLoS ONE* 38: e30–e46.

Merabet, L. B. and Pascual-Leone, A. 2010. Neural reorganization following sensory loss: The opportunity of change. *Nature Reviews Neuroscience* 111: 44–52.

Newell, F. N., Ernst, M. O., Tjan, B. S. et al. 2001. Viewpoint dependence in visual and haptic object recognition. *Psychological Science* 12: 37–42.

Olzak, L. and Thomas, J. P. l986. Seeing spatial patterns. In *Handbook of Perception and Human Performance: Vol. 7*, eds. K. R. Boff, L. Kaufman and J. P. Thomas., pp. 7-1–7-56. New York: Wiley.

O'Regan, J. K. and Noë, A. 2001. A sensorimotor account of visual consciousness. *Behavioral and Brain Sciences* 11: 939–973.

Pascual-Leone, A., Amedi, A., Fregni, F. et al. 2005. The plastic human brain cortex. *Annual Review of Neuroscience* 28: 377–401.

Pascual-Leone, A. and Hamilton, R. 2001. The metamodal organization of the brain. *Progress in Brain Research* 134: 427–445.

Pascual-Leone, A. and Torres, F. 1993. Plasticity of the sensorimotor cortex representation of the reading finger in Braille readers. *Brain* 116: 39–52.

Perrott, D. R. and Saberi, K. 1990. Minimum audible angle thresholds for sources varying in both elevation and azimuth. *Journal of the Acoustical Society of America* 87: 1728–1731.

Phillips, F., Egan, E. J. L., and Perry, B. N. 2009 Perceptual equivalence between vision and touch is complexity dependent. *Acta Psychologica* 132: 259–266.

Poirier, C., Collignon, O., Devolder, A. G. et al. 2005. Specific activation of the V5 brain area by auditory motion processing: An fMRI study. *Cognitive Brain Research* 253: 650–658.

Poirier, C., Collignon, O., Scheiber, C. et al. 2006. Auditory motion perception activates visual motion areas in early blind subjects. *Neuroimage* 311: 279–285.

Pollok B., Schnitzler I., Mierdorf T. et al. 2005. Image-to-sound conversion: Experience-induced plasticity in auditory cortex of blindfolded adults. *Experimental Brain Research* 167: 287–291.

Pratt, C. C. 1930. The spatial character of high and low tones. *Journal of Experimental Psychology* 13: 278–285.

Proulx, M. J. 2010. Synthetic synaesthesia and sensory substitution. *Consciousness and Cognition* 19: 501–503.

Putzar, L., Goerendt, I., Lange, K. et al. 2007. Early visual deprivation impairs multisensory interactions in humans. *Nature Neuroscience* 10: 1243–1245.

Rauschecker, J. P. 1995. Compensatory plasticity and sensory substitution in the cerebral cortex. *Trends in Neuroscience* 181: 36–43.

Renier, L., Collignon, O., Poirier, C. et al. 2005 Cross-modal activation of visual cortex during depth perception using auditory substitution of vision. *NeuroImage* 26: 573–580.

Ricciardi, E., Vanello, N., Sani, L. et al. 2007. The effect of visual experience on the development of functional architecture in hMT+. *Cerebral Cortex* 1712: 2933–2939.

Rieser, J. J., Ashmead, D. H., Ebner, F. F. et al. eds. 2008. *Blindness and Brain Plasticity in Navigation and Object Perception*. New York: Lawrence Erlbaum Associates.

Rock, I. and Victor, J. 1964 Vision and touch: An experimentally created conflict between the two senses. *Science* 143: 594–596.

Sadato, N., Pascual-Leone, A., Grafman, J. et al. 1996. Activation of the primary visual cortex by Braille reading in blind subjects. *Nature* 380: 526–528.

Sampaio, E., Maris, S., and Bach-y-Rita, P. 2001. Brain plasticity: 'visual' acuity of blind persons via the tongue. *Brain Research* 908: 204–207.

Sathian, K. and Lacey, S. 2007. Journeying beyond classical somatosensory cortex. *Canadian Journal of Experimental Psychology* 61: 254–264.

Sathian, K. and Stilla, R. 2010. Cross-modal plasticity of tactile perception in blindness. *Restorative Neurology and Neuroscience* 28: 271–281.

Sathian, K., Zangaladze, A., Hoffman, J. M. et al. 1997. Feeling with the mind's eye. *NeuroReport* 8: 3877–3881.

Segond, H., Weiss, D., and Sampiao, E. 2005. Human spatial navigation via a visuotactile sensory substitution system. *Perception* 34: 1231–1249.

Siegle, J. H. and Warren, W. H. 2010. Distal attribution and distance perception in sensory substitution. *Perception* 39: 208–223.

Simner, J., Mulvenna, C., Sagiv, N. et al. 2006. Synaesthesia: The prevalence of atypical cross-modal experiences. *Perception* 358: 1024–1033.

Sterr, A., Muller, M. M., Elbert, T. et al. 1998. Changed perceptions in Braille readers. *Nature* 391: 134–135.

Stilla, R., Hanna, R., Hu, X. et al. 2008. Neural processing underlying tactile microspatial discrimination in the blind: A functional magnetic resonance imaging study. *Journal of Vision* 810: 11–19.

Struiksma, M. E., Noordzij, M. L., and Postma, A. 2009. What is the link between language and spatial images? Behavioral and neural findings in blind and sighted individuals. *Acta Psychologica* 132: 145–156.

Strybel, T. Z. and Perrott, D. R. 1984. Auditory distance discrimination: The success and failure of the intensity discrimination hypothesis. *Journal of the Acoustical Society of America* 76: 318–320.

Ungar, S., Blades, M., and Spencer, C. 1996. The construction of cognitive maps and children with visual impairments. In *The Construction of Cognitive Maps*, J. Portugali, ed., pp. 247–273. Dordrecht, The Netherlands: Klüwer Academic Publishing.

Veraart, C. 1989. Neurophysiological approach to the design of visual prostheses: A theoretical discussion. *Journal of Medical Engineering and Technology* 13: 57–62.

Veraart, C. and Wanet, M. C. 1985. Sensory substitution of vision by audition. In *Electronic Spatial Sensing for the Blind*, eds. D. H. Warren and E. R. Strelow, pp. 217–236. Boston: Martinus Nijhoff.

Walker, P., Bremner, J. G., Mason, U. et al. 2010. Preverbal infants' sensitivity to synaesthetic cross-modality correspondences. *Psychological Science* 21: 21–25.

Wall, S. and Brewster, S. 2006. Sensory substitution using tactile pin arrays: Human factors, technology and applications. *Signal Processing* 86: 3674–3695.

Ward, J. and Meijer, P. 2010. Visual experiences in the blind induced by an auditory sensory substitution device. *Consciousness and Cognition* 19: 492–500.

Warren, D. H. and Strelow, E. R., eds. 1985. *Electronic Spatial Sensing for the Blind*. Boston: Martinus Nijhoff.

Watson, A. B. 1986. Temporal sensitivity. In *Handbook of Perception and Human Performance*, eds. K. R. Boff, L. Kaufman, and J. P. Thomas, Vol. 1 (pp. 6-1-6–43). New York: Wiley.

Watson, J. D., Myers, R., Frackowiak, R. S. et al. 1993. Area V5 of the human brain: Evidence from a combined study using positron emission tomography and magnetic resonance imaging. *Cerebral Cortex* 32: 79–94.

Weeks, R., Horwitz, B., Aziz-Sultan et al. 2000. A positron emission tomographic study of auditory localization in the congenitally blind. *Journal of Neuroscience* 207: 2664–2672.

Welch, R. B. and Warren, D. H. 1980. Immediate perceptual response to intersensory discrepancy. *Psychological Bulletin 88:* 638–667.

Wertheim, T. 1894. Über die indirekte sehschärfe. *Zeitschrift für Psychologie,* 7: 172–189.

Westheimer, G. 1987. Visual acuity. In *Adler's Physiology of the Eye: Clinical Application*, eds. R. A. Moses and W. M. Hart, pp. 530–544. St Louis, MO: Mosby.

White, B. W. 1970. Perceptual findings with the vision-substitution system. *IEEE Transactions on Man-Machine Systems* MMS-11: 54–59.

White, B. W., Saunden, F. A., Scadden, L. et al. 1970. Seeing with the skin. *Attention, Perception, & Psychophysics* 7: 223–227.

Wijntjes, M. W. A., Lienen, T. van, Verstijnen, I. M. et al. 2008a. The influence of picture size on recognition and exploratory behaviour in raised line drawings. *Perception* 37: 602–614.

Wijntjes, M. W. A., Lienen, T. van, Verstijnen, I. M. et al. 2008b. Look what I have felt: Unidentified haptic line drawings are identified after sketching. *Acta Psychologica* 128: 255–263.

Wijntjes, M. W. A., Volcic, R., Pont, S. C. et al. 2009. Haptic perception disambiguates visual perception of 3d shape. *Experimental Brain Research* 193: 639–644.

Winkler, S. 2005. *Digital Video Quality—Vision Models and Metrics*. Chichester, UK: John Wiley and Sons.

Wolbers, T., Wutte, M., Klatzky, R. L. et al. 2011a. Modality-independent coding of spatial layout in the human brain. *Current Biology* 2111: 984–989.

Wolbers, T., Zahorik, P., and Giudice, N. A. 2011b. Decoding the direction of auditory motion in blind humans. *Neuroimage* 56: 681–687.

Zangaladze, A., Epstein, C. M., Grafton, S. T. et al. 1999. Involvement of visual cortex in tactile discrimination of orientation. *Nature* 40: 587–590.

Zue, V. and Cole, R. 1979. Experiments on spectrogram reading. In *ICASSP 1979. Proceedings of the IEEE International Conference on Acoustics, Speech and Signal Processing* pp. 116–119.

9

Tactile Reading: Tactile Understanding

Yvonne Eriksson

CONTENTS

Introduction

As pointed out already by the French philosopher Dennis Diderot in the late 18th century, sight is a very efficient and elegant sense (Diderot, 1749). It is possible to see great distances and very close-up views. By looking, we can quickly get an idea of an environment or a specific milieu. Through pictures on the Internet, nonfiction books, storybooks for children or magazines, we get information about, for example, different parts of the world or fashion. Sight is used to orient us in many different ways, socially and geographically. It is possible to perceive space entirely from vision, but it could be apprehended from haptic experience as well as hearing. For sighted people, hearing and haptic understanding support the visual impression, while people with visual impairment have to depend on them. This chapter will address questions about how blind children learn to use touch for a better understanding of the environment. I will here focus on how tactile pictures in storybooks can support further discussions about everyday objects and episodes, and more abstract conversations. I will also address theories about tactile and multimodal reading processes that are involved in tactile decoding, and how they relate to visual perception and visual literacy.

Pictures and text from their first day of life orient sighted children, but not blind children. To stimulate children's interest in Braille letters, parents of blind children frequently put Braille letters on furniture and on daily objects as a way to enable their blind child to encounter Braille by chance. However, tactile pictures are less frequent. Pictures for visually impaired people have been controversial over time. Both sighted and blind people themselves have been critical. Sighted people have in many cases found it provocative that pictures can be read by touch, and visually impaired people comprehend the offer of tactile pictures as an abuse by the sighted since they recognize them as visual phenomena. However, I have found that the enthusiasm for and belief in tactile pictures have been related to pictures concerning education in general. Whereas the negative expectations in relation to tactile pictures are to be found in the discussion about pictures as sensual and misleading, something that stimulates children to dream away instead of focusing on the actual subject (Eriksson, 1998).

I will discuss tactile picture books from a multimodal perspective focusing on three different sites that give meaning to pictures: *production* of the images, the *image itself*, and the *audience*. Those methodological tools are from Gillian Rose (2007), and I have chosen to use them to summarize my involvement in tactile picture production, earlier as a project leader in the production of tactile pictures and later as a researcher (Eriksson, 1998, 1999; 2003). I will stress three different perspectives: first, the production of tactile pictures; second, the analysis of some tactile picture books, scientific illustrations for tactile reading, and maps; third, I will discuss the audience by giving examples from two research projects. One is about how a blind girl performs while her mother reads a tactile picture book with her, the other is an example of how adult Braille readers read and interpret tactile pictures.

Braille has a relatively short history compared to written text. Braille has been used since the late 19th century; before the invention of Braille, several efforts were made to develop different kinds of embossed letters. The most successful of the embossed letters was the so-called Moon, which is still in use. Braille consists of a cell with six raised dots that can be combined in 64 different ways. Every letter in the alphabet is represented by a combination of dots. For mathematics and for music notations, the same Braille alphabet is used, but to distinguish regular Braille from mathematic and music, Braille symbols are used (see also Chapter 14). Before a number there are always four dots that look like a reversed L. Braille is read by the fingertips, and Braille readers have different reading styles. Some use the index finger, others use two or three fingers, and some use one hand while others use both hands. Braille reading has been studied from many points of view and for different reasons, such as reading strategies, speed, and understanding; the results of those research projects have taught us that there is no best hand or finger for efficient reading (Millar, 1997). Their functions vary according to the task to solve. Other researchers have found the same results; the reading technique and reading rate in Braille depend on the kind of reading tasks (Knowlton and Wetzel, 1996). Bertelson et al. (1985) have divided the reading styles into three categories: conjoint, disjoint, and mixed exploration. Conjoint means that both index fingers proceed along the line and more or less evenly during line shifting. On the contrary, a disjoint technique means that the two hands explore different parts of the line, for example, one hand reads while the other navigates to the next line and starts reading until the other hand assembles and takes over the reading. The most common style is a mixed pattern such that the left hand starts reading when the right hand is finishing the previous line, and then the hands meet and read together in the middle of the line before they separate again (Breidegard et al., 2006).

Since there was no tactile writing when Valentine Haüy initiated the first organized education for the blind in 1784, tactile pictures and maps were central teaching tools. All teaching was oral. In the late 18th century and early 19th century, schools and asylums for the blind appeared in almost every European country. From written sources it is possible to follow the pedagogical ideas of those schools. Many of the teachers recommended tactile pictures and maps. Maps and pictures from that time were made of high quality paper with embossed shapes representing objects. The content of the tactile pictures was mainly depictions of objects and phenomena from natural science. The maps showed cities, parts of countries, countries, and continents. Often, the maps were divided into political and geographical maps (Eriksson, 1998).

From a Producer's Perspective—Why Tactile Pictures?

Tactile pictures have been produced since the late 17th century. However, no pictures remain from that time, only written sources that discuss the advantage of pictures for the blind. The oldest example that has been found is a map from 1800, made for the blind singer Maria Therese von Paradise. The aim of the map was to give the singer an overview of her singing tours around Europe. It is a printed map on which the borders and rivers are embroidered to be tactile; buttons represent towns.

Tactile pictures are still used in education for children who are blind, as well as adults, to provide information about the appearance of things. But to be able to talk about information, the concept of *information* has to be defined. Information can be explained as "something that describes an ordered reality and has some knowable, or at least idealized, isomorphic relation to that reality" (Dervin, 1999, p. 36). Furthermore, "information is a tool designed by human beings to make sense of a reality assumed to be both chaotic and orderly" (Dervin, 1999, p. 39). Tactile pictures are tools for information that can be used to describe reality in a tangible way.

Pictures are often necessary to describe concepts that are not verbal. In contrast to language, pictures are symbols that can look similar to the concept. A picture of a dog looks like a dog, while the word *dog* does not. For sighted people, pictures are frequently valued for their aesthetic aspects, often related to artworks. Interestingly, the definition of aesthetics that derives from the late 18th century concerned *sensuous perception* rather than focusing on beauty in a traditional way. The philosopher Alexander Gottlieb Baumgarten defined the term *aesthetics* in the 18th century. He used the Greek term "aesthesis" (which means "sensuous perception") to designate aesthetics as the autonomous science of sensitive knowing (Baumgarten, 1954, p. 78; Carlsson, 2010). Baumgarten focused on sensuous perception in general, not only in art. The most famous and quoted scholar in this context is Immanuel Kant. His use of the term "aesthetic" became of great importance for the succeeding aesthetic paradigm. In *Critique of Judgment* (1790), he writes that an aesthetic judgment does not have to do with objectivity, but with the feeling of pleasure and pain in relation to beauty and the sublime in nature. He associates the aesthetic judgment's beauty with disinterestedness (Kant, 1952, p. 479).

The interest in tactile perception developed in the late 18th century. It must be elucidated in relation to Enlightenment and empirical epistemology. John Locke had already in 1690 published the so-called Molyneux problem in *An Essay Concerning Human Understanding.* That is: *Would a man, born blind, but who regained vision later, recognize by sight alone objects and shapes that he had previously known only through touch?* Dennis Diderot, in *Lettre sur les aveugles* (1748), discussed the conditions for tactile perception. Followed by psychologists and practitioners within pedagogy, the discussion and systematic research in the area of tactile perception was intense during the 19th century. The teachers of the blind wanted to find the most efficient way to teach tactile decoding, while the psychologists focused on what could be perceived via touch.

Theodor Heller (1895) and David Katz (1925) were the most influential scholars and teachers dominating the international arena of that time, and others picked up from the results of their research. Teachers who were active in schools for the blind were internationally organized and met regularly, often every other year. New ideas concerning pedagogy or results from studies in relation to blind children's capacities or limitations spread out among practitioners in a very efficient way. In this context it is important to mention that teachers in schools for the blind during the 18th and 19th centuries were reformists and radical.

In my doctoral thesis *Tactile pictures. Pictorial representations for the blind 1784–1940,* I proposed that tactile pictures and maps, even when they are made for tactile perception, follow more or less the same rules of representation as those that apply to visual pictures and maps, since tactile pictures are normally based on visual originals. How is it that qualified knowledge about tactile perception is often invisible in tactile representations? Tactile pictures and models for the blind emanate from the second part of the 18th century

and have enabled people with visual impairment to learn how their surroundings may be understood visually and to become aware of the different
methods used in visualization. When two- and three-dimensional representations for the blind were made, the aim was to clarify, in a tangible and
concrete way, objects and certain concepts and phenomena. In the early education for the blind, that is in the late 18th century, the debate about what
could be perceived by touch was flowering. Later, research into tactile perception gave additional knowledge, and the printing technique allowed
"mass-production" of tactile material. The main producer, Martin Kunz, produced more than 100,000 embossed pictures in the late 19th and early 20th
centuries. The interest in tactile perception and tactile material ebbed away
in the context of education after the World War II. This could be explained by
the fact that the interest in and knowledge of what is called *Anschaung-
sunterricht*, outlook education, declined. And the logocentric culture dominated pedagogy in schools, except for demonstrations in science subjects
(Eriksson, 1998). However, tactile picture production continued in Europe
and USA during the following decades, although the teachers did not really
know how to introduce them to the children.

In the discussion of the use of pictures for the blind during the 18th and
19th centuries, the literature rarely discusses aesthetic values. Instead, the
discussion is focused on the value of pictures as an entity for knowledge,
that is, how pictures can contribute to a further understanding of the environment. There was a great belief in pictures as an entity that could generate
knowledge, and no discussion about the readers' role or about the fact that
the picture could be interpreted in different ways and have different meanings for different children. The teacher never expected the reading act to be
interactive. However, nowadays, when discussing tactile pictures in storybooks, the aesthetic aspects of the pictures are often brought up. But how are
the aesthetics valued in tactile pictures? Is it their tactile or visual qualities
that are treasured? I will argue that in the early days of tactile picture production, the aesthetic qualities were taken into consideration, and thus the
tactile quality was good. As I will discuss later, the quality of contemporary
tactile pictures is not as good as in the old days.

Tactile Perception

Since Molyneux raised the question of the relation between tactile and visual
perception, scholars have been interested in research into the capacity of tactile perception and into what can be interpreted by touch. Very simply, tactile
perception can be defined in the following way: Everything that is tangible
can be perceived by touch, but perceiving significance, and especially understanding the picture's overall meaning, is more complex. It is one thing to

feel the shape of an object and another to interpret it. This is generally in analogy with picture interpretation: being able to identify single elements in a picture does not mean being able to interpret it as a meaningful whole (see also Chapter 8). To enable correct interpretation, a tactile picture should be made with distinct shapes, and the object should preferably be depicted from the front, from the side, or from above or below. Tactile reading is rarely something that children discover spontaneously; usually children have to learn how to touch to derive some information from the pictures.

However, outline pictures explored by touch follow the same principles as outline pictures examined by the eye; the line stands for surface boundaries (Kennedy, 2000, p. 67). Furthermore, results indicate that blind people are able to use mental representations to analyze visuospatial patterns, although their performance may be less effective in complex tasks and the process may take longer (Cornoldi and Vecchi, 2000, p.148). Consequently, graphics displaying visuospatial phenomena and those portraying objects can be represented in tactile pictures. However, sighted and blind people have similar mental images, since mental images are generated by integration of linguistic, haptic, and visual information. Blind people compensate for the lack of sight by using touch (Klintberg, 2007). I suggest that tactile pictures help blind people to create mental images just as visual pictures stimulate mental images for the sighted.

Tactile Pictures

Tactile pictures for blind people are simple outline drawings made by raised lines or with surfaces in different textures or materials that form a relief perceivable by touch. In a tactile picture, details have to be eliminated and things such as light, shadows, and perspective cannot be represented. Therefore, sighted people often experience tactile pictures as unattractive compared to visual pictures. To be able to value tactile pictures from an aesthetic point of view it is necessary to take their tactile qualities into consideration. But what are tactile aesthetics? As mentioned before, tactile aesthetics result when the picture is made to carry tactile perception.

Pictures can be divided into two kinds: those that portray things that are essentially visuospatial and those that represent things that are not inherently visual. Maps, molecules, and architectural drawings belong to the first group; organization charts, flow diagrams, and graphs belong to the second group. In pictures for the blind, there has been a predominance of pictures that portray objects, and fewer abstract pictures that do not directly refer to something concrete in the environment. This could be explained by the fact that tactile pictures originally were meant to give blind children a deeper understanding of actual objects. In written sources from the early

20th century, teachers often express how they use tactile pictures to control the perception of objects and phenomena—in the sense that they have access to something tangible that could be used by teachers as a building block for further explanations. The ideas about a direct correlation between reality and its representation are very well represented in the dominant pedagogy for teaching to blind children. It is very rare that a teacher would let blind children explore tactile pictures by themselves and make their own interpretation. Teachers often correct the children and tell them what is in the picture, regardless of whether misinterpretations are important or not.

Technology for Production of Tactile Figures and Tactile Picture Books

The technology for production of tactile pictures has varied and so has the material used. The technology is partly dependent on technological development, and that has affected the material and style of the pictures. But tactile pictures follow the tradition from the late 19th century in many ways. When production of tactile pictures was initiated in the late 18th century, the pictures consisted of embossed figures made of paper. The tactile pictures were printed on heavy, good quality paper. Molds of various shapes were used; early molds were carved out of wood. Later this method was developed so that different materials could be used for the molds, and so a more distinct relief was achieved. These molds produced relief pictures with several levels and unbroken surfaces. Other producers of relief pictures only made contour drawings (Eriksson, 1998). Later, during the 1960s, paper was replaced by plastic. The molds looked pretty much the same, and a thermoform was used to shape the plastic around the mold.

Today there are mainly three kinds of techniques for tactile picture; swell papers, silk screen, and application books. Swell paper is a paper that is covered with an emulsion. The paper can be put in a regular ink printer; to get raised lines and surfaces one has to expose the paper to infrared light. The parts that have ink on them will rise. The silkscreen method is the same as for regular silkscreen printing, the only difference being that one has to use a thicker film and a paint that dries quickly, so the paint will remain thick in order to give a raised surface or line. In tactile pictures for young children, silkscreen print is often combined with motifs made by applications, where different materials are used to make the pictures more exciting to touch.

Tactile books for children are mainly made in the application technique in combination with silkscreen. Large sheets are printed in silkscreen with color and transparent ink that gives raised surface or lines. The large sheets are cut into the required size. The figures are designed and cut with computer-controlled laser cutting techniques. Therefore the designer has to draw the pictures digitally. Since different parts of an object or figure are represented in different materials, the figures are cut out in different pieces. The laser cutter can handle several layers of a material at the same time, which allows for numerous editions, and the pieces are arranged on the sheet so as to use up most of the material. The next step is accomplished by the designer, who glues the single parts on the printed carbon sheet. The last step is to bind the book with a wire. This is an expensive and demanding production compared to swell paper. To stimulate the interest in tactile pictures among children, the Swedish Library of Talking Books and Braille has decided to give priority to application books.

Tactile Story Picture Books

To break the tradition of only offering tactile pictures in the educational context, production of tactile picture books for preschool children was initiated at the Swedish Library of Talking Books and Braille in the early 1990s (Eriksson, 1997a,b). Since the library's policy is to make printed books accessible for people with reading disabilities, the tactile storybooks have to be made from already existing books. So there was never a discussion about producing books specifically made for blind children. From the beginning there was a demand from teachers that the content of the storybooks should be naturalistic so that the objects in the pictures could be found in the environment. The preschool teachers with whom the library collaborated emphasized the importance of a direct relation between the representation and the represented object or phenomenon. The books are made in different materials and in bright colors so that individuals who have some sight can read them.

Since the late 1950s, Swedish children's books have focused on the children's perspective and to a great extent omitted stories with a moral. In the 1970s, books for very young children became popular, and Gunilla Wolde was a pioneer with books about the boy Totte. In 2006, one of the books was transformed into the tactile picture book *Totte bakar* (Totte bakes). I will here analyze the tactile picture book without consideration to the visual book.

The cover of the book shows a bowl and a whisk in silkscreen relief. The title and the author's name are written in transparent Braille, printed in silkscreen. The book starts with a presentation of Totte (Figure 9.1). The tactile picture is made of different materials and with laser-cut details; this makes for a sharp and clear outline. The scale in which the boy is made is unnecessarily small. A larger representation of the boy would have facilitated tactile reading. It is very hard to recognize details such as eyes, mouth, and ears. But since Totte will be shown later in the book together with other objects, there is no room for a bigger figure. However, in my research I have found that scale does not matter in the same way for tactile perception as for vision (Y. Eriksson, unpublished). But this is in relation to other objects; it is not possible to change the scale of an object from page to page within a book. That is because touch gives a physical experience of the object and affects the

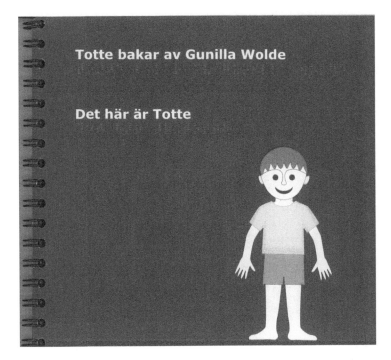

FIGURE 9.1
From the tactile picture book: Totte bakar (Totte Bakes) by Gunilla Wolde. Tactile pictures by
Annica Norberg. Produced by the Swedish Library of Talking Books and Braille.

bodily memory. Therefore, Totte has to appear in a small size in this first
picture.

From the text we can read that Totte put an egg, a package of sugar, flour,
and butter on the table before he starts. All these things are represented in
the picture. However, the scale differs from object to object. Children are
often more concentrated on interpreting the actual object, and very rarely
compare the sizes of the objects; otherwise the exercises focus on size comparison. In the next pictures the equipment is shown. The bowls and the cup
are represented in cross-section, because a bowl and a cup are things to fill
up (Figure 9.2). In the following pictures we follow Totte while he is putting
on his apron, cracking the egg, whisking, tasting the cake mixture, and putting it in the oven. The door of the oven can be opened and closed, and the
bowl in the oven is represented in cross-section, which is a great mistake
because it is shown empty and not with the cake mixture. I will consider this
mistake as an example of the producer's and the actual designer's inconsistent understanding of tactile perception. They use conventions for tactile
representations worked out from research based on blind children's own
drawings. But they have not carefully thought of the meaning of bodily
experience that is offered from touch. In tactile picture making there must be

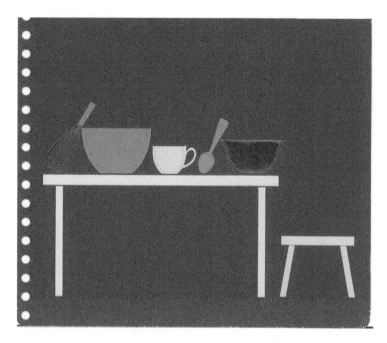

FIGURE 9.2
From the tactile picture book: Totte bakar (Totte Bakes) by Gunilla Wolde. Tactile pictures by Annica Norberg. Produced by the Swedish Library of Talking Books and Braille.

a triangular experience from touch, conventions from visual pictures, and the combination of touch and visual references. When those three aspects are fulfilled we have a high quality and aesthetic tactile picture.

Transferring visual pictures into tactile ones is challenging. The challenge could be divided or identified on different levels, the producer's perspective level and the image level. What happens to the visual quality when the pictures are adapted to tactile perception? Since there is an essential difference between the conditions for visual and tactile perception, the pictures must be changed. The visual qualities can hardly be kept, but the tactile pictures can still have considerable artistic qualities based on the original pictures. But the question is: how much, and in which ways? How to maintain the visual qualities in the tactile version? If the tactile version of a visual picture is regarded as a map of the original image, the comparison between the two will affect how we interpret the tactile version. We will probably accept the picture as an overview of the visual illustration and appreciate its appearance. From the producer's or the designer's perspective, it will be helpful to use the map metaphor. I will illustrate this by discussing an example from a book by the Swedish artist Ivar Arosenius (1878–1909), who wrote and illustrated the book *Kattresan* (The Cat's Journey, Arosenius, 1909), a classic children's book, very well known and read in Sweden for many decades.

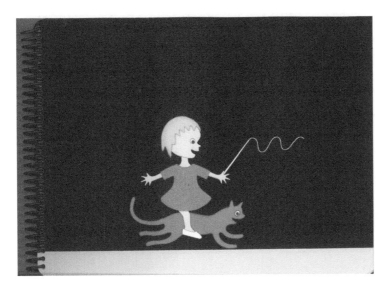

FIGURE 9.3
From the tactile picture book: Kattresan (The Cat's Journey) by Ivar Arosenius. Tactile pictures by Eva P. Eriksson. Produced by the Swedish Library of Talking Books and Braille.

The designer has painstakingly tried to be faithful to Arosenius' artistic expression. The tactile pictures are also made in a playful and abstract style. But there is hardly any resemblance between the original version and the tactile book (Figure 9.3). How come? An easy answer would be: because of the adaptation to the tactile perception. This is not true; it has to do with an inconsistent imitation of the illustrations. If the producer and the designer had used the map metaphor, they would have found the crucial nodes for the figures. The two main figures in the book are the little girl and the cat. The cat is depicted in an abstract manner in the original book and in the tactile book, but not in the same way. Arosenius kept the characteristics of a cat, while the tactile picture is missing that point (Figure 9.4). The cat in the tactile picture book is not anchored in its body; it is a flat figure sailing around in the book sheet. That is because the legs are incorrectly depicted. The designer and the producer used Arosenius' pictures of a cat as a model, but they did not stick to the original figure. It is, in fact, an interpretation of the visual pictures that is represented in the tactile book. If they had considered the tactile picture as a map of the visual picture, details such as the angle of the legs and the shift in the tail from situation to situation throughout the book would have been taken into consideration. From the reader's point of view, it should have been possible to get an experience of a relaxed, deeply sleeping cat in the book's last picture. Now the tail of the cat is in the same position as if the cat were hunting. From the producer's (and the designer's) perspective, the ambition was to make it possible for the reader to recognize the cat throughout the story, but from an image perspective the cat in the

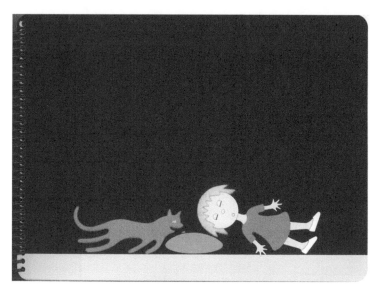

FIGURE 9.4
From the tactile picture book: Kattresan (The Cat's Journey) by Ivar Arosenius. Tactile pictures by Eva P. Eriksson. Produced by the Swedish Library of Talking Books and Braille.

tactile picture has no similarity with the original cat, and from the readers' perspective, one would hardly experience any differences in relation to shift of mode or expressions in the different pictures.

The storybook *Historien om någon* (Story about Someone) is one of the first modern Swedish storybooks for children presented from a child's point of view, rather than a story with a moral. The book has been republished and is still on the market. The pictures represent everyday objects that are familiar to children, sighted and blind. In the book there is a main theme that runs through the whole story, from page to page. There were two reasons for making this book into a tactile picture book: first, the pictures contain objects that can easily be recognized by blind children, and second, it is a classic storybook and therefore will stimulate inclusion in contemporary children's culture. It is not just the story in *Historien om någon* that transmits a modern cultural heritage: the pictures refer to 1950s Swedish design and specifically to one of the more dominant and influential designers at that time, Stig Lindberg. In the book's second page we see his well-known porcelain on the table. The interiors represented in the book are typical of that time, a mixture of modern and traditional. But what is left in the tactile picture book of visual culture history? Hardly anything, I would say. Yet, the tactile picture book has a lot of aesthetic qualities that appeal to the pleasure of touch. I will here give some examples.

I start with the opening with the overturned table and the knitting on the floor, since the knitting is crucial for the story (Figure 9.5). We can see how the yarn crosses the room and continues through the door. The interiors, as

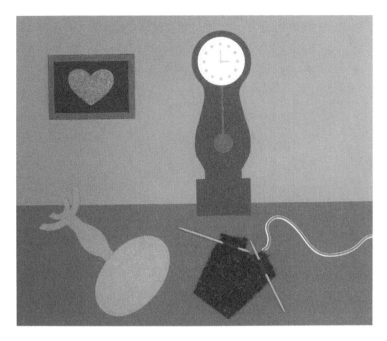

FIGURE 9.5
From the tactile picture book: Historien om någon (Story about Someone) by Åke Löfgren. Tactile pictures by Eva P. Eriksson. Produced by the Swedish Library of Talking Books and Braille.

mentioned before, are rich in details. In the corresponding opening in the tactile picture book, a lot of the interiors are left out to facilitate the tactile perception. We see the overturned table, the grandfather's clock, and a simple picture on the wall. The grandfather's clock is easy to interpret tactually because of the very distinct relief marks and hands. The shape of the clock does not correspond to that in the original book, but it could easily have been made similar. The designers of the tactile picture book made up the motif of the pictures, because they wanted to present something that could be easily read by touch. The table in the tactile picture book is more or less a copy of the one in the original book, and so is the knitting. For tactile reading, the table is hard to interpret since it is shown in an atypical shape, and children today do not have much experience with that kind of table design—especially blind children, because they never had access to visual representations of older furniture. The picture elements that have been chosen are mentioned in the text, except for the grandfather's clock. Many blind children have interpreted the knitting as a carpet.

The reader follows the yarn into the kitchen and finds that two fishes have been eaten. The interiors show a 1950s kitchen with a checkered floor, cupboards with sliding doors, a stove, and a pantry. Visually, the picture is simple, but tactually it is full of details that are hard to interpret. Therefore, the picture is divided in two parts. In the first part we see the stove with a pan on the top.

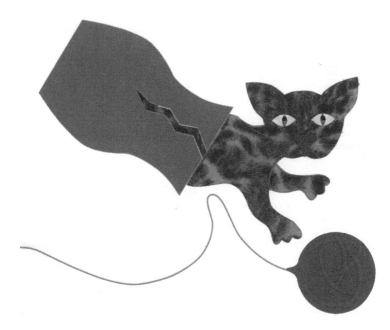

FIGURE 9.6
From the tactile picture book: Historien om någon (Story about Someone) by Åke Löfgren. Tactile pictures by Eva P. Eriksson. Produced by the Swedish Library of Talking Books and Braille.

On the floor there are the remains of two fish. In the next picture, the yarn continues into the pantry, and a carafe is shown overturned.

In the last part of the storybook, the reader follows the yarn up to the loft where there is disorder and a lot of old lumber, before the cat is found in a closet (Figure 9.6). If we compare the visual picture with the tactile one, we find that the disorder has been transformed into order. In a picture storybook, text and pictures interact. If we change the pictures we somehow change the story. In a tactile book, the reader misses all the additional information.

How Does the Reader Understand the Book?

In a reading situation with an adult reading together with a child, the actual storybook often has two functions. First, the book tells a story read by the adult, and second, the pictures support the tale and stimulate discussion about the content of the book. In addition, the story and the illustrations also inspire dialogues about the child's previous experiences. Compared to verbal representations, pictures have a unique ability to stimulate a child's memories and associations and hence generate possibilities for reflection on emotions and incidents or events. According to Vygotskij, the child perceives details in the environment that are familiar (Vygotskij, 1981). The same condition is to be found in picture perception; if a child is familiar with oranges, he or she will interpret a round orange object as the fruit. This does not contradict the fact that pictures encourage children's personal interpretation of a visual artifact.

Historien om någon has been studied in a situation with a congenitally blind girl reading the tactile picture book together with her mother (Domincovic et al., 2006). We, a teacher of Braille and a teacher specialized in teaching by reading aloud, met the girl and her mother four times and let them read the same book. The reading session was videotaped and analyzed from the data collected. When we taped the reading session, the girl was 4.5 old and had had some previous experience of tactile picture books from a daycare center. The reading session took place in their home. Mother and daughter were sitting in a sofa side by side.

The read-aloud session begins with the mother asking the girl, named Anna, if she wants to hear *Historien om någon*. When Anna says yes, the mother takes her hands and shows her the Braille letters on the cover and the upraised red yarn. Anna takes the initiative to start reading by turning over to the first page in the book. Anna starts to touch the coat on the hanger. Anna asks her mother: What is this? The mother takes the opportunity to start reading. By putting Anna's fingers on different parts of the page when they are mentioned in the text, the mother makes Anna aware of different details in the picture. When Anna is told that the object she first recognized was a coat, the following discussion took place:

The mother:	What is this?
Anna:	What is it?
The mother:	A coat.
Anna:	With buttonholes.
The mother:	Yes.
Anna:	But there are no buttons in the coat.
The mother:	It only feels like buttonholes.
Anna:	Turn over the next page.

Because of production technique reasons, we could not make buttons on the coat. But as we can see, we were naïve when we thought that a hole could appear as a button to the touch.

Anna often rests her hands on the tactile pictures while listening to the story read by her mother. When the mother finishes a page she starts asking about different details in the picture. Anna always initiates turning the page. The first time they read the book she comments on the yarn and says: Here

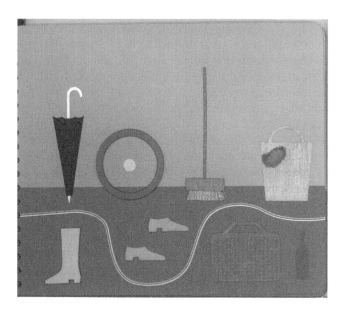

FIGURE 9.7
From the tactile picture book: Historien om någon (Story about Someone) by Åke Löfgren. Tactile pictures by Eva P. Eriksson. Produced by the Swedish Library of Talking Books and Braille.

is different yarn. After they have read the first part of the book, Anna corrects herself and says: Here the yarn continues.

Anna is exposed to the picture showing the loft with a lot of things—a bicycle wheel, bags, a broom, an umbrella, shoes, and a bottle (Figure 9.7). When the mother has finished reading the accompanying text, the girl starts to investigate the picture page. She begins with the wheel, and spontaneously interprets it as a tunnel. For those who are not familiar with spatial training of blind children, it may seem odd to interpret the wheel as a tunnel. But for the girl this is very logical, because in preschool she experienced crawling in a circular tunnel in the playroom, and she immediately recognizes the shape of the entrance. Her experience of bicycle wheels is scarcer. But when the mother tells her that it is a bicycle wheel, she can recognize the object as a wheel. The other picture element that she paid attention to was the broom. She first discovered the brush and then the broomstick, and spontaneously exclaimed, "Broom."

How come she could recognize and identify elements in the picture as representations of objects? First of all, the objects are represented in such a way that the perceptual and the physical shapes are very similar, which of course is paramount for recognizing a tactile representation as a representation of a familiar object. Second, she used her experience and, we assume, organized her thinking into different domains or categories. Categories can be defined according to their properties. The property the girl recognized was the circular shape:

1. When she first discovered the wheel, she thought of it as a circular shape.
2. The circular shape made it distinct from the umbrella to the left (which she could not identify).
3. The circular shape of the bicycle wheel reminded the girl of the entrance to the tunnel she had experienced; the tunnel resembled the element in the picture.
4. She put the object into the category of circular shapes.

When talking about visual images, we need to be aware of the interplay between categories and singular representations. We need to use this interplay in order to create images of objects depicted in such a way that they simultaneously can represent a specific object and function as a representation of a specific category. From the very beginning, children with visual impairment (blindness) need to learn what characterizes different categories of objects, animals, and human beings. Otherwise they will not be able to identify specific objects by touch.

There is great hope and belief in visual communication to overcome language obstacles and to provide overviews. Pictures are valuable tools in the learning process, for communication between teachers and pupils and between mates. The enthusiasm for all kinds of pictures rests on the belief that they benefit comprehension and learning and foster insight. As Barbara Tversky (2004, 2005) shows, visual representations relieve the pressure on memory because they externalize memory and reduce the processing load by allowing the assembling to be done on external representations rather than internal representations. That reduces the use of working memory. But we do not know whether tactile pictures have the same function concerning working memory. Pictures and illustrations have long been used for instructions. Research shows that action-oriented instruction from the user perspective is the most effective way of representing instructions, since the reader can identify with the acting subject. The picture book *Totte bakar* shows a user perspective. For sighted children who regularly learn from imitating, the action-oriented user perspective is customary. For blind children it is not. Therefore I argue that the representation of Totte in the tactile picture book is unnecessary. For a young blind child, his representation in the actual situation does not relate to the different parts of the story. He or she will understand the story from what could be defined as an egocentric perspective. If the designer had focused on the representation of the objects, the tactile aesthetics could have been fulfilled. Now the details are far too small to suite tactile perception. Blind children are more used to meeting the represented environment as presented in *Historien om någon*, that is, an object spread over a picture surface and no action orientation. There are several fields of applications for tactile pictures, but there is very little research published about their design.

In the reading situation discussed in this chapter, it is clear that the girl refers to previous experience when she interprets the pictures, and that the pictures work as a platform for further discussion about the object and about emotions. The third time we met Anna and her mother, Anna stopped at the picture showing a broken bowl. She was upset and started to ask if someone had been angry about the broken bowl. The mother tried to hide Anna's interest in the picture by ignoring her question and urged her to turn to the next page. It was clear that something had happened since the last reading session; probably Anna had broken something and the picture of the smashed bowl brought up memories. She wanted to talk about the occurrence, but her mother did not want to continue the discussion in front of us. However, this small episode indicates that tactile pictures as well as visual pictures can stimulate memories and interest, foster insight about how objects look and relate to each other, and arouse pleasure.

Scientific Tactile Pictures and Maps

Scientific illustration belongs to the category of instrumental images, pictures that have an intended function. The aim could be to portray things or to show relations or functions. The purpose of the illustration often determines the character of the picture. In order to portray an object, the picture has to be naturalistic, while relations are often represented in abstract graphs or diagrams. The tradition of making instrumental tactile pictures follows the same rules as for visual pictures. Most scientific illustrations for tactile reading have been produced for textbooks in subjects like biology, botany, physics, chemistry, and geometry. Illustrations in biology and botany require naturalistic depictions. In subjects like physics, chemistry, and geometry, the illustrations represent relations and objects or phenomena that could not be perceived by the eyes, or by touch. Those pictures are often abstract. There has been a discussion of the benefits; the discussion has blossomed anew many times over the last 100 years, and has affected the frequency of tactile pictures in textbooks and in Braille books over the years (Eriksson, 1998). But still there has been a continuity of scientific tactile picture production from the late 19th century.

It is obvious that there has been a great interest in tactile pictures of the body in textbooks, nonfiction books, and books for professionals such as physiotherapists and chiropractors. Tactile pictures showing the body must be considered as a map of the body; this is pretty much the same as in illustrations of the body for sighted people. The pictures illustrate where organs, muscles, bones, and so on are placed in the body. However, as in a map, the different parts of the body should be indicated either by the name on the actual part of the body or by a number or letter explained in an accompanying list. The full name is preferred since it gives a direct experience and understanding of the location and relations to other parts of the body. But Braille is very space consuming, and it is often impossible to place the full name of an organ or a body part on the part depicted. The Braille will break up the shape of the depicted part, which makes interpretation difficult. There have been different solutions for that problem; one has been to make two copies, one with Braille, one without. The reader can interpret the entire picture and its parts, and learn the appearance of details and the relations between different parts. In the second picture it is possible to read the names of the different parts. From interviews with Braille readers (Y. Eriksson, unpublished) we know that this solution is not successful. Many readers experience two different contents; they find it hard to relate the two versions to each other. This could be explained by the fact that the shapes, or the outlines, of the different parts of the body change when the Braille is added. Therefore it is preferable to indicate the name(s) with the initial letter(s), which provides direct association to the name. When the readers have learned the contractions, they can easily remember the full name. Reading tactile pictures is a bodily experience, and the interpretation act is related to the body axes, and from those the reader remembers and recognizes different parts in the tactile picture (Millar, 1997, 2008).

The body is something we all have a relation to since we are the body. Therefore a map of the body is easier to relate to than a topographical map. However, many maps that are produced for Braille readers have been requested by the users. They want a map of the actual surroundings, to use either as a mobility map or to get an overview. Others want to have a map of travel destinations, a place they are going to visit on vacation. It is common for tactile maps to be simplified as compared to visual maps. Even a tactile map that looks very simplified could be hard to interpret. One has to keep in mind that interpreting and using a map is a multilayered activity; first the person has to define his or her position in the surroundings, then find the spot on the map that represents the area, and third, interpret and understand the relation between the environment and the map. Finally, the person should be able to navigate in the surroundings with help from the map. The map in Figure 9.8 was made on demand from a Braille reader in Stockholm. It shows a limited area of one of the central parts of the city. The building blocks are marked with dotted surfaces, and the streets in-between are left open. The open space between the blocks facilitates tactile reading, allows one to easily follow the smooth surface, and makes it possible to put Braille letters on the actual streets. Since the street names include many letters, only the initial letters are represented on the map. The map is accompanied by a key with full names. The crossroads with traffic lights are indicated by a circular shape with a Braille symbol in it.

Strategies for Braille reading and for interpretation of tactile pictures have mainly been studied separately. A project called "Tactile reading" was

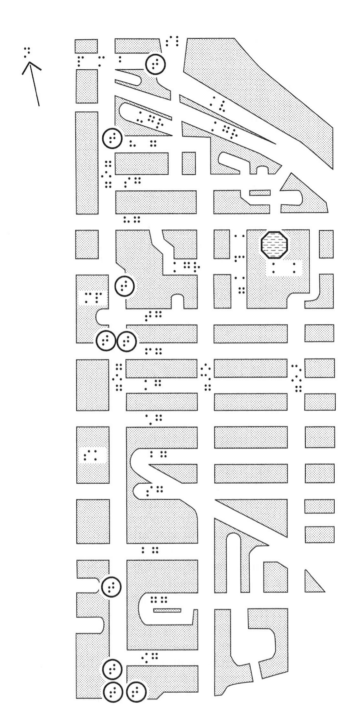

FIGURE 9.8
Tactile map of the area Slussen in Stockholm.

launched in the Centre for Languages and Literature at Lund University*—integrated in a new multidisciplinary laboratory environment for the study of languages, culture, communication, and cognition (Breidegard et al., 2006). The aim of this project was to study Braille reading, the interaction between Braille and tactile pictures, comparisons of tactile reading behavior in children and adults, and a contrastive study of tactile and visual reading. Twenty-six Braille readers were tested and registered in the whole project. A new registration technique called "motion tracker" was used. The technique has been used before in linguistic research to register gestures, for instance when people are talking. The motion tracker that was used in the project had up to eight infrared cameras that filmed the measurement area from different angles. Small markers were applied on the subjects' fingers reflecting infrared light emitted from lamps inside the cameras. By viewing these markers from different positions, the system is able to create a 3-D measurement of the movement of each reflector. Markers were attached on each fingernail on both hands of the subject except for the thumbs, and also on the knuckles, in order to register the movements of the height of the hand during reading. The data have then been processed by an interactive program and visualized for analysis. The collected data include finger and hand movements when reading different tactile materials in Braille. One of the tasks given to the 26 subjects who participated in the study was a typical school task for third graders including a tactile map followed by multiple-choice answers in Braille. The tactile map in the test was a modified version of the map in the reading test for sighted children. In our test the fictive map of the island was made considering tactile perception (Eriksson et al., 2003). The map was made in swell paper; it had a headline with the following text: "The Island. Use this map to answer the questions." In the upper left, a compass card is represented by a cross with arrows showing the four cardinal points. The island is surrounded by a texture used for representing water. A distinct contour line defines the shape of the island, and different textures are used to symbolize different areas of the island: a park, a forest, a lake, and a marsh. A squared pattern is used to indicate the town in the island. A farm is indicated by a single square. Three distinct roads connect the different parts of the island; two of the roads are named and indicated in Braille. For the registration, all pages had to be fastened to the table, which resulted in a rather unnatural reading position. The map was placed on the top of the table, and the questions in Braille in two columns were located under the island. The participants were asked to follow the instructions (i.e., to solve the exercises). Some of the participants started to explore the map carefully, and some of them noticed the map symbols and their interrelations. Others focused only on the Braille, and a few of them spent a long time exploring the map but did not notice the spatial relations. One of the results from the study was clear: problem solving was facilitated when the participant noticed

---

* www.sol.lu.se

the spatial relations, the map symbols, and the Braille from the beginning. They used less time to answer the questions, all of which were about relations and locations in the map.

Tactile Pictures for Pleasure and Decoration

The Swedish Library for Talking Books and Braille publishes wall calendars for sale. The calendar for 2012 has motives from nature. It contains flowers and one insect. Each flower has a connection with a classic novel, from different ages, presented on the back of the calendar's page that represents it. The ambition was to find plants that are more or less of the same size to be able to represent them in the same scale. This idea was inspired by representations for plants in the early education of the blind (Eriksson, 1998). The plants are produced in swell paper with colored ink (Figure 9.9). One new plant is presented each month, except for December when a door beetle is represented (Figure 9.10). This is because of the literature tip of the month, which is a Christmas story about a door beetle. The characteristic of the tactile pictures in the wall calendar is their relation to the tradition of handbooks of plants, insects, and birds. Every detail is named, such as leaf, flower, berry, fruit, and so on. This makes it possible to get an idea of the plants'

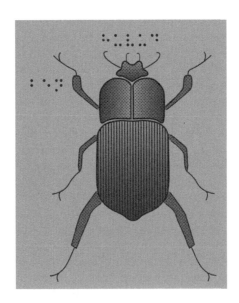

FIGURE 9.9
From the Swedish Library for Talking Books and Braille wall calendar 2012, door beetle, for the month of June.

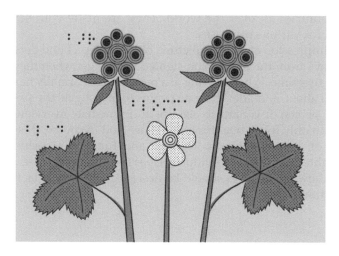

FIGURE 9.10
From the Swedish Library for Talking Books and Braille wall calendar 2012, cloudberry, for the month of April.

different stages, from bud to flower to seed. The colored ink makes the calendar attractive for sighted people, but would be less accessible for partially sighted people because the colors are represented by shadings. The calendar will fulfil a need among many people with visual impairment, to decorate their wall with something that is enjoyable both by sight and by touch.

Conclusions

The relation between the producer, the picture book, and the reader has been analyzed in this chapter. If by visual communication we mean visual artifacts, architecture, gestures, and mimicry, unmediated visual communication is not possible for blind persons. But via tactile pictures it is possible to gain access to visual symbols that are used for pictorial representations. Tactile pictures have two main functions for congenitally blind persons: first, to give access to the appearance of objects that would otherwise not be perceivable; second, to gain knowledge about the way a picture of an object appears and thus to mediate the visual culture. Furthermore, tactile pictures are often necessary in many school subjects—especially at the university level. Therefore, it is important that blind children have access to tactile pictures at an early age. In addition, tactile maps are the only way for a blind person to get a topographical overview. Today, different kinds of tactile images and maps are produced in many countries all over the world. They are made with several techniques and for various purposes.

The first impression of a tactile picture, observed by a blind person, differs in many ways from the impression sighted people get when they see a picture for the first time. When looking at a picture, one normally has an idea of what it is all about, and after that one begins to investigate the single details. For a blind person, it is hard to acquire an immediate overview by touch, since one can only touch one thing at a time. And of course, this affects the perception of a representation. The use and function of pictures differs between sighted and blind individuals. Does the difference make sense? Yes, in terms of how the pictures should be designed and of how tactile reading should be stimulated.

References

Arosenius, I. 1909/2004. *Kattresan: Bilderbok*. Stockholm: Bonnier Carlsen. http://karlsson.ownit.nu/kattresan/

Baumgarten, A. G. 1735/1954. *Reflections on Poetry: Alexander Gottlieb Baumgarten's Meditationes philosophicae de Nonnullis Ad Poema Pertinentibus*. Translation by Karl Achenbrenner & William B. Holter. Berkeley: University California Press.

Bertelson, P., Mousty, P., and D'Alimonte, G. 1985. A study of Braille reading, 2: Patterns of hand activity in one-handed and two-handed reading. *Quarterly Journal of Experimental Psychology* 37:235–256.

Breidegard, B., Jönsson, B., Fellenius, K., and Strömqvist, S. 2006. Disclosing the secret of Braille reading: Computer-aided registration and interactive analysis. *Visual Impairment Research* 8:49–59.

Carlsson, A-L. 2010. The aesthetic and the poetic elements of information design. *Information Visualization (IV)* 14th International Conference. London.

Cornoldi, C. and Vecchi, T. 2000. Mental imagery in blind people: The role of passive and active visuospatial processes. *Touch, Representation, and Blindness*. Ed. M. A. Heller, pp. 143–182. Oxford: Oxford University Press.

Dervin, B. 1999. Chaos, order, and sense-making: A proposed theory for information design. *Informationon Design*. Ed. R. Jacobson, pp. 35–58. Mass.: MIT Press.

Diderot, D. 1749. *Lettre Sur les Aveugles, à l'usage de Ceux Qui Voyent*. Paris: Gale ECCO.

Domincovic, K., Eriksson, Y., and Fellenius, K. 2006. *Högläsning för Barn*. Lund: Studentlitteratur.

Eriksson, Y. 1997a. *Att Känna Bilder*. Solna: SIH Läromedel.

Eriksson, Y. 1997b. *Från Föremål Till Taktil Bild*. Solna: SIH Läromedel.

Eriksson, Y. 1998. *Tactile Pictures. Pictorial Representations for the Blind*, Diss. Göteborg: Acta Universitatis Gothoburegensis.

Eriksson, Y. 1999. The mythology of the blind and womens place in history. Deuxième confeérnce internationale sur les aveugles dans l'histoire et l'histore des aveugles, Paris: Institute de Valentin Haüy.

Eriksson, Y. 2003. *What Is the History of Tactile Pictures? Art Beyond Sight. A Resource Guide to Art, Creativity, and Visual Impairment.* New York: AFB Press.

Eriksson, Y., Jansson, G., and Strucel, M. 2003. *Tactile Maps. Guidelines for the Production of Maps for the Visually Impaired*, Enskede: Punktskriftsnämnen.

Heller, T. 1895. Studien zur Blinden-Psychologie. *Philosophische Studien*, Ed. Wilhelm Wundt. Leipzig: Verlag von Wilhelm Engelmann.

Kant, I. 1787/1952. *The Critique of Judgment.* Translation by James Creel Meredith. Chicago: Encyclopedia Britannica.

Kennedy, J. M. 2000. Recognizing outline pictures via touch: Alignment theory. *Touch, Representation, and Blindness.* Ed. M.A. Heller, pp. 67–98. Oxford: Oxford University Press.

Katz, D. 1925/1989. *The World of Touch.* New Jersey: LEA.

Klintberg, T. 2007. *Den översvämmade Hjärnan.* Stockholm: Natur&Kultur.

Knowlton, M. and Wetzel, R. 1996. Braille reading rates as a function of reading tasks. *Journal of Visual Impairment and Blindness* 3:227–236.

Millar, S. 1997. *Reading by Touch.* London: Routledge.

Millar, S. 2008. *Space and Sense.* Oxford: Psychology Press Ltd.

Rose, G. 2007.*Visual Methodologies: An Introduction to Interpreting Visual Materials*, second edition, London: Sage.

Tversky, B. 2004. Semantic, syntax, and pragmatics of graphics. *Language and Visualization.* Eds. Y. Eriksson and K. Holmqvist, pp. 141–158. Lund: Lund University Press.

Tversky, B. 2005. Functional significance of visuospatial representations. *Handbook of Higher-Level of Visuospatial Thinking.* Eds. P. Shah and A. Miyake, pp. 1–34. Cambridge: Cambridge University Press.

Vygotskij, L. 1981. *Psykologi Och Dialektik.* Stockholm: Norstedts Förlag.

10

Camera-Based Access to Visual Information

James Coughlan and Roberto Manduchi

CONTENTS

Introduction

Computer vision (also known as machine vision) is a form of artificial intelligence that strives to make computers able to "see" like normally sighted persons. The basic approach consists of analyzing visual information taken of a scene—either a static image or a video sequence, acquired by one or more cameras—and using software algorithms to infer important visual elements in the scene, including the presence, location, and appearance of various objects and the three-dimensional (3-D) scene layout.

While computer vision is far from a solved problem, and is in fact the subject of intensive research, the last several decades of progress have led to a variety of successful algorithms, including OCR (optical character recognition), object recognition (including face recognition), 3-D reconstruction of objects and other structures, and video analysis and event recognition. As we describe in more detail below, such algorithms drive a wide range of practical applications, many of them used in commercial products and equipment. Moreover, as computers become ever more powerful and compact, they make possible mobile platforms that deliver the power of computer vision to the fingertips of any smartphone (such as an iPhone or Android) owner.

The potential to harness computer vision to provide access to visual information that is otherwise inaccessible to visually impaired persons is extremely exciting and promising. However, important limitations of computer vision technology make it challenging to provide this kind of access. First, computer vision is successful in restricted domains but is often unreliable outside these domains, under the various types of highly variable and uncontrolled conditions that are commonly encountered by users "in the field." (For instance, OCR often fails unless the text to be read is a standard font that has been imaged clearly, which is often a problem for reading text printed on signs, which we discuss below.) Second, it is not yet capable of the truly high level of inference that would be desirable to many users—such as taking a picture of a scene and asking the computer "How do I get to the conference room?" or "Is there a place to sit nearby?" Finally, various hardware and processing constraints such as the limited field of view of the camera (which makes it difficult for a visually impaired user to locate an object of interest) and delays incurred by computer vision processing pose additional challenges to the design of an effective user interface for any computer vision-based assistive technology. The aim of this chapter is thus to provide an overview of what computer vision does well, to survey the applications that have been most successful for visually impaired users, and to discuss the most important usability issues that must be considered in developing these applications. Similar material, but aimed more specifically at a computer science audience, is discussed in Manduchi and Coughlan (2012), and is the topic of an ongoing workshop series organized by the authors, Computer Vision Applications for Visual Impairment (CVAVI), which was previously held in 2005 in San Diego,* in 2008 in Marseille,† and in 2010 in San Francisco.‡

---

* http://users.soe.ucsc.edu/~manduchi/CVAVI/
† http://www.ski.org/Rehab/Coughlan_lab/General/CVAVI08.html
‡ http://italia.cse.ucsc.edu/~CVAVI10/

Success Story: Optical Character Recognition

Some History

Without a doubt, the most successful image-based assistive technology to date is OCR. An OCR system uses an imaging sensor to access text (typically, printed on paper) and some "intelligence" to translate the image content into letters and words. The output of OCR can then be recorded as a text file in various formats (e.g., PDF), and/or read aloud by a text-to-speech system. Thus, OCR allows a person with visual impairment to access printed information—a tremendous achievement, considering the paramount role of printed matter in human communication. In fact, OCR may also help persons who can see but have other forms of reading disabilities.

It is remarkable that the first fully electronic OCR system ever demonstrated was intended for use by blind people. The system was built in 1946 by a research group under the direction of Flory and Pike at RCA Laboratories, with sponsorship by the Veteran Administration and the wartime Office of Scientific Research (Mann 1949). The "reading machine" would read text, spelling it out letter by letter; the machine was also able to read a few whole words. Its "eye" was a scanner moved over the text by hand, with eight spots of light aligned in a column flashing on and off 600 times a second, and a photoreceptor that would read the light reflected off the printed paper. When illuminating a text character, only a few of these spots of light would be reflected by the paper; analysis of the pattern of reflected light by a system composed by more than 160 vacuum tubes produced the character, which would then be read aloud by activating one of 40 magnetic tape phonographs.

Although this initial prototype did not find practical use (due, among other things, to its cost and size), it spurred a whole new industry with important applications. The first OCR company, Intelligent Machines, was founded by Shepard and Cook in the early 1950s. The Reading Machine, developed by Rabinow while at the National Bureau of Standards, showed improved performance through a "best match" procedure—essentially, by optically correlating each character of text against all possible alphanumerical characters. Image correlation (by digital means) has been a mainstream procedure for OCR for many years, especially for standard fonts. More recently, approaches based on pattern matching, for example, via neural networks (Le Cun et al. 1990), have been used successfully in more complex situations, such as handwritten text.

OCR quickly found extensive application in automatic document processing for business transactions and postal service (Hull et al. 1984). The development of accessible OCR systems with text-to-speech capabilities made this technology available to the visually impaired community. Two commercial products had a pivotal role in making OCR a widely used assistive technology device: the Kurzweil Reading Machine and Arkenston's OpenBook.

In 1974, Kurzweil Computer Products developed the first commercial OCR that could recognize multiple fonts. (Previous systems used standardized fonts, such as the fixed-width mono-spaced format called OCR-A.) In his book *The Age of Spiritual Machines* (Kurzweil 2000), Ray Kurzweil recalls that an encounter with a blind person on a plane flight convinced him that the best use of this technology would be to support the blind community. The Kurzweil Reading Machine, which integrated omni-font OCR with a flat-bed scanner and a text-to-speech synthesizer, was introduced with much fanfare in 1976, and made commercially available in 1979. Extensive preproduction user testing supported by the National Federation of the Blind (NFB) were undertaken to ensure that this product would really be usable by visually impaired persons. Kurzweil Computer Products was later integrated in ScanSoft (a Xerox spin-off), which eventually merged with Nuance Communication.

Arkenstone, a nonprofit organization founded in 1989 by Jim Fruchterman, also developed reading tools for people with disabilities. Arkenstone's reading system was originally based on technology by Calera Recognition System (an OCR company started by Fruchterman in 1982). It delivered OCR systems to more than 35,000 visually impaired individuals before it sold its business operations to Freedom Scientific in 2000. Arkenstone's OpenBook Scanning and Reading software (which utilizes both Nuance OmniPage and ABBYY FineReader OCR engines) is currently marketed by Freedom Scientific.

OCR by Sensory Substitution: Optacon

OCR systems translate printed text into a computer-accessible format that can then be accessed via text-to-speech. One commercial product sidestepped the middle link of this chain, seeking to provide a blind user with more direct access to text via sensory substitution. The Optacon, developed by John Linvill and marketed by Telesensory Systems from 1971 to 1996, used a 24 by 6 pixel optical sensor that was manually moved across the text line to be read. A matching array of vibrating pins was used to "feel" the text, letter by letter, with one's fingertip, from the images taken by the optical sensor. (For more information about sensory substitution systems, see Chapter 8.)

The Optacon found success with a community of devoted users, who were not intimidated by the relatively long (2 weeks) recommended training period. Typical reading speeds varied between 5 and 15 words per minute (Schoof 1975)—much lower than the typical Braille reading speed of approximately 125 words per minute. However, the Optacon provided an unprecedented level of access to printed text and to the nuances of typographic styles (Stein 1998).

Mobile OCR

While early OCR systems were very bulky and included a flat-bed scanner to image the desired text and a desktop computer to perform the necessary software analysis, vast increases in computing power have recently enabled the development of portable OCR systems. As a result, a variety of OCR smartphone apps are now available for normally sighted users, including the ABBYY TextGrabber + Translator* and the Prizmo,[†] as well as Word Lens,[‡] an "augmented reality" OCR app that reads all text visible in the camera's field of view, translates it to another language and graphically rerenders it on the viewfinder in place of the original text in the scene.

The first commercial mobile OCR system designed for visually impaired users, the knfb Reader Classic, was released in 2005 by K–NFB Reading Technology, Inc.[§] (a joint venture between Kurzweil Technologies and the NFB). This handheld system consisted of a PDA (personal digital assistant) bundled with a separate digital camera, and was soon succeeded by smartphone versions, the knfbReader Mobile and kReader Mobile. Similar functionality is provided by the Intel Reader,[¶] which is a portable tablet device intended for a variety of special needs populations, including the visually impaired and persons with dyslexia.

It is important to understand the great challenges that mobile OCR applications for visually impaired persons impose compared with standard desktop OCR, which was designed for use with high-quality images of printed documents obtained using a flat-bed scanner. First and foremost, it may be difficult or impossible for the user to know where to point the camera so as to properly frame the text of interest in the camera's field of view. Indeed, the kReader Mobile/knfbReader Mobile User Manual has an entire section on "Learning to Aim Your Reader," which includes instructions on practicing aiming the smartphone camera with a special training page. The aiming problem is especially severe if the user is unsure as to whether a sign (or other printed matter) is even present in the vicinity, as when searching a corridor for a particular room number.

Second, even if the camera is pointed toward the desired text, if it is too close then the text may be partly cropped and/or out of focus; if it is too far then the text may be too small to read clearly, and/or the OCR may be confused by the expanse of nontext scene clutter surrounding the text. Third, images of text acquired by mobile devices are often poorly resolved because the text of interest is too far away, poorly illuminated, motion blurred (often exacerbated by a long camera exposure due to low light levels, see Figure 10.1), or appears on a curved surface (e.g., the label on a can of food). Finally, much text printed on informational signs is rendered in nonstandard fonts—often combined with special symbols and commercial logos—which is difficult for OCR to read.

A large body of ongoing research is focused on addressing these challenges, illustrated in the following examples. The problem of detecting text

---

* http://www.abbyy.com/textgrabber/
[†] http://www.creaceed.com/prizmo/iphone
[‡] http://questvisual.com/
[§] http://www.knfbreader.com/
[¶] http://www.careinnovations.com/Products/Reader/Default.aspx

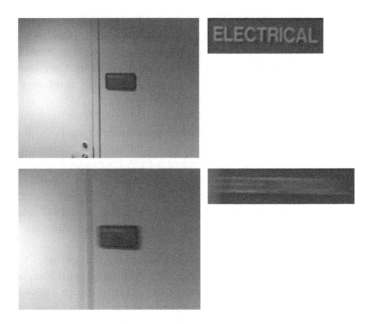

FIGURE 10.1

OCR and motion blur. Top row: clear smartphone camera image taken of indoor sign on left; zoomed-in portion on right shows that text is legible, and OCR reads it correctly. Bottom row: motion-blurred image taken by same camera on left; zoomed-in portion on right shows that text is unreadable, and OCR is unable to read it.

in cluttered scenes is an increasingly popular topic of research in computer vision and document analysis (for samples of recent work, see Epshtein et al. 2010; Chen et al. 2011; Lee et al. 2011), including work on finding text that may be too small or poorly resolved to read (Sanketi et al. 2011). Related work (Coates et al. 2011; Wang et al. 2011) seeks approaches that integrate text detection with reading to improve performance on natural scenes. Finally, specialized techniques for detecting and reading text shown in LED and LCD displays—which are becoming increasingly common in household appliances such as microwave ovens and DVD players—are being developed (Tekin et al. 2011) to provide visually impaired persons with access to these displays. Despite the considerable progress that has been accomplished in these areas, much work remains in making mobile OCR systems practical for use by visually impaired persons.

Other Semantic Information

The previous section on OCR focused on the recognition of printed text, which is the ubiquitous building block of an enormous range of documents and informational signs. However, many forms of semantic information are represented by visual patterns other than text, including stand-alone icons or signs primarily identified by the icons they bear (such as traffic signs and commercial signs), paper currency, and barcodes, which cannot be read by OCR and are therefore inaccessible to blind and visually impaired persons.

Reading Signs and Signals

Compared with OCR and text detection, relatively little research has focused specifically on the detection and recognition of nontext semantic information. Many important commercial signs (e.g., labeling stores and restaurants) are identified by distinctive nontext icons or logos, sometimes with accompanying text (which is often in a highly nonstandard font that is difficult or impossible for OCR to read). Rather than attempting to recognize such signs individually and out of context, most work on sign recognition (Mattar et al. 2005; Silapachote et al. 2005) simplifies the problem by matching an image of an unknown sign to a database of known signs, thereby constraining the recognition problem to a smaller number of possible interpretations.

An important component of research on reading nontext signs addresses the need for robots and autonomous vehicles to recognize traffic signs and signals in order to safely navigate, negotiate roads, and avoid contacting pedestrians. Of greater relevance to blind and visually impaired persons is the closely related problem of designing computer vision algorithms to find and recognize pedestrian signs and signals, including painted crosswalk patterns (Se 2000), Walk lights (Aranda and Mares 2004), or other traffic lights (Park and Jeong 2009), which are of paramount importance for pedestrian safety at traffic intersections. As discussed in Chapter 3, crossing a street is a challenging (and dangerous) undertaken without sight. In particular, one needs to be well aware of the crosswalk layout and of the flow of traffic; figure out exactly where the crosswalk begins, and align himself or herself toward the correct crossing direction; estimate the precise time for crossing; and, once starting to walk, maintain the correct direction without drifting out of the crosswalk. Walk light timing information from Accessible Pedestrian Signals is helpful in those intersections where they are installed (and some people can also use these signals to help align themselves correctly to the crosswalk), but unfortunately these signals are lacking at most intersections (Figure 10.2).

Image-based technologies may be used to both estimate the precise geometry of the crosswalk (allowing one to align correctly with it) and access information about the timing of the Walk lights, by extracting information from the signs, painted patterns, and signals that are already present in traffic intersections. Prototypes of this kind of software have been ported to smartphones, including the "Crosswatch" system for recognizing crosswalks and Walk lights in real time (Ivanchenko et al. 2009, 2010), and tests with blind users have demonstrated the feasibility of this system. However, the challenge of performing the necessary pattern recognition reliably and swiftly, under a

(a)

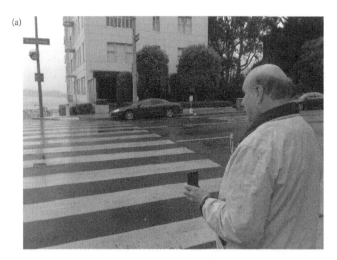

(b)

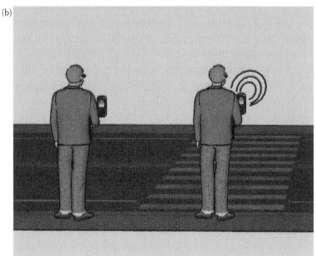

FIGURE 10.2
Crosswatch, computer vision-based smartphone system for providing guidance to visually impaired pedestrians at traffic intersections. (a) system in use by blind tester. (b) schematic shows how system provides audio cues to signal proper alignment of user to crosswalk.

wide range of operating conditions (and accommodating many variations in the appearance of pedestrian signs, signals, and crosswalks), makes the solutions proposed so far unsuitable for wide adoption.

Barcodes

The last category of nontext semantic information we consider is the barcode. The most common barcodes are one-dimensional (1-D) patterns (such as the

UPC, or "Universal Product Code," in widespread use in North America) labeling the vast majority of commercial products, which were designed to permit rapid product identification by a laser scanner. Several dedicated barcode readers have been designed for visually impaired users, such as the i.d. mate OMNI and Summit talking barcode readers (from Envision America),[*] but the growing power of smartphone technology has led to the development of barcode reader smartphone apps, such as the Red Laser iPhone app[†] intended for normally sighted users and the Digit-Eyes iPhone app[‡] designed expressly for visually impaired users. As mentioned earlier, a major challenge imposed by any barcode reader is the difficulty of a blind or visually impaired user having to find the barcode on a package before it can be read; this difficulty motivated the development of smartphone barcode readers that interactively guide the user to the barcode (Tekin and Coughlan 2010; Kutiyanawala et al. 2011). An additional difficulty of the smartphone platform is the fact that the barcode is analyzed from an image taken by the smartphone camera, which is noisier and thus harder to decode than intensity data acquired using laser scanners (for which the 1-D barcode was originally designed); as a result, research (Gallo and Manduchi 2011) has focused specifically on improving the accuracy of barcode recognition in challenging images.

Two-dimensional (2-D) barcodes (such as the QR code and Data Matrix) were designed to be read by camera-based systems rather than laser scanners, and are superior to 1-D barcodes in that they are more easily read by camera-based systems and encode more data in a smaller area. Most modern smartphones come equipped with one or more apps capable of reading QR codes, which are increasingly used in magazines, tickets, signs, billboard advertisements, and other printed matter to encode Internet links to provide additional information about the printed content. While most QR codes are targeted at normally sighted smartphone users—who find it much less difficult to locate the codes and point their cameras accurately at them than do visually impaired users—there is ongoing work on using QR codes in applications intended for visually impaired persons, such as annotating objects in a museum and identifying product packages labeled with QR codes (Al-Khalifa 2008).

Signs for Wayfinding

Another intriguing application of nontextual signs is to support blind wayfinding. Sighted persons, when in unfamiliar places, routinely use available signage for understanding their location in the environment, and for determining how to reach a destination. Signs are particularly important in environments with complex layouts such as airports, where one needs to quickly find their way in stressful and potentially confusing situations. Unfortunately,

---

[*] http://www.envisionamerica.com/products/idmate/
[†] http://redlaser.com/
[‡] http://www.digit-eyes.com/

signage is an inherently visual feature, and cannot be accessed without sight. (Braille or raised print signs are indeed accessible, but one first needs to physically reach them, which makes them useless for wayfinding in many situations.)

It is conceivable, though, that a camera may work as the "eye" of a blind person to detect existing signs. In fact, special signage that can be read efficiently by a machine may also be used for this purpose. For example, as mentioned earlier, 2-D bar codes (e.g., QR codes) are increasingly being used for smartphone-accessible information embedding. These signs are designed to pack as many bits of information as possible in a small amount of space. Similar types of signs have been used for wayfinding applications (Tjan et al. 2005). Another type of nontextual marker, with information embedded through colors, was developed by the authors (Coughlan and Manduchi 2009) and used for experiments in guided mobility (Manduchi et al. 2010; Figure 10.3). Color markers have the advantage that they require minimal computation for detection, and can be seen from a long distance even under relatively difficult light conditions (Bagherinia and Manduchi 2011).

In some cases, camera-based sign detection can also be used to estimate one's location and orientation ("pose") with respect to the sign. ARToolkit (Poupyrev et al. 2000), a 2-D barcode design standard with accompanying software developed at the University of Washington, has been employed extensively in "augmented reality" applications that use the estimated camera location to create special graphics effects visible through the viewfinder. The ability to compute and track one's relative position is an intriguing feature of image-based sign detection. This information could potentially be used to provide some local guidance to a blind person to reach a specific destination.

Other approaches currently being investigated for assisted wayfinding include embedding radio-frequency identification (RFID) tags in the environment (e.g., under carpet tiles). RFID tags, which can be accessed by a suitable device at an appropriate distance, are thus equivalent to "signs" that can be placed throughout the environment (Kulyukin et al. 2004; Ross and Reynolds 2010).

Camera-accessible signage is a promising approach to provide location-based information to persons without sight. It represents a sensible and cost-effective way to render information perceptible to all—regardless of whether one can see or not. As such, it fits well within the framework of "Universal Design," a concept that has gained increasing popularity over the past decade. Universal Design (Preiser and Ostroff 2001) aims to produce buildings, products, and environments that can be used by all (with or without disabilities), rather than having to be adapted to one's particular needs. One of the principles of Universal Design is "Perceptible Information," which states that the design should communicate "necessary information effectively to the user, regardless of ambient conditions or the user's sensory abilities." Signage that can be accessed via mobile imaging represents one sensible way to achieve this goal.

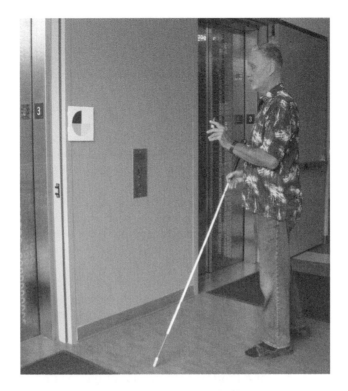

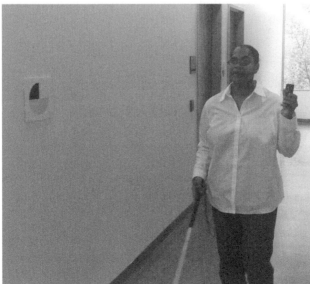

FIGURE 10.3
Wayfinding experiments using a color marker that is easily detectable by a camera-equipped smartphone.

Computer Vision for Mobility

As discussed at length in Chapter 3, mobility (the ability to move around safely and efficiently) and orientation (the ability to find a path to destination) are critical skills for a visually impaired traveler. The long cane and the dog guide are the standard mobility tools. Several ultrasonic or light-based mobility devices (electronic travel aids or ETAs) have been proposed in the past; their features and limitations are described in Chapter 3. It is only natural that researchers would consider applying image-based techniques to orientation and mobility.

Much of this effort derived from experience acquired research in autonomous robotics. After all, an autonomous robot is a "blind" agent: it needs sensors for obstacle detection, along with some level of intelligence for path planning and navigation. Reliable autonomous navigation with both wheeled and legged platforms has been demonstrated in recent years, owing much to the use of imaging and depth sensors. It would be a mistake, though, to think that by simply augmenting a sensory system with some sort of acoustic or tactile interface, a usable mobility tool for a blind traveler would be created. Humans are not robots; what works well on an autonomous navigation platform may be totally inadequate for a blind traveler. The reader is referred to the "Recommendations for the Design Process" section in Chapter 8 for a thorough discussion of the "engineering trap"— developing technical solutions without proper consideration of the end user, which all too often results in lack of adoption.

Vision-Based Electronic Travel Aids

A number of vision-based ETA prototypes have been developed in recent years. It should be noted that very few of these systems have undergone thorough testing with visually impaired users in realistic situations. Hence, the following exposition should be considered more as an indication of recent research trends, rather than a list of tools ready for adoption.

Sensory systems for mobility support are normally designed to detect and possibly characterize environmental features that are important for safe ambulation: different types of obstacles, steps or curbs, or points of access (doors or passages). In most cases, detection is based on depth perception, achieved either by stereo vision or by active triangulation. Stereo vision is based on the triangulation principle: if a surface point is seen by two cameras at a certain distance from each other, it projects onto two different locations in the two cameras' focal planes. The distance between the locations of the projections ("disparity") is inversely proportional to the distance of the point from the cameras. Thus, by matching each point in the image produced by one camera to the corresponding point in the image produced by the other camera, one may obtain a "depth image"—effectively, a 3-D representation of the whole scene (see Figure 10.4).

Active triangulation systems operate on a similar principle but do not need two cameras. Instead, light is produced by a source (typically, a laser or LED source) that is geometrically calibrated with the camera. By locating the return of the light reflected by a surface point on the image, the depth of this point is estimated. Active triangulation systems may use a single point source (producing only one depth measurement), a "striper" light source (producing readings over a plane in space), or a pattern of points that sample the space (as with the Microsoft Kinect* system). Although stereo and active triangulation systems produce the same type of data, there are important technical differences between the two. Stereo requires the visible surfaces to reflect light from a light source (and thus cannot work in the dark), and does not work well with untextured surfaces (e.g., a white wall), because it is difficult to match points in the two images in these situations. Active triangulation, conversely, does not work well under full sunlight, because the light from the environment overwhelms the light irradiated by the source, thus making detection of the return from the light source difficult. Both systems fail in front of a transparent surface such as a glass door.

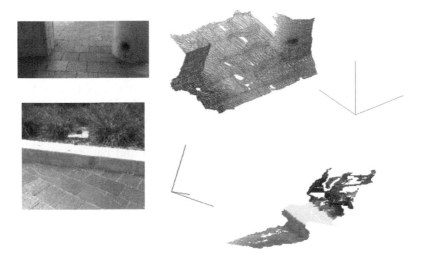

FIGURE 10.4
Stereo camera system estimates 3-D structure of scenes. Top row: scene shown on left, 3-D reconstruction on right clearly shows wall and column protruding from ground plane (*xyz*-axes drawn with green line indicating the camera's line of sight). Bottom row: scene of curb shown on left, 3-D reconstruction shows step structure, which is clearly present despite distortion of reconstruction.

---

* http://www.xbox.com/en-US/kinect

Other types of depth sensors are based on computing the "time of flight" (TOF), that is, the time that it takes for a pulse of light (or a modulated light signal) emitted by a source to reach a surface in the scene, reflect back from the surface, and return to the sensor. The distance to the surface is thus proportional to the TOF. Systems that use the TOF principle (LIDARS) require that the light source be mechanically rotated to span the desired section of the scene. Imaging TOF systems have recently been marketed; these "3-D cameras" have great potential for mobility applications.

An example of an ETA based on active triangulation is the "Teletact" system (Farcy et al. 2006). This device, normally clipped on a long cane, measures the distance to a surface using a single point light source (a laser pointer), and communicates it to the user using a simple tactile or acoustic interface. The device can reliably measure distances up to 6 m with a very narrow "field of view" angle. According to Farcy et al. (2006), Teletact has been tested with more than 200 users. Note that the narrow field of view angle achieved by the laser beam represents an important difference with respect to the ultrasonic ETAs mentioned in Chapter 3, which typically have a much broader receptive field.

In general, safe ambulation requires awareness of multiple environment features, such as steps or drop-offs that, if undetected, could lead to a fall. Recognizing these features by means of point distance measurements may be difficult or impossible, and thus other techniques that use multiple measurements or depth imaging may be needed. For example, Yuan and Manduchi (2004) developed a prototype active triangulation system that not only measures distance, but also analyzes the time profile of distance as the user moves the device (pivoting it around a horizontal axis) to detect depth discontinuities that could signify steps or drop-offs. This system was later extended to use a laser striper, which allows for detection of surface features from a single image (Ilstrup and Manduchi 2011).

Stereo-based detection of curbs and steps for blind navigation was first proposed by Molton et al. (1998). If 3-D information about the environment is available (from a stereo camera or other depth imaging device such as the Kinect), this data can be integrated through time using a technique called "simultaneous localization and mapping" (SLAM). This allows for the geometric reconstruction of the environment, and at the same time enables self-localization. This technique was recently proposed as a means to support blind mobility (Pradeep et al. 2010).

Image-based techniques can produce a very rich representation of the environment geometry, which makes it possible to identify features of interest for safe mobility. This approach may also support orientation, by computing paths to destination. One should be very careful, however, when considering how this technology can be used to effectively help a visually impaired traveler. As discussed at length in Chapter 8, communicating geometric descriptions to a person without sight can be very challenging, and there is no clear agreement as yet about what level of information should be communicated (whether only high-level, semantic information, or some sort of general description), and what type of interface should be used (speech, sound, spatialized sound, or tactile).

But the main challenge for a developer of assistive technology for mobility is to prove that a proposed new device is superior to the baseline tool—the long cane. The cane is economical; it always works and never runs out of power; when not in use, it can be folded and put in one's pocket; and it signals the presence of a blind person to other people. Expert users of the long cane are naturally reluctant to the idea of giving it up for something that is less tried and tested (or even augmenting it with any kind of new technology). Thus, a developer may have to work hard (and provide strong experimental results with adequate user studies—see Chapters 6 and 7) to convince more than a few enthusiastic "early adopters" to convert to a new technology.

It should be noted, however, that the long cane cannot detect all types of obstacles. In particular, the user is not protected against obstacles at head height. In a survey with 300 blind and legally blind individuals (Manduchi and Kurniawan 2011), 13% of the respondents reported experiencing collision with head-level obstacles at least once a month, often with traumatic consequences. Hence, technology that could reliably detect obstacles at head height (Jameson and Manduchi 2010) may have good potential for acceptance at least by a portion of blind and low vision travelers.

Recognizing Stuff

It is often difficult or impossible for a blind or visually impaired person to determine the identity of an object even when it is within reach; in some circumstances, it may be inconvenient to seek this kind of information by simply asking someone for help, as when a blind person wishes to learn who is standing nearby at a party or other gathering. For such problems, computer vision object recognition algorithms, which recognize an object in an image as an instance of an object category, are a promising tool.

Object recognition is a fundamental problem in computer vision (see Szeliski 2010 for a recent overview), and has become powerful enough for widespread use in visual online search engines. Many smartphone apps enabled by object recognition have recently emerged. Perhaps the best-known example is Google Goggles,* a smartphone app which automatically recognizes many types of objects, including landmarks, book covers, and artwork as well as text and logos. Other similar apps include oMoby, A9's SnapTell, and Microsoft's Bing Mobile, most of which are optimized for

---

* http://www.google.com/mobile/goggles/

commercial product visual searches. These apps are intended for normally sighted users, who can easily center the object of interest in the camera viewfinder, snap a photo, and wait for a response. Unfortunately, such a user interface is impractical for many blind and visually impaired persons, who may have great difficulty knowing which objects are visible to the camera—and in some cases may not even know whether an object of interest is even present. For this reason, few object recognition systems are used by this population (unless one categorizes OCR as a type of object recognition).

Some important exceptions to this general rule are object recognition systems that employ user interfaces tailored to the needs of blind and visually impaired users, typically focusing on a specific problem domain rather than attempting completely general object recognition. One such domain is the problem of grocery product identification, which Winlock et al. (2010) approach by matching the packaging of an unknown product—which can include any combination of text, logos, and other graphics—against a database of known products. This approach circumvents the problem of attempting to identify a product solely through OCR, which is unreliable for the types of nonstandard fonts (and inhomogeneous backgrounds) that are typically printed on grocery products; moreover, unlike product identification based on barcodes, it does not force the user to locate the barcode on a package, which can be a difficult task in itself. The user interface in Winlock et al.'s system also alleviates the problem of knowing where to aim the camera through the use of a "mosaicing" technique that combines multiple views of the shelves taken in video over time to assemble a single coherent image of the entire scene.

Another object recognition-based system tailored to the needs of blind and visually impaired users is the currency reader, which determines the denomination of American paper currency (unlike paper bills in other countries, whose denominations may be distinguished simply by the size of the bill)—information that is vitally important to a visually impaired person anytime he/she conducts a cash transaction. Stand-alone currency readers have been available for many years (such as the Note Teller*), but smartphone-based currency readers (Liu 2008) have become commercially available, including the knfb Reader Mobile and the LookTel Money Reader† smartphone app (see Figure 10.5). The LookTel system is distinguished by its ability to recognize currency in real time, as the user is aiming the camera toward the bill, rather than having the user take a photo, wait for the results to be read aloud, and possibly repeat the process until a suitable photo has been taken.

The ability to recognize faces is another specific object recognition task that would be very valuable for blind and visually impaired persons in some social contexts. Not only is it awkward to have to ask people around you who

---

* http://www.brytech.com/noteteller
† http://www.looktel.com

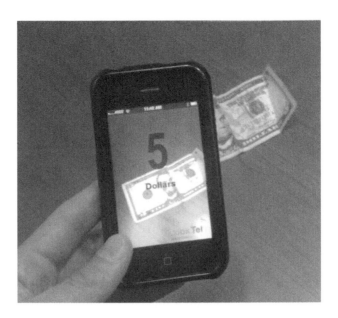

FIGURE 10.5
LookTel Money Reader, a currency reader app for the iPhone. System detects and reads aloud the denomination of the bill (in this case, $5) in real time.

is near, but a partially sighted person whose visual impairment is not immediately obvious to others may risk offending people by failing to recognize them. In addition, people with otherwise normal vision who suffer from prosopagnosia (face blindness) could also benefit from a face recognition system. Face recognition is an active topic of research in computer vision (see Li and Jain 2005 for an overview) that is especially challenging because of the enormous variability that a person's facial appearance undergoes due to varying facial expressions, lighting conditions, viewing angles, and the placement of hair, glasses, clothing, and so on. Because of these challenges, relatively little research has been done on practical face recognition systems for blind and visually impaired persons. However, Kramer et al. (2010) implemented a successful prototype smartphone-based face recognition system that announces with text-to-speech the names of people identified by the system. Going beyond basic face recognition, other research (Krishna et al. 2005; Gade et al. 2009) explores a wearable interaction assistant system to identify and interpret facial expressions, emotions, and gestures, which are another important form of information (in addition to identity) that may be inaccessible to people with vision loss.

Finally, in some circumstances, a blind or visually impaired person (possibly someone with color blindness) may know the identity of an object but not its color, as when choosing an article of clothing to wear or selecting a color-coded file folder. In such cases, a system that automatically recognizes color can be helpful. Color identifiers (also known as color recognizers) such as the ColorTest (from Caretec), Brytech's Color Teller, or Cobolt Systems' Speechmaster speak aloud the color of a surface that the device is pointed to; not surprisingly, a "Color Identifier" app* is now available for the iPhone with similar functionality. Research on the related but more difficult problem of matching patterns according to both color and texture may be useful for helping visually impaired people match multiple items of clothes (Yang et al. 2011).

Image Enhancement for Low Vision

In previous sections, we have emphasized assistive technology systems that harness computer vision to provide audio or tactile feedback about a visually impaired person's environment. Some people with sufficient partial vision, however, may prefer user interfaces that make the most of their residual vision by using computer vision or image processing to *enhance* images of the scene, which are presented on a computer/smartphone screen or via a head-mounted display. As discussed in Chapters 2 and 4, there are many different types of functional vision loss, and we will outline approaches to image enhancement according to some of the more common types.

A relatively minor form of vision impairment is color blindness, which is a reduced ability to perceive color or color differences (and which often occurs in people with otherwise normal vision). As an alternative to the types of color identifier systems discussed at the end of the previous section, which announce (using text-to-speech) the color pointed to by a camera or similar light probe, the colors in an entire image (or electronic document) can be remapped to a new color palette and rerendered, so as to make the colors appear as perceptually distinct as possible to the viewer while preserving the approximate contrast between different colors that would be perceived by a normally sighted viewer. (The most appropriate mapping depends not only on the range of colors present in the image but also on the particular type of color blindness.) "Postpublication" techniques (Jefferson and Harvey 2006) address the problem of how to rerender a static image, webpage, or entire document on a computer screen or printed page. The same approach can also be applied to video, and when it is implemented in real time, it constitutes an augmented reality system, such as the DanKam,[†] an experimental app iPhone app (designed for the most common form of color blindness, anomalous trichromancy) which continuously rerenders the scene acquired by the camera on the smartphone's viewfinder.

---

* http://www.greengar.com/apps/color-identifier/
[†] http://dankaminsky.com/dankam/

Much more serious functional vision impairments include poor acuity, poor contrast sensitivity, and tunnel vision, which arise from multiple causes. Poor acuity is a particularly debilitating problem because it can impair a person's ability to read and to find and recognize objects, even under good lighting conditions and at high contrast. Magnification is a standard technique for addressing this problem (Wiener et al. 2010), using either an optical telescope (for distant targets) or a screen magnifier (for print). Unfortunately, as discussed in Chapter 4, a fundamental limitation of magnification is that it reduces the field of view—in effect, causing a type of functional tunnel vision, which makes it harder to find a target of interest, or to interpret an extended pattern larger than the field of view. (The problem is exacerbated with poorer acuity, which requires the use of higher magnification.) One computer vision-based attempt to mitigate this problem in the context of reading signs is the "Smart Telescope" SBIR project from Blindsight Corporation,* which automatically detects text regions in a scene acquired by a wearable camera and presents the regions one at a time to a partially sighted user, using a head-mounted display that zooms into the text to enable him/her to read it.

Many systems that magnify scenes for people with poor acuity also enhance contrast (Harper et al. 1999), such as the head-mounted system created by Li et al. (2011), since poor acuity due to central field loss is often associated with low contrast sensitivity. While simple contrast enhancement techniques are often adequate for improving the readability of text (typically characterized by a single foreground color against a single background color)—techniques that are available in many video magnifiers (Sardegna and Paul 1991)—enhancing the visibility of an entire natural scene with a multitude of objects and textures is a complex problem. Eli Peli and his collaborators have investigated this problem using a variety of contrast enhancement techniques, including narrowband contrast enhancement (Peli and Peli 1984), contrast enhancement in the JPEG and MPEG domains (Tang et al. 2004; Kim et al. 2004) in which images and video are compressed, and wideband enhancement (Peli et al. 2004), which adds highly visible edge and bar feature contours to the image.

Finally, the restricted field of view associated with tunnel vision has inspired the development of novel techniques for processing and displaying images, most involving some form of minification (the opposite of magnification, used to compact a large field of view into the much narrower field of view of the person's eyes). A promising approach due to Peli (2001) uses a head-mounted display to superimpose minified edge images of the entire scene over the user's natural vision. The key to the approach is the fact that the edge pixels comprise a small fraction of pixels in the original images, so that the superimposed edge image interferes minimally with what the user already sees unaided. Experiments with tunnel vision patients showed that

---

* http://www.blindsight.com/

the system increased the speed with which they are able to conduct search tasks (for targets outside their natural field of view).

Many experiments have demonstrated statistically significant benefits to users of these types of image enhancement systems to perform real-world tasks (Luo and Peli 2011). However, for many applications such as image enhancement for viewing TV and video (Peli and Woods 2009), the determination of quantitative measures to objectively evaluate the benefits of image enhancement is a major challenge in itself. Indeed, given the extremely variable and multidimensional nature of functional vision deficits among persons with visual impairments, coupled with the highly individual needs of this population, this challenge is likely to be a research enterprise as great as the development and improvement of the image enhancement techniques themselves.

Usability

There are several aspects of a camera-based system that need to be addressed before it can be considered usable by visually impaired persons. In the following we discuss a few issues related to the physical placement of the system, the quality of the task being performed, the communication of relevant data to the user, and the distribution of processing tasks between the local platform and remote (or even human) resources.

Wearable or Portable?

One important issue is how exactly the visually impaired user will carry the camera or cameras. The camera needs to have an adequate clear field of view, and thus cannot be placed anywhere the view could be occluded. At the same time, cosmetic considerations may discourage the placement of cameras in highly conspicuous locations. The availability of miniaturized cameras, which could be embedded, for example, in someone's eyeglasses, may help reduce some of these concerns. An alternative solution to "wearable" cameras is the use of a hand-held device such as a camera-equipped smartphone. Using a widely available commodity such as a smartphone has many advantages with respect to customized solutions, in terms of cost, availability of support, and convenience. In addition, a smartphone carries none of the stigma normally attached to assistive technology devices. Assistive technology "apps" are currently being created for both the Android and iPhone platforms. Of course, all aspects of accessibility need to be considered: if a blind user cannot start or control the application on the smartphone because this requires visual feedback, then even the most powerful application would be useless! Thankfully, accessibility interfaces (e.g., VoiceOver for Apple devices) are available to enable nonvisual interaction even with touchscreen-based smartphones (see also Chapter 11).

In spite of their attractive features mentioned above, hand-held smartphones may not be the most desirable choice for all applications. A smartphone is ideal for things like checking the value of a banknote or for reading a bill or a menu via OCR and text-to-speech. However, holding a smartphone by hand and pointing it around for an extended period of time while walking in search of a sign (indicating, for example, the location of a restroom or of the elevator) may be unwieldy, especially considering that the user would normally have one hand already occupied with handling the long cane or holding the dog guide. For this type of application, a wearable camera system that does not need to be constantly held may prove a more convenient solution.

Performance

Simply stated, if an assistive technology solution does not work well enough, it will not be used. How to quantify "acceptable performance," however, is not always clear.

A camera-based system can be characterized by a number of parameters, including the field of view of the camera, the image resolution (the number of pixels in the image), and the effective frame rate (the number of images that can be processed per second). In addition, there are application-specific performance measures. Consider, for example, a device used to find a particular sign in the environment. This system may be evaluated in terms of its detection rate (the percentage of times the sought sign is correctly detected in an image) and of its false-positive rate (the percentage of times that the system declares a detection when in fact there was no sign visible). Detection and false-positive rates are normally related to each other via specific parameters in the algorithms (e.g., a threshold in the classification algorithm). By tweaking such parameters, one may be able to increase (or decrease) the detection rate, but this will necessarily come at the cost of an increased (or decreased) false-positive rate. Fixing the "operating point" of the system (i.e., tuning the parameters to obtain a certain detection/false-positive rate pair) is a difficult art. One may, for example, decide on a maximum acceptable value for the false-positive rate, under the assumption that if the system produces too many false alarms, the user will decide to turn it off.

The resulting detection rate depends on a number of factors, including the size of the sign, the distance at which it is seen, the field of view of the camera, and the image resolution. A sign of a certain size, seen at a certain distance, will be easier to detect if the image resolution is high or if the field of view angle is small (e.g., using a telephoto lens). Increasing the image resolution, however, typically leads to longer processing time, which may reduce the effective frame rate. By contrast, a narrow field of view implies that a smaller portion of the environment is visualized at each frame. Low frame rate and narrow field of view may both hamper the visual exploration task if one is using the system to "scan" the environment in search of the sign, perhaps by rotating the camera around a vertical axis (see Figure 10.3). If the camera is moved too fast, there may be portions of the visible space that will not be processed because they happen to appear between two consecutive frames. Thus, the user may have to apply extra attention while exploring the space with the camera, possibly repeating the scanning operation several times to make sure that the entire scene is correctly analyzed.

It should also be noted that fast camera motion may produce blurred pictures and thus complicate processing by the computer vision algorithm. This effect is particularly noticeable with low ambient light, as in this case the system needs to increase the exposure time of each image, which is liable to increase the risk of motion-induced blur.

As this simple example suggests, the performance of a camera-based system is a function of multiple interconnected components. Ultimately, the system should accomplish the task it was designed for in a reasonable amount of time and without requiring too much effort of the user. Optimizing the system for best performance, and quantifying the overall quality of the user-mediated application, is a difficult but critical component of the design process.

User Interface

A camera-based system implicitly performs some sort of sensory substitution. The visual data is "digested" by the computer vision algorithm, and the output of this processing (be it the detection of a step 2 m away, the OCR decoding of a piece of text, the brand of a can of food, or the presence of a sign on a wall) is communicated to the user via one or more of his or her remaining senses. Clearly, the modality for this communication should be application-dependent. In some cases, a few bits of information is all that is needed (e.g., to communicate the presence of a head-level hazard in time for the user to stop and avoid it). In other cases (e.g., OCR access to text), more data needs to be communicated, in this example via text-to-speech.

Specific to the case of camera-based systems are situations in which a stream of geometry-related information needs to be communicated to the user as he or she is maneuvering the camera. Consider, for example, the case of a smartphone used for mobile access to text, for example, to read a bill received in the mail. As mentioned earlier, one of the challenges of using such a system is that the smartphone needs to be positioned so that the camera has a clear view of the entirety of the text (an operation that may be challenging without sight). The system may provide continuous information to the user as to how to move the camera to improve framing of the desired text (e.g., up/down, left/right, closer/farther). As another example, a wayfinding application may inform the user of the distance and bearing angle of a detected sign.

There is no general rule about what combination of speech, sound, spatialized sound (if the user is wearing headphones), or tactile signal (vibration) is preferable for communicating geometry-related information, in part because each application has its own specific requirements. Precious little published research has performed comparative evaluation of multiple interfaces in this context (Ross and Blasch 2000; Walker and Lindsay 2005; Marston et al. 2006). Indeed, user interface design often winds up being "the afterthought at the end of the project" (Miele 2005), receiving less attention than other technical components of the device. Yet, the interface, from the user's standpoint, is one of the most important aspects of the sensory substitution system: a poorly designed interface may make an otherwise impeccable algorithm practically unusable.

From Local to Cloud to Crowd

As pointed out earlier, the processing speed (measured, e.g., by the effective frame rate) is a critical component of a camera-based system. There is no universal rule for what the minimum acceptable response time of a system should be. For example, if a smartphone is used to determine the brand of a can of food, it may be acceptable to wait for a few seconds from the time a snapshot is taken to the time the response is uttered by the text-to-speech system. The situation is different if the computer vision system is supposed to provide a stream of signals, for example, to help the user point the camera correctly in order to take a well-framed picture that will then be OCR-processed. In this case, a system that takes more than 1 or 2 s to process an image at each individual camera pose may be cumbersome to operate. Other applications (e.g., detection of a particular sign or of a hazard as one is walking) may have even more stringent frame rate requirements.

Image processing is notoriously time consuming. An image is composed of hundreds of thousands or millions of pixels, and the computer vision algorithm may require multiple iterations of complex routines involving possibly large neighborhoods of each pixel. Miniaturized platforms (e.g., smartphones), in spite of technological innovations such as multiple core processors and graphics processing units (GPU), are not as powerful as desktop computers. Thus, in order to increase processing speed, it may be sensible to use remote servers ("the cloud") to perform operations that would require too much time on the local processor. Of course, this requires that a good wireless Internet connection be available between the local platform (e.g., the smartphone) and the remote server. Indeed, transmitting streams of high-resolution images to the server may wind up taking more time than performing some simple local processing! Thus, a more effective strategy may consist of distributing the processing load between the local processor and the remote server. For example, input images may be analyzed locally to extract relevant features, which are then transmitted (using much less data than the original image) to the remote server for further analysis (Chandrasekhar et al. 2009).

Another intriguing possibility offered by the increasing availability of ubiquitous wireless connection is to do away with computer vision altogether, and rely instead on input from remote human assistants looking at images taken by the blind user and sent to them via Internet. One example of this approach is Sight On Call, a product being developed at Blindsight with funding from the NIH. Sight On Call is an on-demand assistance service for blind and moderate low-vision persons. The user of this service contacts specially trained operators who, based on sensor data (e.g., GPS location) and images taken by the user's cell phone, can provide specific assistance as regards wayfinding and object recognition. A different approach is taken by VizWiz, developed by Bigham's group at the University of Rochester (Jayant and Bigham 2010). VizWiz uses "crowdsourcing" mechanisms (specifically, Amazon's Mechanical Turk*) to enable the user to ask and get answers to queries about an image taken with his or her cell phone.

Using "human intelligence" rather than computer vision is attractive for multiple reasons. Humans are much more reliable than computers for most tasks that require image analysis. More important is the fact that humans can answer complex and generic questions such as "Where am I?" or "What is close to me?" At the same time, this approach has some intrinsic limitations in terms of latency. The image taken by the user's cell phone needs to be transmitted to a server and analyzed by one (or more) human operators, before the answer to the user's query is sent back and uttered via text-to-speech. This chain of operations may take up to a few seconds. As mentioned earlier, this delay may be irrelevant for some applications, yet unacceptable for other tasks that require close to real-time feedback.

Acknowledgments

Coughlan acknowledges support by the National Institutes of Health from grants No. 1 R21 EY021643-01, 2 R01EY018345-04, 1 R01 EY018210-01A1, and 1 R01 EY018890-01, and by the Department of Education, NIDRR grant number H133E110004.

Manduchi acknowledges support by the National Science Foundation (NSF) from grants No. IIS-0835645 and CNS-0709472, and by the National Institutes of Health under grant No. 1R21EY021643-01.

---

* http://www.mturk.com

References

Al-Khalifa, H. 2008. Utilizing QR code and mobile phones for blinds and visually impaired people. In *Proc. International Conference on Computers Helping People with Special Needs (ICCHP '08)*. Linz, Austria.

Aranda, J. and Mares, P. 2004. Visual system to help blind people to cross the street. In *Proc. International Conference on Computers Helping People with Special Needs (ICCHP '04)*. Paris, France.

Bagherinia, H. and Manduchi, R. 2011. Robust real-time detection of multi-color markers on a cell phone. *Journal of Real-Time Image Processing*, 6, 1–17.

Chandrasekhar, V., Takacs, G., Chen, D. M., Tsai, S. S., Grzeszczuk, R., and Girod, B. 2009. CHoG: Compressed histogram of gradients—A low bit rate feature descriptor. In *Proc. IEEE Conference on Computer Vision and Pattern Recognition*. Miami, Florida.

Chen, H., Tsai, S. S., Schroth, G., Chen, D. M., Grzeszczuk, R., and Girod, B. 2011. Robust text detection in natural images with edge-enhanced maximally stable extremal regions. In *Proc. IEEE International Conference on Image Processing (ICIP 2011)*. Brussels, Belgium.

Coates, A., Carpenter, B., Case, C., Satheesh, S., Suresh, B., Wang, T., and Ng, A.Y. 2011. Text detection and character recognition in scene images with unsupervised feature learning. In *Proc. International Conference on Document Analysis and Recognition (ICDAR 2011)*. Beijing, China.

Coughlan, J. and Manduchi, R. 2009. Functional assessment of a camera phone-based wayfinding system operated by blind and visually impaired users. *International Journal on Artificial Intelligence Tools, Special Issue on Artificial Intelligence Based Assistive Technologies: Methods and Systems for People with Disabilities*, 18, 379–397.

Epshtein, B., Ofek, E., and Wexler, Y. 2010. Detecting text in natural scenes with stroke width transform. In *Proc. Conference on Computer Vision and Pattern Recognition (CVPR 2010)*. San Francisco, California.

Farcy, R., Leroux, R., Jucha, A., Damaschini, R., Gregoire, C., and Zogaghi, A. 2006. Electronic travel aids and electronic orientation aids for blind people: Technical, rehabilitation and everyday life points of view. In *Proceedings of the International Conference on Assistive Technologies for Vision and Hearing Impairment*. Kufstein, Austria.

Gade, L., Krisha, S., and Panchanathan, S. 2009. Person localization using a wearable camera towards enhancing social interactions for individuals with visual impairment. In *Proc. 1st ACM SIGMM International Workshop on Media Studies and Implementations That Help Improving Access to Disabled Users (MSIADU '09)*. ACM, New York, NY, USA, pp. 53–62.

Gallo, O. and Manduchi, R. 2011. Reading 1-D barcodes with mobile phones using deformable templates. *IEEE Transactions on Pattern Analysis and Machine Intelligence (PAMI)*, 33(9), 1834–1843.

Harper, R., Culham, L., and Dickinson, C. 1999. Head mounted video magnification devices for low vision rehabilitation: A comparison with existing technology. *British Journal of Ophthalmology*, 83(4), 495–500.

Hull, J. J, Krishnan, G., Palumbo, P. Srihari, S.N. et al. 1984. Optical character recognition in mail sorting: A review of algorithms. Technical report 214, CS Department, State University of New York.

Ilstrup, D. and Manduchi, R. 2011. Return detection for outdoor active triangulation. In *Proc. SPIE 3D Image Processing (3DIP) and Applications.* Paris, France.

Ivanchenko, V., Coughlan, J., and Shen, H. 2009. Staying in the crosswalk: A system for guiding visually impaired pedestrians at traffic intersections. In *Proc. Association for the Advancement of Assistive Technology in Europe (AAATE 2009).* Florence, Italy.

Ivanchenko, V., Coughlan, J., and Shen, H. 2010. Real-time walk light detection with a mobile phone. In *Proc. International Conference on Computers Helping People with Special Needs (ICCHP '10).* Vienna, Austria.

Jameson, B. and Manduchi, R. 2010. Watch your head: A wearable collision warning sensor system for the blind. *IEEE Sensors 2010 Conference.* Waikoloa, Hawaii

Jayant, C. and Bigham, J. 2010. VizWiz::LocateIt—Enabling blind people to locate objects in their environment. In *Proc. IEEE Workshop on Computer Vision Applications for the Visually Impaired.* San Francisco, California.

Jefferson, L. and Harvey, R. 2006. Accommodating color blind computer users. In *Proc. 8th International ACM SIGACCESS Conference on Computers and Accessibility (Assets '06).* ACM, New York, NY, USA, pp. 40–47.

Kim, J., Vora, A., and Peli, E. 2004. MPEG based image enhancement for the visually impaired. *Optical Engineering,* 43(6), 1318–1328.

Kramer, K. M., Hedin, D. S., and Rolkosky, D. J. 2010. Smartphone based face recognition tool for the blind. In *Proc. IEEE Engineering in Medicine & Biology Society.* Buenos Aires, Argentina.

Krishna, S., Little, G., Black, J., and Panchanathan, S. 2005. A wearable face recognition system for individuals with visual impairments. In *Proc. 7th International ACM SIGACCESS Conference on Computers and Accessibility (Assets '05).* ACM, New York, NY, USA, pp. 106–113.

Kulyukin, V., Gharpure, C., Nicholson, J., and Pavithran, S. 2004. RFID in robot-assisted indoor navigation for the visually impaired. In *Proc. IEEE/RSJ International Conference on Intelligent Robots and Systems (IROS 2004).* Sendai, Japan.

Kurzweil, R. 2000. *The Age of Spiritual Machines.* London, UK: Penguin.

Kutiyanawala, A., Kulyukin, V., and Nicholson, J. 2011. Toward real time eyes-free barcode scanning on smartphones in video mode. In *Proc. 2011 Rehabilitation Engineering and Assistive Technology Society of North America Conference (RESNA 2011).* Toronto, Canada.

Le Cun, Y., Boser, B., Denker, J. S. et al. 1990. Handwritten digit recognition with a back-propagation network. In *Proc. Advances in Neural Information Processing Systems (NIPS).* Denver, Colorado.

Lee, J. J., Lee, P. H., Koch, C., and Yuille, A. L. 2011. AdaBoost for text detection in natural scene. In *Proc. International Conference on Document Analysis and Recognition (ICDAR 2011).* Beijing, China.

Li, S. Z. and Jain, A. K. (eds). 2005. *Handbook of Face Recognition.* London, UK: Springer.

Li, Z., Luo, G., and Peli, E. 2011. Image enhancement of high digital magnification for patients with central field loss. In *SPIE-IS&T Electronic Imaging, SPIE Vol. 7865, Human Vision and Electronic Imaging XVI.*

Liu, X. 2008. A camera phone based currency reader for the visually impaired. In *Proc. International ACM SIGACCESS Conference on Computers and Accessibility (ASSETS 2008).* Halifax, Nova Scotia.

Luo, G. and Peli, E. 2011. Development and evaluation of vision rehabilitation devices. In *Proc. 33rd Annual International Conference of the IEEE Engineering in Medicine and Biology Society (EMBC '11)*, Boston, Massachusetts, USA, August 30–September 3. pp. 5228–5231.

Manduchi, R. and Coughlan, J. 2012. (Computer) vision without sight. *Communications of the ACM*, 55(1).

Manduchi, R. and Kurniawan, S. 2011. Mobility-related accidents experienced by people with visual impairment. *Insight: Research and Practice in Visual Impairment and Blindness*, 4(2), 44–54.

Manduchi, R., Kurniawan, S., and Bagherinia, H. 2010. Blind guidance using mobile computer vision: A usability study. *ACM SIGACCESS Conference on Computers and Accessibility (ASSETS)*. Orlando, Florida.

Mann, M. 1949. Reading machine spells out loud. *Popular Science*, February.

Marston, J. R., Loomis, J. M., Klatzky, R. L., Golledge, R. G., and Smith E. L. 2006. Evaluation of spatial displays for navigation without sight. *ACM Transactions on Applied Perception*, 3(2), 110–124.

Mattar, M. A., Hanson, A. R., and Learned-Miller, E. G. 2005. Sign Classification using local and meta-features. In *Proc. Computer Vision Applications for the Visually Impaired (CVAVI)*, San Diego, CA.

Miele, J. 2005. User interface: The afterthought at the end of the project. Unpublished presentation at the *IEEE Workshop on Computer Vision Applications for the Visually Impaired*. San Diego, California.

Molton, N., Se, S., Brady, J. M., Lee D., and Probert, P. 1998. A stereo vision-based aid for the visually impaired. *Image and Vision Computing*, 16(4), 251–263.

Park, J. H. and Jeong, C. S. 2009. Real-time signal light detection. *International Journal of Signal Processing, Image Processing and Pattern Recognition*, 2(2), 139–142.

Peli, E. 2001. Vision multiplexing—An engineering approach to vision rehabilitation device development. *Optometry and Vision Science*, 78, 304–315.

Peli, E., Kim, J., Yitzhaky, Y., Goldstein, R. B., and Woods, R. L. 2004. Wide-band enhancement of television images for people with visual-impairments. *Journal of the Optical Society of America A*, 21(6), 937–950.

Peli, E. and Peli, T. 1984. Image enhancement for the visually impaired. *Optical Engineering*, 23, 47–51.

Peli, E. and Woods, R. L. 2009. Image enhancement for impaired vision: The challenge of evaluation. *International Journal on Artificial Intelligence Tools*, 18(3), 415–438.

Poupyrev, I., Kato, H., and Billinghurst, M. 2000. *ARToolkit User Manual*. Human Interface Technology Lab, University of Washington.

Pradeep, V., Medioni, G., and Weiland, J. 2010. Robot vision for the visually impaired. In *Proc. IEEE Workshop on Computer Vision Applications for the Visually Impaired*. San Francisco, California.

Preiser, W. and Ostroff, E. 2001. *Universal Design Handbook*. London, UK: McGraw-Hill Professional.

Ross, D. A. and Blasch, B. B. 2000. Wearable interfaces for orientation and wayfinding. In *Proc. ACM Conference on Assistive Technologies (ASSETS '00)*. Arlington, Virginia.

Ross, D. A and Reynolds, M. S. 2010. RFID floors to provide indoor navigation information for people with visual impairment. In *Proc. 23th Annual International Technology & Persons with Disabilities Conference (CSUN)*. San Diego, California.

Sanketi, P., Shen, H., and Coughlan, J. 2011. Localizing blurry and low-resolution text in natural images. In *Proc. IEEE Workshop on Applications of Computer Vision (WACV 2011)*. Kona, Hawaii.

Sardegna, J. and Paul, T. O. 1991. *The Encyclopedia of Blindness and Visual Impairment*. Facts on File, Inc. New York.

Schoof, L. T. 1975. An analysis of Optacon usage. *American Foundation for the Blind Research Bulletin*, 29, 33–50.

Se, S. 2000. Zebra-crossing detection for the partially sighted. In *Proc. Conference on Computer Vision and Pattern Recognition (CVPR 2000)*. Hilton Head, South Carolina.

Silapachote, P., Weinman, J., Hanson, A., Weiss, R., and Mattar, M. 2005. Automatic sign detection and recognition in natural scenes. In *Proc. Computer Vision Applications for the Visually Impaired (CVAVI)*. San Diego, CA.

Stein, B. K. 1998. The Optacon: Past, present, and future. *DIGIT-EYES: The Computer Users' Network News*.

Szeliski, R. 2010. Computer vision: Algorithms and applications. Springer, New York.

Tang, J., Kim, J. H., and Peli, E. 2004. Image enhancement in the JPEG domain for people with vision impairment. *IEEE Transactions on Biomedical Engineering*, 51(11), 2013–2023.

Tekin, E. and Coughlan, J. 2010. A mobile phone application enabling visually impaired users to find and read product barcodes. In *Proc. International Conference on Computers Helping People with Special Needs (ICCHP '10)*. Vienna, Austria.

Tekin, E., Coughlan, J., and Shen, H. 2011. Real-time detection and reading of LED/LCD displays for visually impaired persons. In *Proc. IEEE Workshop on Applications of Computer Vision (WACV 2011)*. Kona, Hawaii.

Tjan, B. S., Beckmann, P. J., Roy, R., Giudice, N., and Legge, G. E. 2005. Digital sign system for indoor wayfinding for the visually impaired. In *Proc. IEEE Workshop on Computer Vision Applications for the Visually Impaired*. San Diego, California.

Walker, B. N. and Lindsay, J. 2005. Navigation performance in a virtual environment with bonephones. In *Proc. International Conference on Auditory Display (ICAD 2005)*. Limerick, Ireland.

Wang, K., Babenko, B., and Belongie, S. 2011. End-to-end scene text recognition. In *Proc. International Conference on Computer Vision (ICCV 2011)*. Barcelona, Spain.

Wiener, W. R., Welsh, R. L., and Blasch, B. B. 2010. *Foundations of Orientation and Mobility*, Third edition. New York, NY: AFB Press.

Winlock, T., Christiansen, E., and Belongie, S. 2010. Toward real-time grocery detection for the visually impaired. In *Proc. Computer Vision Applications for the Visually Impaired (CVAVI)*. San Francisco, CA.

Yang, X., Yuan, S., and Tian, Y. 2011. Recognizing clothes patterns for blind people by confidence margin based feature combination. In *Proc. 19th ACM International Conference on Multimedia*. Scottsdale, Arizona.

Yuan, D. and Manduchi, R. 2004. A tool for range sensing and environment discovery for the blind. In *Proc. IEEE Workshop on Real–Time 3D Sensor and Their Use*. Washington, D.C.

11

Screenreaders, Magnifiers, and Other Ways of Using Computers

Alasdair King

CONTENTS

Introduction

People who are blind or have a visual impairment have problems using computers since computers are designed for mouse users who can see the screen. But computers offer so much to blind people that it is worth using computers anyway even if it is hard.

The solution is to use *access software*: a screenreader, a magnifier, a nonstandard application, or what native capacity there is in the operating system. Most blind people use some combination of all these strategies, knowingly or not. This chapter describes these categories of access software for blind people; how screenreaders work; the state of the art in access software; and a review of some of the big challenges facing access software.

Categories of Access Software for Blind People

Access software for blind people can be categorized into three categories: *screenreader/magnifier software*, which lets users use the standard computer applications like Word or a web browser; *dedicated software*, which means users use a specially designed bit of software; and *adaption and customization*, which means users take advantage of whatever users can do in the operating system or existing applications to make them work better.

Screenreaders and Magnifiers (e.g., JAWS)

A *screenreader* works out what is happening on the screen and sends its output either to synthesized speech or, far less commonly, to a Braille display (Evans and Blenkhorn, 2003). (Braille has some considerable advantages, is politically contentious, and is very rare.) Generally, users use a screenreader if they cannot see anything at all. A *magnifier* magnifies the screen so that if users have some vision they can use the mouse (Blenkhorn et al., 2003). Generally, users use a magnifier if they have some sight. In fact, most screenreader software provides both screenreading and magnification because most blind people have some sight, and being able to peer at the screen and make an attempt at working out what is going on can be very useful at times. Traditionally, magnifiers did not have an offscreen model but screenreaders did, but the distinction has blurred.

Using a screenreader effectively is hard. Screenreaders are trying to communicate quite heterogeneous user interfaces: Microsoft Word is quite different from a web page. The user cannot scan around the screen to try to spot the right function or the content he or she wants to read; he or she has to explore slowly and carefully. To compensate and speed things up, screenreaders have acquired dozens of shortcut keys, which are useful for power users but mean lots more to learn. And many things will not work at all (buttons with images but no text, for example).

It would therefore seem natural that magnification is better for anyone who can see the screen to some degree. However, using magnification is really hard since it is easy to get confused with the location of the mouse pointer and where one is on the screen, especially at high levels of magnification, and the quality of the display is often poor because of the pixilation of the magnified bitmap display (Blenkhorn et al., 2003).

Dedicated Software: Self-Contained Alternatives to Standard Applications (e.g., Guide)

Screenreaders are powerful general-purpose access software solutions suitable for users who seek to use their machine just as a sighted person does. But sighted users, the success of the iPad suggests, seek to use their machines for a relatively limited set of uses: web browsing (though that means so much more, now), email, chat, video and music, and a little occasional word processing. Why cannot blind people access a similarly limited but customized system that suits their particular modality? If a non-PC interface is good enough for sighted people, why not for blind users?

These systems do exist. The main commercial PC system is Guide from Dolphin in the United Kingdom. It allows a user to do email, web browsing, and other essential applications with self-voicing menus. This is not dissimilar to some of the expensive dedicated portable notetaker or notebook devices that are sold with Braille input and output interfaces, or speech, and are often based on Windows machines: dedicated bookreaders might also be regarded as simplified user interface machines dedicated to blind users.

The situation is less clear-cut and more positive on non-PC platforms. The Mobile Accessibility for Android from screenreader.net replaces the essential features of a tablet or phone with a fully accessible customized interface. The iPhone, or iPad especially, allows users to browse the web, listen to the radio, read and write email, and the other essentials of normal computer use, with a self-voicing application that is both fashionable and works well. If blind people did not have to work in offices with standard desktop applications like Excel, then the iPad might have "solved" the screenreader problem for good (cost of the device aside—although with the cost of the access software taken into account, the iPad is actually inexpensive).

This leaves the option of using nonstandard applications: rather than struggling to use applications designed primarily for mouse and screen users, why not employ applications that are specifically written for blind screenreader users? These can be designed to work well with any screenreader—for example, always placing a caret in a text area, keeping the number of controls on a form to a minimum, and including access and shortcut keys. Or they can replace the screenreader for that application, self-voicing: generating their own speech (or in theory Braille). The WebbIE suite of applications (web browser, RSS news reader, podcatcher, eBook reader) for Windows falls into the former category. The SpeakOn application includes a similar set of functions (play CDs, live radio, BBC stations from the last week) but also synthesizes its own speech (and has no visible user interface!) Both are free projects. Less all-encompassing products include Qwitter, an accessible Twitter client, and PowerTalk for reading PowerPoint presentations using synthesized speech: when few screenreaders could handle the web, IBM's HomePage Reader filled the gap (Asakawa and Itoh, 1998). In 5 years, many of these will have stopped being developed, and many more will have appeared: this is a rich but temporary ecosystem.

However, many blind users prefer to use standard common applications over nonstandard applications. There are good reasons: skills and techniques learned from using normal, fairly inaccessible applications may be more transferable to novel situations when they are encountered. Nonstandard applications are often free, or not the main commercial product for a company, and therefore lack support and often lag behind in features. Simplified user interfaces are great, but often functions are cut. But most important perhaps is the sentiment that nonstandard applications present a crippled, fake experience, and deny blind screenreader users the authentic status of being users of the same applications as "normal" people. Even if their screenreader employs three nonvisual accessibility APIs and a script and an offscreen model to communicate to the end user, the user still feels that he or she is using the standard application directly.

Adaption and Customization of Existing systems (i.e., Native OS/app Accessibility Settings)

Everyone approaches applications with their own set of needs and wants. People with disabilities are no different, but they add "works with my disability" to their criteria. Users gravitate where possible to applications that work with their access technology. "Which BitTorrent client should I use?" can be answered with "the one that works with your screenreader." It is harder when the application is one that cannot be replaced, like Microsoft Outlook in corporate user mode. Users themselves, or carers or experts, swap tips on "accessible" applications on email groups or websites. Simple tools of limited utility to people without disabilities are often pressed into service. For example, TextAloud from NextUp provides text-to-speech facilities, ostensibly for anyone who wants to create audio from text. In practice, this provides both a simple, low-cost way for blind people to generate audio for listening to later and a set of good speech synthesizers that can be employed in other applications. These are not applications intended for people with disabilities but they have a strong following in these communities because of their longevity, simple interfaces, and low cost.

There are also applications that are of particular use to people with disabilities, such as optical character recognition (OCR) programs or speech recognition programs. Adding these to an otherwise standard build can make all the difference.

Users can also employ the built-in accessibility features of operating systems or applications (Kurniawan et al., 2006). These have gradually improved over the last 15 years, with notable milestones, including the Microsoft developments from 2000 of the Narrator screenreader, a magnifier, on-screen keyboards and system customization; the free VoiceOver screenreader in the Apple operating system; and the touch-based screenreader in the iPhone and iPad. The story is quite different on Windows desktop machines, where the operating system access software (Narrator, Magnifier) has traditionally been very limited compared to the commercial access software (Narrator supports neither Internet Explorer nor Microsoft Word, for example) and has been quite unsuccessful, versus Apple machines, especially the iPad and iPhone, where VoiceOver has been more successful, helped by the lack of commercial competition and the greater homogeneity of the Apple environment.

How Screenreaders Work

It is important to have an idea about how screenreaders work to understand their limitations and the politics and technology behind them.

Screenreaders communicate to the blind user what is happening on the screen. To do this they hook into keyboard input and hook into system events, such as new windows or menus being activated. This allows them to echo back what the user types and make the user aware of changes to the screen, such as pop-up windows or web browsers loading a new page. They also have to communicate the contents of windows—user interfaces and the contents of documents like web pages or Word documents. So the key techniques for screenreaders are to communicate with other applications to identify when they change and what they are now displaying.

Crudely, there are three ways for a screenreader to access another application and communicate its contents to the user. First, through an *offscreen model*. Second, through an application-specific *application API*. And third, through an operating system *accessibility API*.

The offscreen model could be regarded as the "traditional" screenreader mechanism (Evans and Blenkhorn, 2003). Every application has to draw UI components, text, and graphics on the screen, which usually means they call low-level operating system routines like DrawText on Windows. The operating system updates the video display driver, and the text and windows appear on the screen. An offscreen model is built by intercepting these calls and, if possible, querying the operating system for the current state of the screen display. The screenreader can then communicate the contents of the offscreen model to the user as appropriate. This approach can be immensely powerful: the screenreader has access to the whole visible contents of the screen, as text, and can use sophisticated heuristics to do things like work out the caption for a text field by checking for text above or to the left of it (or the right in Arabic or Hebrew), or watch for the redrawing of the caret graphic to spot focus changes. However, there are three drawbacks to the offscreen model: first, such low-level interaction with the operating system can lead to system instability; second, they are really hard to build and maintain; and third, some applications use their own internal mechanisms to render text and graphics and hence are blank voids to the offscreen model (Java applications using Swing are a classic example, but DirectDraw applications like Internet Explorer 9 or Firefox 7 are increasingly common). For these reasons, newer screenreaders like NVDA have elected to go with application-specific and operating system APIs.

Application-specific APIs allow a screenreader developer to write code to connect to and query an application about its current state. For example, on Windows machines a developer can use COM to talk to Microsoft Word to find out the current line, the formatting, the caret position, and launch the spellcheck—all through the Word Object Model API. These APIs are powerful but application-specific: a developer must write code to support each one. And the API content does not necessarily reflect the application experience for a blind user—menus activity is not generally reflected in the API, for example—so the application cannot be completely supported through the API alone.

Operating system accessibility APIs were developed starting with Microsoft Active Accessibility (MSAA) in 1998. An application that complies with an accessibility API guarantees that screenreaders and other access software will be provided with information on the current control, the window, activity and anything else that is needed. For example, it might say that all buttons will announce themselves as type "button" and provide the caption and whether the button has, or can take the focus. Now, no matter how the button is actually drawn on the screen and made to operate—whether Windows API, .Net, Qt, GTK, Java, or any other graphical toolkit or underlying programming language—a button looks and works the same to a screenreader. So the screenreader no longer has to maintain an expensive and unreliable offscreen model: instead it can interact with this parallel representation of the program. The accessibility API draws the user interface to a screenreader just as the conventional code draws the user interface to the screen for a mouse user. In theory, accessibility APIs are the best solution for access software operation.

There are three problems, however, with accessibility APIs. First, the interfaces they represent are complex and designed for visual and mouse use: these alternative representations are not equal in terms of task profile (Bennett and Edwards, 1998). If the user presses a button that makes text in another control bold, the sighted user can see the change and understand it. A screenreader could announce that the button has been pressed, or announce the text that has been bolded, or play a tone and move the user focus to the selected text—it is not trivial to communicate the change nor for the user to understand it. The accessibility API may announce different events—button pressed, text changed, selection changed—depending on the implementing application. A naïve screenreader relying only on the accessibility API will still encounter different behavior and characteristics of common controls, where the similarities in function are obvious to a sighted user—between Microsoft Word and OpenOffice, for example. Screenreader developers must still write application-specific code despite the accessibility APIs.

The more significant problem with accessibility APIs is that, like many standards, different people use a different standard. Sometimes there are political reasons: it is unsurprising that Sun never supported the Microsoft MSAA in Java applications written for Windows, or that Microsoft Office on the Apple Mac does not support the Apple Mac OSX Accessibility Model. Sometimes there are engineering reasons: the simple MSAA API cannot handle the complexity of the Microsoft Word document area, so Microsoft has had to introduce a new accessibility API, user interface automation (UIA). Sometimes there are pragmatic reasons: accessibility API support usually comes later on in the development of an application, maybe in the second or third release, and lags behind commercially important user interface developments. So, while, in theory, accessibility APIs reduce screenreader development requirements and obviate the need for offscreen models, in practice, the workload is still significant. To support a reasonable "minimum specification" for a screenreader on Windows, supporting Windows Explorer, Notepad, Microsoft Word, Internet Explorer, Firefox, and Java applications on a Windows machine users would need to handle MSAA, the Microsoft Word Document Object Model, the Internet Explorer Document Object Model and/or UIA, IAccessible2, and the Java Access Bridge. In this area, homogeneity and monopoly is a great boon: if everyone still used exclusively Internet Explorer 6 and Microsoft Office, then the work of the screenreader vendors would be greatly eased!

Finally, the existence of a defined accessibility API for a technology does not mean that complying with it is automatic or trivial. It is not a panacea. Developers must still attend to the use of their application by a screenreader user (e.g., can users tab around the whole user interface with the keyboard, or do users need to use the mouse?) and work around any problems encountered in user testing: this work is often not done, although automated tools to identify accessibility problems like Accessibility Checker for Windows can help. The requirements of complying with the API may be at odds with other requirements, such as the appearance or security concerns. An interesting example is Windows Explorer. The Folder Options dialog contains a list of checkbox options, which one would assume would work well with MSAA or UIA by default. However, Microsoft contains a "screenreader flag," a global internal setting which when set indicates to applications that they should make themselves accessible if they were not before, shown in Figure 11.1. If this is set then the checkbox list in Windows Explorer suddenly gains explicit text in the label for each textbox that shows the checked state. Clearly, either the MSAA/UIA interface for this dialog could not be correctly implemented or the testing indicated that it could not be used. Such design compromises are both necessary and infrequently the top priority for application developers.

Here, then, is how a new screenreader without an offscreen model might enable a user to work with Microsoft Word:

1. The screenreader uses the Windows API to identify the foreground window as Word.
2. The screenreader uses MSAA to get the currently selected control in Word. It turns out to be the document area (where users type, as opposed to the ribbon control area).
3. The screenreader queries the Word Document Object Model to get the caret position and the surrounding text.
4. The screenreader hooks a low-level keypress by the user indicating that the current line in Word should be read aloud.
5. The screenreader queries the Word DOM and gets the text.
6. The screenreader sends the text to the speech synthesizer or the Braille display.

Screenreaders tie together a profusion of interfaces and techniques to try to present a coherent audio/Braille user interface for a blind user. It is a difficult task, made more so by the incompatible standards employed and the rapid changes in applications and operating systems common on modern machines.

How the Desktop User Experiences a Screenreader

A desktop screenreader user is using a nonvisual modality—touch or more usually speech. This means that he or she cannot quickly grasp the contents of the screen—what is happening? How many buttons? What can I click on right now?—but must explore the current application to find buttons, controls, and other features. It is much more a process of learning how a particular application works with the user's screenreader than is the more obvious mouse/screen interface. Screenreader users therefore need to build accurate mental models of applications, and to use them efficiently, they often employ dozens of keyboard shortcut keys. This is cognitively challenging, for a start. It needs good keyboard skills: multiple-key combinations can be a challenging combination of keys to hit and most blind people

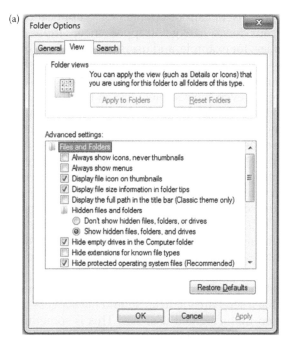

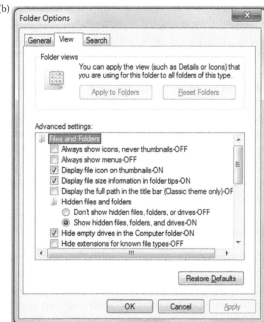

FIGURE 11.1
Windows Explorer with the screenreader flag off (a) and on (b) showing how text is added to support screenreaders.

cannot touch-type. Users cannot operate some applications with the keyboard alone—your focus can get trapped in an input field in a badly designed web page, for example, and users cannot tab out of it. And changes in applications—for example, the introduction of the ribbon in Microsoft Office 2007—can mean the loss of painstakingly acquired knowledge of how to do things or even the complete loss of the ability to use an application (if the changes are major). Blind screenreader users therefore often hate change even more than most users, and are loath to migrate from one screenreader to another, or even to update their software, operating system, or screenreader if they can avoid it. Using a full screenreader is therefore difficult and for some people too unrewarding: they stop using a computer at all, or rely on squinting or magnification. Using a screenreader is not the same as using the screen and mouse, no matter how skilled a screenreader user becomes. Their task profile, what is easy and what is not, and the fundamental interfaces they are using, keyboard and API rather than mouse and window, means their user experience is very different—even if they do not know it.

The fact is that the dominant paradigm for screenreader use is functional completeness: that a screenreader user should have access to all the information on the screen that a sighted user has. This is sometimes an idea more strongly held by sighted people than actual screenreader users, who are forced to be more pragmatic. In consequence, the idea of eliding content to improve aspects of usability is regarded with suspicion. Rather than the concept of "maximum output for minimum time" (Blenkhorn and Evans, 2001)—truncating or simplifying user interfaces to permit screenreader users to operate them faster, at the cost of some theoretical "full" understanding—the philosophy is to make sure that every element is made available somehow, if only the user has the patience. This is not unreasonable given the history of incomplete and outdated "accessible versions" of web pages and other products. But this is not an accurate task analysis for screenreader users employing a different modality from sighted mouse users: prioritizing completeness over speed of operation may reduce operational efficiency to the point where the user may simply give up on the screenreader (King 2007).

How a Screenreader Vendor Experiences the Desktop

Even if every application fully complied with the operating system accessibility API, the nuances and complexities of real-world usage in anything beyond the most trivial user interface means that the chances of a screenreader working efficiently "out of the box" with a given application are small. Decisions that have no impact on the standard sighted mouse user are very important to screenreader users. When users open an email in your email client, where is focus placed first—the From field, the Subject field, or the body of the email? Is there a caret? Are the From/Subject fields fixed labels, or are they text areas? Even if a developer attempts to comply with the accessibility API requirements, he or she is unlikely to provide the same quality of user experience to a screenreader user. This requires that a screenreader vendor (or a third party) writes code (or a script) to handle the application. For example, when an email is opened the screenreader may detect this event, read the From/Subject fields, then instruct the application to place the focus and a caret in the email body. This can be very effective, but the burden of work is thus placed on the screenreader vendor, and there are hundreds of applications in common use and thousands upon thousands in general use on each platform. Each represents an investment of time by the screenreader vendor. Unless a competitor is claiming better support for a popular application, or your existing customers are insisting on support, users will have little incentive to do more work to support yet another application, now and in future, and especially with ever-faster-changing user interfaces. What this means is that with any given fixed resource of developers, a screenreader vendor can support and maintain only a limited set of applications. With bigger commercial products able to support more developers (JAWS), this set can be bigger. With fewer developers (NVDA, other screenreaders) it will be smaller. So, if users need email, word processing, web browsing and a media player, and do not mind what application users use to achieve these ends, then anything from VoiceOver to JAWS will suit users, and users can use one of the free screenreaders: home users like this have many possibilities. But if users need to use a particular specialized application for work, then users will probably need to use JAWS on a Windows machine—and pay for the latest version too.

State of the Art of Access Software (Screenreaders and Magnifiers)

Just as there are other office suites apart from Microsoft Office but relatively few people use them, there are other screenreaders apart from Freedom Scientific's JAWS. JAWS dominates the screenreader market. It is the gold standard against which everything else is measured: alternative screenreaders must work like JAWS, applications must work with JAWS, documents must be formatted to be usable in JAWS, and HTML accessibility standards must be based on how JAWS operates. Freedom Scientific provides a 40 min free demo version, which although strictly forbidden is widely used by sighted people to test their application or website. Cracked versions are widely available and used, especially in the developing world. With the ubiquity of JAWS in mind, here is the current state of screenreader and magnification technology.

Access Software for Microsoft Windows

Windows remains the main platform for accessible desktop machines because it has the most access software, is the most widely used and available operating system, and is used in work. Access software in its current form also developed in the late 1990s/early 2000s, when Windows was almost unchallenged, and since no one ever likes updating or changing their access software, much access software is still Windows-based.

Native Applications and APIs in Windows

Windows Narrator has provided a basic screenreader since Windows 2000 and is essentially unaltered in function since then: it does not support, for example, Microsoft Word or Internet Explorer (or any standard web browser) although the Developer Preview version for Windows 8 Metro has been beefed up. Regulatory, commercial, and practical concerns have probably kept Microsoft from building a capable screenreader—that may change in Windows 8. Windows Magnifier provides a basic magnifier, and has been greatly improved in Windows 7, but it lacks smoothing: this was to have been provided by the graphical display system used in Windows Presentation Framework, but this ran into the delayed Windows Vista problems and has never been supported. In theory, the next version of Windows after XP was to launch in 2005 with vector graphics, which of course can scale perfectly in magnification. This eventually arrived in Windows Presentation Foundation, so for a brief period, smooth magnification worked. Then, WPF was changed to remove this functionality to meet requirements in the underlying operating system. This may change again in Windows 8 in 2012 with the move to HTML applications rendered using DirectDraw and accelerated graphics.

The operating system also allows for font sizes and colors and the screen resolution to be changed to make text and graphics larger and easier to see. Microsoft's own applications now generally support this well, but third-party applications usually fail, leading to (for example) overlapping text in list boxes or dialogs that will not fit on the screen. Screenreaders usually enable these changes when they are installed, and AT professionals and some organizations proselytize about these features, but their relative complexity and inconsistent application makes them less popular than they might be. For example, users can make text bigger in Microsoft Outlook, but Outlook will not notice that users can no longer make use of the preview pane and turn it off or place it below your Inbox rather than beside it. The cascade of configuration and changes users need to make lead to a level of complexity such that only experienced volunteers for blind charities—usually retired IT workers—employ these techniques, being technical, poor, and having the time. (There is a general problem with access software: first, users have to realize users have a problem. Second, users have to realize there are solutions. Third, users have to be able to get them and operate them.)

Microsoft also provides two Windows operating system accessibility APIs. The first, MSAA, was developed for Windows 2000 (it worked on Windows 98 with an update). The second, UIA appeared in Windows Vista. Crudely put, MSAA is good for buttons, checkboxes, and plain text, and is accessible through COM and the Windows API, while UIA adds support for rich text areas, like the document area in Microsoft Word or web pages, and is accessible through the .Net framework. UIA always falls back to MSAA, so in practice, developers use the MSAA interface and various nonaccessibility COM interfaces for complex applications like Microsoft Word (Word DOM) or Internet Explorer (the W3C DOM or DHTML DOM). Third-party accessibility APIs on Windows include IAccessible2 API (Firefox) and the Java Access Bridge (Java).

The summary for Microsoft Windows might be good accessibility APIs, the dominant operating system for accessibility for PCs, and a wide range of access software; but a heterogeneous and fast-changing environment of programs leaves access software vendors struggling to make their screenreaders work everywhere on the latest products. If Internet Explorer 9 is coming out in a new version every year, users have to run to stay still.

Commercial Access Software

Windows provides the widest range of commercial access software for blind users. The ubiquitous JAWS from Freedom Scientific is dominant as a screenreader and is the *de facto* standard. Other important screenreaders include WindowEyes from GW Micro and SuperNova from Dolphin in the United Kingdom. Most screenreaders now can be *scripted*. That is, third-party developers can make and sell sets of instructions that enable screenreaders to operate with and support other applications. This widens the range of supported applications and provides an ecosystem of people interested in developing for the platform. For example, Jawbone is a script that enables JAWS to operate with Nuance's Dragon NaturallySpeaking, a speech recognition program. Without it, the utility of Dragon is greatly reduced: with it, there is yet another reason to use JAWS.

These products all fit the model of "standard computer plus software." However, many people use Windows machines with expensive hardware Braille displays, especially in Germany and other countries with good state support through medical insurance. The manufacturers of these Braille displays may use JAWS—all the commercial screenreader products are able to drive Braille displays—but often use their own screenreader software or reuse products under license from commercial vendors. These users are a tiny minority—very few blind people know any Braille, and even fewer can afford a Braille display—but they are often influential advocates for technology and blind people.

Free Software

For 30 years, from the 1980s onward, screenreaders and other access software were commercially available and usually expensive. There are now several free pieces of software.

The Thunder screenreader from screenreader.net launched in 2006 and is freeware—no cost, but copyright. It is aimed at novice blind users. However, its failure until recently to work with a web browser directly (it relied until 2010 on the WebbIE text browser), its copyright status, and its limited feature set compared to JAWS have limited its support among advocates.

The NVDA screenreader, by contrast, is a free software under the GNU Public License. Developed by two blind Australian developers, it has acquired a positive reputation and a strong following, even if most users may still also use JAWS and other commercial applications. It relies commercially on grants from large companies, attracted by the good publicity, eager to do something charitable, and perhaps also interested in annoying their competitors. For example, the Mozilla Foundation has funded NVDA to provide support for the Firefox web browser, which enables Mozilla to proclaim that their browser is "more accessible" than Microsoft's Internet Explorer and helps them to break down the Microsoft lock on access software. NVDA, like many good open-source products, is strongly influenced by the market leader, JAWS, so it is familiar and useful for experienced blind users and receives their approval. After 4 years, NVDA is looking increasingly mature and has enabled many users to move away from the commercial software upgrade cycle.

Finally, System Access To Go is a commercial screenreader that is delivered over the web. Users navigate to a simple small download that runs without installation and starts speaking: this operates on the whole machine, not just in the web browser that ran the download.

Access Software for Apple Mac OSX

Apple shipped the 10.4 version of its Apple Mac operating system in 2005 with the new built-in VoiceOver screenreader. Superficially, this operates in a similar manner to Microsoft's built-in Narrator, in that it relies on applications complying with the Apple operating system accessibility API, the Mac OS X Accessibility Protocol, just as Narrator relies on applications complying with MSAA/UIA. However, while Narrator is generally unpopular, VoiceOver has received favorable attention and has a following. There are two reasons for this.

First, VoiceOver is a fully featured screenreader, with all the shortcut and hotkeys that blind screenreader users expect and can use to maximize their productivity. It works with dozens of Braille displays out-of-the-box, and has multiple high-quality voices (as of the Lion OS 10.7 update) in many languages.

The second, more important reason for VoiceOver's success is the wide-spread correct adoption of the Mac accessibility API. In Window, few applications have been written to support MSAA/UIA fully. On the Apple platform, applications such as Safari (web browsing), Pages (word processing), iTunes (media), and Finder (file explorer) all work very well with VoiceOver "out of the box" and are all standard applications. A blind screenreader user with an Apple Mac can enjoy the use of the same applications as his sighted peers because they have been written to support the Mac accessibility API.

There is a significant caveat, however. All these applications support the Mac accessibility API because they have been developed by Apple itself. Other non-Apple applications, like Mozilla Firefox, or OpenOffice, or Microsoft Office, fail to do so or do so as an afterthought. This is not uncommon: Apple's iTunes for Windows appeared in 2003, but blind users had to wait until iTunes 8 and the threat of legal action in 2008 to get MSAA support. Blind people on the Mac therefore find themselves in a walled garden. They are fine so long as they are happy with the Apple applications, but if they need to step outside that garden, then their screenreader breaks down. For home users, this is perhaps not a problem: the Apple applications are robust, powerful, and inexpensive. For business users unable to use Microsoft Office this is unsatisfactory and perhaps prevents more widespread adoption of VoiceOver.

It is interesting to compare the Windows ecosystem, where competing third parties create screenreaders, and the Mac ecosystem, where now only VoiceOver exists (at least since the end of OutSpoken from Berkeley Accessibility). On Windows, the Mozilla Foundation was able to grant the NVDA project money to support Firefox: Apple was able to persuade Window Eyes to develop iTunes support. The screenreader developers could then trumpet their new feature—"works with Firefox/iTunes!"—and the application developer could claim accessibility and avoid lawsuits, negative publicity, and potential loss of sales from corporate and government customers. On Apple, there is no such leverage: Microsoft is unlikely to pay Apple to make VoiceOver work with Office, Apple is unlikely to take the money and do it. The situation on the Mac—VoiceOver with Apple products, or nothing—is therefore unlikely to change.

Access Software for GNU/Linux

On the face of it, the GNU/Linux environment ought to be a good one for access software: all the underlying technologies from the kernel upward are available as source code, the high costs that are alleged to be a significant barrier to the deployment of access software are missing, and the ability to review, reuse and redistribute code means developers can cooperate rather than employ the patents and trade secrets of the commercial screenreader vendors. In practice, however, the free-wheeling development environment is at odds with access software development, which requires consistency and compliance with agreed standards. The situation is better when developers are interested in "scratching their own itch," developing solutions for their own needs, or corporations are willing to pay for development to meet some corporate or political goal, such as Mozilla funding for NVDA.

Discussing Linux accessibility is hard without going into distros and window managers (e.g., GNOME vs. KDE). A few general points: Linux, like Unix, has a greater emphasis on command line usage than OSX or Windows, which may be more accessible for screenreader users—it is at least linear and text-only—and the Speakup screenreader has been available to read shell windows in GNU/Linux since 1998. Like OSX and Windows, GNU/Linux has system-wide accessibility settings for font size, color, contrast, and magnification: like them, too, applications may or may not respect these settings. There are three interfaces analogous to MSAA, the widely supported Assistive Technology Service Provider Interface (AT-SPI), the Accessibility Toolkit (ATK) used in GNOME applications, and the IAccessible2 interface used in Firefox (as in Windows), and the situation is further confused by different approaches of the two main desktop environments, KDE and GNOME. But all the fundamentals are there.

The current mainstream screenreader for GNU/Linux is Orca (continuing a tradition of naming screenreaders after sea animals) taking over from *Gnopernicus*. It is installed by default with the GNOME desktop, used in the Ubuntu distribution, but various system and applications settings have to be changed to best employ it. The Vinux distribution addresses this by creating an Ubuntu distribution in which Orca and other accessibility settings are enabled by default. Another GNU/Linux system of note is the Emacspeaks application, which enables the mighty Emacs text editor to control an entire system, read the web, and do email, all with speech.

One significant issue for GNU/Linux systems is that high-quality speech synthesizers are not so readily available as on the Windows and Apple platforms. MBROLA voices and eSpeak voices are free, and commercial voices are available, but generally human-sounding voices are the preserve of the commercial platforms. However, screenreader users often prefer the more "robotic-sounding" voices as being more reliably understandable and amenable to being speeded up to an astonishing degree.

Access Software on Tablets and Mobile (Cell) Phones

These two types of device are being taken together because they share operating systems: in 10 years time when we all are using tablets instead of PCs, this may seem a ludicrous aggregation. It is certainly the case for sighted people that a tablet is not the same as a phone: for a blind user it may or may not be more similar.

Texting and using an address book on a cellphone has been a problem for blind people. Nuance's Talks&Zooms for the Symbian phone operating system from Nokia enabled users to use a cellphone and provided an enormous degree of independence. However, it has since been eclipsed by the hugely influential iPhone from Apple, using the iOS operating system and including the free VoiceOver screenreader. Apple has built VoiceOver right into the heart of how the iPhone (and the later iPad) operates, so every application developed by Apple for the iPhone/iPad works with VoiceOver—including the web browser, Safari, which allows the blind user to explore a webpage by touch in two dimensions (speaking what is under the finger), quite different from the traditional re-presentation in a screenreader as a linear stream of text items. In addition, the control that Apple exercises over the applications permitted in the Apple App Store and the constrained environment in which they operate means that most applications are accessible by default to an extent that is not the same on the Apple OSX desktop, let alone in Windows. The iPad, which is larger and therefore requires less fine control and dexterity to operate by touch, also allows people with some sight to easily bring the display up to their face, and zoom web pages and other content easily with gestures, so people can take advantage of what sight they have. Both can drive Braille displays by Bluetooth. Taken together they represent a revolution in accessibility for blind people—at least those able to afford the hardware and to understand and utilize the powerful features. Anyone seeking to use a different screenreader from VoiceOver, however, will be disappointed because of the structure of iOS: only one application can run at once, so users cannot run a screenreader at the same time as your email program or web browser. Self-voicing applications are possible, and eBook readers on the iPad often have this feature, but third-party screenreader development on the iOS platform is currently impossible.

Until Windows 8 Mobile comes out in 2012, the only other serious player in the cellphone space is Android from Google. Android has a screenreader developed by Google, Talkback, and Android 1.6 "Donut" in 2009 introduced an accessibility API for third-party applications. At present, iOS has the momentum and popularity, but Android is selling in greater absolute numbers and becoming more powerful with each new version. Its more open architecture may allow for more third-party technology, such as the Safe & Sound applications from screenreader.net.

Big Specific Issues for Access Software

It is useful to review some key challenges for access software that will shape new and existing products over the next 5 years.

New Web (HTML5, The Cloud)

It is possible that everything in this chapter about screenreader applications running on desktop systems will be as redundant in 20 years as the green-screen terminal. The current fashion is for applications to be written as web pages—that is, HTML plus JavaScript and CSS, variously known as "HTML5" or "Web 2.0" or "Ajax" or "DHTML" or "web applications." These applications can now be as fully featured, complex, and hence unusable for screenreader users as desktop applications.

How does the blind user approach a web application? At present, of course, he or she uses his or her screenreader to access the standard browser that is rendering the web application. At a superficial level, then, this is a problem of degree, not of kind: web applications are web pages rendered in browsers, and screenreaders know how to read web pages in browsers, so all is well. There are two problems with this optimistic view.

First is the degree of complexity. Microsoft Word is more than a text box with a toolbar stuck on it, and Google Docs is more than a TEXTAREA element in a web page with some links. Saying that the individual components are accessible does not mean that the whole is usable in any practical sense. In effect, the problems of supporting applications described above now extends to websites: if your screenreader vendor can support 10 applications, but now must consider Facebook and Microsoft Office 365 and Google Docs all as fully featured applications in their own right, with all the scripting and thought and work required to support them fully, then the number of native nonweb applications on your machine that can be supported is reduced by three. This would not be such a problem if the web application market were as dominated by a few major players as the desktop market: if everyone on the web used Google Docs, and no one used Microsoft Office 365, then users needed only write the code to support Google Docs. But the web is in a state of flux: we do not know which web applications will win out, or even if the monocultures enjoyed by screenreader users in the past will ever be achieved again. So, in effect, the access software industry must suddenly support dozens of innovative new online applications; new ones are being developed at a rapid rate, and applications are able to change literally overnight without user resistance.

The second problem is that the technology employed in building web pages is changing. Microsoft's domination of the market with Internet Explorer 6 has ended, and the result is a sudden rate of change in HTML and associated technologies not seen for a decade. It is not just the extent of the changes but their nature, for example, input elements, like buttons, which are correctly identified for screenreaders by browsers, can now be replaced by other arbitrary elements (e.g., DIV elements) with the appropriate click and focus events. For the mouse user, they look and work the same way as a "real" button. For the web developer, new exciting features can replace the old boring button. For the screenreader user, however, the identifiable button element has disappeared, and suddenly he or she cannot use the web application at all. Of particular note is the HTML5 CANVAS element, which completely abandons the idea of HTML rendering content and JavaScript providing only functionality. This may never have been true in practice—try turning off JavaScript in your browser and going to Facebook or the BBC iPlayer—but the general principle was that a static, accessible HTML page should fulfill all the tasks for which the page was written, without recourse to the complicated and inaccessible features of JavaScript. A CANVAS element by contrast is a blank, textless area on which images and text are drawn by JavaScript—exactly like desktop applications before the accessibility APIs, when screenreaders had to rely entirely on offscreen models and intercepting drawing messages. CANVAS is already being employed for games and graphical applications, and browser developers have committed to developing graphic acceleration techniques to make it more responsive. As graphical toolkits are developed for CANVAS, just as toolkits like GTK or Qt or Java Swing have been developed for desktop operating systems, we can expect to see more applications employ user interfaces built entirely with CANVAS. It seems almost certain that these applications will be inaccessible or at least unusable without further web browser and screenreader development.

The situation on HTML5 is analogous to the position of desktop machines in the 1990s before MSAA but it is not identical. We start from a position of advantage. Desktops have progressed from offscreen models and inaccessible applications to accessibility APIs and the assumption that accessibility should be expected. This route provides a roadmap and an example for HTML5 development. The accessibility API for the web has been created, the WAI-ARIA standard, which defines buttons and roles and events in much the same way as the MSAA/UIA/Apple guidelines. Operating system vendors have mapped WAI-ARIA to their particular operating system accessibility APIs. As HTML5 matures, graphical toolkits like the Yahoo! User Interface Library will produce user interface widgets that comply with WAI-ARIA standards, just as Windows toolkits like Qt have produced UI widgets that comply with MSAA. Accessibility, although too-often defined as "works for JAWS users," has won the argument and is regarded as something that vendors and developers must support, and is also a good way for developers to demonstrate their expertise. Web developers will therefore work to support accessibility—assuming that they get it right. The increasing complexity of the accessibility guidelines would suggest that we have become better at using them, but this is not necessarily the case. For example, after 15 stable years, the simple alt attribute is still widely misused by HTML writers: the new accessibility elements in HTML5 and the WAI-ARIA attributes are more complicated. It seems unlikely they will be correctly used, if they are used at all. Huge arguments have erupted in the HTML5 specification process at the dropping of the little-used LONGDESC element, for example; the sorry truth is that it is almost never employed correctly.

The problem is that traditional HTML web pages, limiting as they were for developers and designers, were fundamentally accessible "out of the box." It is hard to write an inaccessible HTML3 web page if users populate the alt attributes on your images. By contrast, it is surprisingly easy to write an inaccessible HTML5 web page: there is so much more opportunity to get things wrong, from using the wrong mechanism to hide error text to trapping the caret in a text area while users try to validate form input. WAI-ARIA assumes that this situation will be resolved by the developer doing more work to add back in the "this is a button" kind of information to allow screenreaders to operate, but experience suggests that this often fails to happen. Since we are moving from enforced accessibility (thanks to the limitations of HTML4) to optional accessibility (the more powerful HTML5), then initially at least HTML5 will be a retrograde step for accessibility. A prosaic online example of this for screenreader users is Macromedia Flash, which like HTML5 can be made accessible but usually is not: it seems likely that this will be the case for much of the HTML5 web in future.

It remains the case that individual sites can now be as complex as applications, and will now require as much investment as individual applications by screenreader vendors, so much of the web will become less accessible. However, highly used applications like Facebook or Google Mail (or their future incarnations) will be made accessible just as Microsoft Word is now. The general idea that just by mastering your web browser and screenreader users can access every website may be lost. But our experience with the desktop environment helps us to know how to proceed, and although the process will be painful, we can hope to achieve yet more accessible and powerful applications delivered through the web to blind users.

Media (Radio, Podcasts, Television)

One of the enormous advantages of the Internet is the sheer quantity of media available. Films, TV, and radio can all be obtained by the blind user from their machine. Audio description can be provided for online formats by the media author or by third parties.

The obstacles that exist are primarily political and economic, not technical. Commercial sources of media, such as the BBC or NetFlix, restrict the user interfaces and media available for licensing reasons: they seek to prevent users from being able to copy media or access it in unapproved ways. For example, the BBC makes television programs available to PC users only through a Flash interface that is difficult for many blind people to use rather than making available their existing H.264 video streams for iPhone, and has taken legal action against anyone attempting to make these streams available for non-iOS users. Blind users therefore receive a less-accessible service.

The obvious question is why blind users do not simply pirate content. Piracy software is often inaccessible, pirate sites even more so, and the high level of fakes and malicious virus-infected content may be off-putting for many blind users who struggle with security issues. However, the true answer is probably demographic: blind people tend to be older, and for technical and social reasons are less likely to pirate. This may change with time, as a quick search for illegal cracked copies of JAWS will show.

Finally, the design of the delivery of multimedia content can make it hard or easy to use the content. The YouTube site, for example, autoplays videos as soon as a page is loaded. The BBC iPlayer site requires the user to navigate to and click a button on the page to start the video. While autoplaying content is generally disapproved of, especially by technically skilled screenreader users who want to retain control over when the content plays and how it interferes with hearing the speech from their screenreader, the YouTube solution is much better for many screenreader users—possibly the majority of them. Standards and expert opinions are not necessarily the best guide to the best experience for the majority.

Office and Email (Microsoft and Others)

Consumption of content is relatively simple to define in terms of user interface, but creation of content is far more complex. This makes screenreader support for content-creation programs more challenging.

The challenge for blind people is that the content they create must be of a good standard for sighted consumers of the content. gETTING YOUR CASE WRONG IN wORD will make users look foolish but is easily done with one accidental keystroke if users cannot see the text users are typing. Tabs, font sizes, and other easy traps await. Screenreaders therefore provide mechanisms that allow users to quickly identify their current styles, and to alert them to unexpected content like ALLCAPS passages. Ideally, perhaps, content creation in email or word processing would be more like content creation in online blog interfaces like WordPress. Here, the user may enter only plain text but the rendered final output acquires attractive and consistent styles and the effect is pleasing to both author and consumer. However, users still need some knowledge of styles or even markup, which is fine for technical users but beyond most people, sighted or not. More generally, although sighted people routinely use layout and formatting to communicate semantics (headers, font sizes, layout), blind people are more reliant on third-party help or trusting that their audience will understand their limited repertoire of visual effects. As a sighted person, websites created by blind people are often obvious as soon as they are seen: linear text, no layout, no indentation.

Another problem for screenreader users is spelling. Users who were once sighted have probably learned to read and write English, so the irregular orthography is at least familiar. Users who have never seen the written word find it much harder to communicate using English (users who have never heard English either, being deafblind, face still greater challenges). Homophones like "there" and "their" and "they're" can elude the blind user when reviewing text, and the handy red underline is not so useful for screen-reader users, who must rely on per-application spellchecks or copy and paste text a great deal to and from Word.

PDF (Adobe Reader, PDF Accessibility)

PDF is the *de facto* format for documents to be printed, exchanged or archived, and is increasingly common for eBooks. As a format designed for printing, not electronic consumption, it can easily be completely inaccessible to screenreaders (containing only image data, not text, and requiring an OCR image-to-text step) or accessible but completely unusable (text in the wrong order, big file sizes, very complex user interfaces and options, and an experience based on a per-page model that works really well only with mouse users). PDFs have therefore acquired a reputation for inaccessibility. In amelioration, the *de facto* standard client, Adobe Reader X, has a "save to text" option, built-in self-voicing options, and there is now a widespread understanding that users must create an "accessible" (nongraphics) PDF file for distribution. In recent years, OCR programs have dropped in price, free accessibility tools and client accessibility APIs are become available, and most screenreaders now support Adobe Reader, so the situation is much improved. It is not unfair to say that PDF files now, although still more cumbersome to read than, say, a Rich Text File format document, are now accessible for the majority of users, and suffer from the inherent tension between original print and current electronic function rather than any specific problem.

Printed Words (OCR, Copyright)

Ebooks, like other media, are restricted more by politics than by technology. The latest Harry Potter novel can be pirated in minutes (usually as a PDF file). However, the official legal channels of Bookshare and other organizations dedicated to providing accessible formats are increasingly speedy and the range of material is increasing. Publishers have been loath to provide content in electronic formats, seeing it as enabling piracy, and concerned about the additional costs and difficulties in creating accessible formats. However, it only requires one person to create a PDF and make it available through the Internet, and so eBooks are increasingly available illicitly. In some jurisdictions, it is even legal to make and distribute copies of books for people with disabilities (e.g., the Copyright (Visually Impaired Person) Act, 2002, in the United Kingdom).

The availability of an eBook, perhaps as a PDF, is not the same as having a fully accessible version of that eBook, perhaps in the specially designed DAISY eBook format, with features like shortcuts to chapters, an index, formatting to allow for magnification for people with some sight, and even embedded text-to-speech. These improved formats are especially important where the book is not a linear novel but a textbook where skipping around chapters and referencing particular passages is vital. These truly accessible formats are still rare, but may become less so as more of them are produced by publishers and agencies, now cognizant of how to make these books and seeking to work better with iPads and Kindles.

Security

Computer security is a concern with everyone, but may be particularly worrying for blind people who are older and nervous about computer use. They also find it hard to pick up on visual cues (font, spelling, color, and graphics) that allow sighted people to discriminate between genuine and malicious pop-up messages and other attempts to make users enable malicious code, like "Your machine is infected, click here!" pop-ups. When users have become accustomed to your computer launching unexpected user interfaces at users, and these user interfaces contain little except "OK" buttons, it is unsurprising if users assent to something dubious without meaning to do so.

Voice Output

Most screenreader users employ synthesized speech. It is often surprising to sighted people how some blind users speed up their speech synthesizers to a rate that is almost incomprehensible to someone who is not used to it. This helps blind users to compensate for their low rate of reading compared to sighted people and their inability to scan and quickly analyze information sources or user interfaces. The speech synthesizers that cope with this process often employ techniques that make them sound very regular but very robotic and mechanical. Conversely, some blind people cannot understand how some other, perhaps less technical, blind people find more naturalistic, human-sounding voices more acceptable and will refuse to listen to a system that is "too robotic." Getting the right speech synthesizer to a user may be as big a factor as getting the right support or the right screenreader or other access software.

Free, high-quality text-to-speech voices are more and more readily available for European languages and Chinese, sometimes as part of the operating system (Apple's Lion OSX 10.7 comes with more than 40 voices). However, for screenreader users in non-Western languages, synthesized speech is poor quality, expensive, or nonexistent; the only voices available are often produced by universities, and do not work on commercial platforms like Windows and disappear when the student responsible graduates. This may change as non-Western countries like India further develop their vibrant software industries, or operating system vendors include more high-quality voices in their operating systems for free.

References

Asakawa, C., Itoh, T. 1998. User interface of a home page reader. In *Assets '98: Proceedings of the Third International ACM Conference on Assistive Technologies.* Blattner, M.M., Karshmer, A.I. (Eds.) Marina del Rey, California, USA. ACM Press, New York, USA. pp. 149–156.

Bennett, D.J., Edwards, A.D.N. 1998. Exploration of nonseen diagrams. *The Fifth International Conference on Auditory Display (ICAD98),* Glasgow, U.K.

Blenkhorn, P., Evans, G., King, A., Kurniawan, S.H., Sutcliffe, A. 2003. Screen magnifiers: Evolution and evaluation. In *IEEE Computer Graphics and Applications,* Volume 23, Number 5, September/October 2003, pp. 54–62. http://www.alasdairking.me.uk/research/Blenkhorn2003-ScreenMagnifiers.html.

Blenkhorn, P., Evans, G. 2001. Considerations for user interaction with talking screen readers. *Technology and Persons with Disabilities Conference (CSUN) 2001.* Northridge, California, USA.

Blenkhorn, P., Evans, D. G. 2001. The architecture of a Windows screen reader. In Marinček, C., Bühler, C., Knops, H, Andrich, R. (Eds.) *Assistive Technology— Added Value to the Quality of Life (AAATE 2001),* IOS Press, Amsterdam, pp. 119–123.

Evans, G., Blenkhorn, P. 2003. Architectures of assistive software applications for Windows-based computers. *Journal of Computer and Network Applications* 26, 213–228.

King, A. 2007. Re-presenting visual content for blind people. PhD Thesis, University of Manchester. http://www.alasdairking.me.uk/research/PhD.htm.

Kurniawan, S.H., King, A., Evans, G. Blenkhorn, P. 2006. Personalising web page presentation for older people. *Interacting with Computers* 18, 457–477.

12

Tools for Improving Web Accessibility for Blind Persons

Sri Kurniawan

CONTENTS

Introduction

The increasing provision of web-based information resources has moved from a simple text interface to dynamic and interactive designs. While this move has provided people with a more creative and flexible experience, there are dangers that some people will be excluded because they cannot use standard methods of access. Research has shown that people with disabilities are most at risk of being excluded from access, and in particular, people who are blind or visually impaired and who use assistive technologies such as screen readers (Brophy and Cavern 2007).

There is a growing, worldwide recognition that users with disabilities, including blind and visually impaired persons, have the same right as others to access web-based information. In the late 1990s, web accessibility received broad attention, and regulations and guidelines were published and adopted.

One of the major focuses of these initiatives, because of the visual-heavy nature of the web, is accessibility for blind users.

In the United States, Section 508 of the Rehabilitation Act (29 U.S.C. 794d), as amended by the Workforce Investment Act of 1998 and has been in effect since June 2001 (from here on, for brevity, this set of guidelines will be called "Section 508"), and the Americans with Disabilities Act (ADA), aim at making sure the web and other information technologies do not disadvantage users with disabilities. Section 508 requires that electronic and information technology that is developed by or purchased by the Federal Agencies be accessible by people with disabilities. In addition to providing for enforceable standards, the amended Section 508 established a complaint procedure and reporting requirements, which further strengthen the law. Beginning in June 2001, all government websites were required to conform to these standards. Any contractor doing web development for the Federal government must build websites that conform to these standards. Any company doing business with the Federal government or with states receiving technical assistance funds (Tech Act states) also has to put forth an accessible web presence.

The ADA, which became law in 1990, is a civil rights law that prohibits discrimination against people with disabilities. The ADA generally requires employers, state and local governments, and places of public accommodation to offer reasonable services or tools to insure that people are not discriminated against on the basis of disability.

In other countries around the world, web accessibility has also been enforced by laws and regulations. For example, the Equality Act came into force in October 2010, replacing the Disability Discrimination Act (DDA) in England, Scotland, and Wales (RNIB 2011). In summary, the act states that it may be unlawful for a website to

- Have links on that are not accessible to a screen reader
- Have application forms (for instance, for bank accounts or job application forms) in a PDF format that cannot be read by a screen reader
- Have core service information (for instance, timetables on a public transport website) that is not in a format accessible to screen readers
- Use text, color contrasting, and formatting that make the website inaccessible to a partially sighted service user
- Change security procedures (for instance, on an e-commerce website) without considering the impact of blind and partially sighted customers who use screen readers, such as by using an image-only CAPTCHA*

---

* A CAPTCHA is a program that protects websites against bots by generating tests that humans can pass but current computer programs cannot. It assumes, for example, that humans can read an image of distorted text, but current computer programs cannot. Unless of course the humans are blind, in which case they cannot see the image that is not readable by a screen reader.

In Canada, The Standard on Web Accessibility came into effect on August 1, 2011. This standard applies to all web pages that are public facing and those that are provided through Government of Canada websites.

One very important set of guidelines is the set developed by World Wide Web Consortium's (W3C) Web Accessibility Initiative,* which includes Web Content Accessibility Guidelines (WCAG), currently version 2.0, Authoring Tool Accessibility Guidelines (ATAG) version 1.0, and User Agent Accessibility Guidelines (UAAG) version 1.0. WCAG addresses the information in a website, including text, images, forms, sounds, and so on. ATAG addresses a software that creates websites, while UAAG addresses web browsers and media players, and relates to assistive technologies.

The aforementioned legislations led to the creation of standards, guidelines, and checklists for accessibility. While they vary in their requirements for compliance, the goal is usually to develop a common understanding of what is needed to make web pages accessible, thereby enabling web designers, web developers, site owners, and businesses to meet these requirements. To help web authors determine whether pages they create meet these guidelines, web accessibility validation tools, and professional website accessibility audits were also developed (Richards and Hanson 2004). However, for many web authors and developers, the issue of web accessibility remains a concern. This chapter starts with the problems blind users face with inappropriately designed web-based information, then continues with the tools that can help web designers and developers make their web-based information more accessible for blind users.

How Do Blind People Access the Web?

In brief, most blind people usually use a screen reader for most computing activities, although there are various other methods for accessing computer-based information (discussed in Chapter 7). If the user is using a screen reader, then he or she is also probably using a mainstream browser to render the page. Some screen readers interface with these mainstream browsers to retrieve structure and other information, and therefore they can, for example, cope with frames by reading each frame in turn, including the title of the frames (if available). Or they can separate the links and the text, allowing for faster browsing to check if there are relevant links in the current page. However, some screen readers operate in a linear way, reading the page left to right, top to bottom, the way they read e-mail or word-processed documents, meaning that the navigation links are mixed together with the text.

---

* http://www.w3.org/WAI/guid-tech.html

Some blind web users use a browser designed specifically for blind users (also discussed in Chapter 7). In this case, the browser should be able to pass the structural information on to the user in a meaningful way. The down side to special browsers is that their development typically lags the development of the more popular browsers. So, they may not support the newest animations, security, or other innovations in some sites.

Finally, a small percentage of blind people use a tactile device, such as BrailleNote, to access the web.

It should be noted that most blind persons cannot use a mouse because it is a relative pointing device and therefore any link that requires mouse movements (e.g., activated by hovering over a location in a page) will be difficult, if not impossible, for blind web users.

Problems Faced by Blind Web Users

Di Blas et al. (2004) summarized very nicely the problems that blind web users face because of the nature of how screen readers work (see Chapter 7 for a more detailed description of the strengths and limitations of screen readers). These problems are listed below. Whenever appropriate, a screenshot of a website as read by a screen reader is presented (the screen reader simulation is performed with WebbIE, a web browser for blind persons that we developed).

1. Because screen readers read the screen, some read all the text in a web page when the page is not carefully designed, including elements of HTML that are solely used for visualization only (and do not convey relevant meaning to the listener)

2. Many screen readers read in a linear way: "top-to-bottom/left-to right," forcing the users to wait for the relevant piece of information unless the information is near the top left of the page.

3. Screen readers do not convey the overall organization of the page, with the relative priorities of the different parts. For example, a sighted reader can immediately see an important section of an online newspaper just by looking at the area at the center of the page. A blind user cannot do this easily unless there is a markup that indicated items of higher importance than others.

4. Screen readers interleave the reading of content with the reading of links. Some screen readers can read only the list of links, but out of context these links might not make sense. In addition, some screen readers organize the links in alphabetical order, which can further confuse the users as the context is definitely lost because of the reordering. Figure 12.1 presents a section of BBC News page when

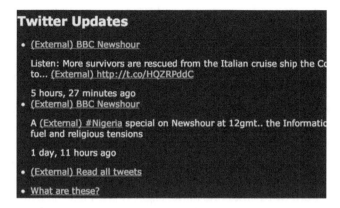

FIGURE 12.1
A section of the BBC website as parsed through a screen reader.

parsed through a screen reader. In this version, because the links are embedded in the text, we know that the link called "What are these" is a link that explains about Twitter updates on BBC News website. However, if the links are grouped together separately from the surrounding text, then this link becomes more difficult to interpret.

5. Because users have to listen to a link being read in its entirety before choosing it, users often miss clicking on that link as the screen readers already move to the next link by the time the users digest the information.

Guidelines for Writing for Blind Web Users

Because of the problems laid out earlier, many organizations had developed guidelines based on Section 508, WCAG, and others. The guidelines presented below are consolidated sets of published guidelines from the Communication Technologies Branch of the United States National Cancer Institute (Theofanos and Redish 2003) as well as the National Federation for the Blind (Chong 2011). The guidelines are summarized below:

1. How to help screen readers read in a more meaningful way:
   a. Write succinctly: Write in short, clear, straightforward sentences. Use bulleted lists. Put the main point at the beginning of a paragraph. Write links that start with keywords.
   b. Use meaningful "ALT" tags to label the images in the site. When a screen reader encounters an image, if the graphic is labeled with an "ALT" tag, it will voice out the text string associated with

the tag. If it does not find any "ALT" tag, it might try to ascertain the name of the file which constitutes the image. If the name is something meaningful such as "company_logo.gif," the blind user may be able to infer that the image is a picture of a company logo. If, on the other hand, the name of the gif file is something like "image01.gif," then there is no way that the blind user can even begin to guess at the nature of the image. Use empty "ALT" text, ALT = "" for pictorial decorative elements on a page.

   c. Make the site structure clear and obvious. Provide site maps.

   d. Make for easy listening. Do not make up unusual names for products, services, or elements of a website. Do not combine two or more words into one name (e.g., "home page" is clearer when read by a screen reader than "homepage"). Figure 12.2 describes an example of a web page with links that could be made clearer when read by a screen reader if the words are separated by spaces (i.e., "wildlife" and "geopolitical").

   e. Make screen readers read an acronym or abbreviation as letters rather than attempting to read it as a word by using the <ACRONYM> and <ABBR> tags.

2. How to help navigation without sight:

   a. Include a skip link at the top of every web page as some screen readers read out all the links before the content.

   b. Make links descriptive by avoiding multiple generic links with the same labels such as "more" or "click here" so that when the links are grouped together, the blind users can still understand which link leads to where.

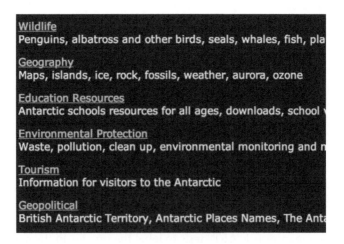

FIGURE 12.2
Two of the links could be made clearer if the words are separated (i.e., wildlife and geopolitical).

c. Do not create many links that start with the same word or phrase (even if the complete link labels are different).

d. Use anchor links in a long page with several topics to allow screen reader users to jump to the desired topic.

e. Be sure that the headings are coded properly in HTML, for example, as <H1> <H2>, and so on. as many screen readers look for the heading tag to indicate important information.

f. In a form, make sure that all fields are coded so that users do not have to switch to and from Edit mode. For HTML documents, this is done through [label] elements. In addition, name each input box and submit button appropriately.

g. Provide an alternative to autorefreshing pages (e.g., a splash screen that changes over time) as screen readers do not cope well with autorefreshing pages.

h. Ensure that the use of tables and multicolumn text does not preclude the ability of screen readers to render the pages in an intelligible and useful manner. Not all screen readers can navigate tables. Moreover, even the most sophisticated screen readers will have trouble with tables that contain many columns, as is the case with bus or train schedules. Figure 12.3 shows how the

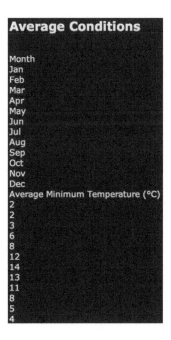

FIGURE 12.3
A linearized table of average temperatures for certain months.

sequence of information that the screen reader reads out loud. Instead of reading the month and the average minimum temperature in pairs (which would be more useful), the screen reader reads all the months followed by all of the average minimum temperatures, which is less useful.

i. Provide an alternative to applets or plug-ins as Java applets, JavaScript, and plug-ins such as Macromedia's Flash can create problems for blind web users.

j. Provide a means to avoid redundant links on a web page. While it is fairly common to place navigation links (e.g., "return to home page" and "contact us") on each page it can be time consuming and unnecessary for blind users to listen to these links multiple times.

Web Accessibility Development Aid and Evaluation Tools

W3C's Web Accessibility Initiative maintains a website that lists the tools that can significantly reduce the time and effort to develop accessible sites and to evaluate websites for accessibility problems.* Because most of these tools check web pages at code level instead of at semantic level (e.g., when there is an image in the page, it can check whether there is an ALT text associated with the image, but it cannot check whether the ALT text is a meaningful representation of the image), they still need to be complemented with manual check (W3C WAI 2006). A manual check was performed on the URL and the tools that were still active were used to either develop or evaluate a web page or (X)HTML file (or a set of web pages or files if the tool has such function).

The following summarizes the different categories of tools that are available for public use. These tools were active as of September 29, 2011 and they share a common characteristic: they are mainly aimed at ensuring web accessibility for blind web users (e.g., tools that check for color contrast are excluded). This list also excludes "services" (i.e., the links that point to a company performing the accessibility evaluation). Because a critical review of the tools and how they work is a part of this chapter, the tools that are not available in English are excluded. This chapter also includes a list of tools that are not in this WAI website, mostly tools that had been developed after 2006 (when the website was last updated).

---

* http://www.w3.org/WAI/ER/tools/complete

Design Helpers

These are tools that are helpful for developing accessible websites. They include tools that generate accessible tables, pop-up windows, and so on. Examples of this category of tools are

1. Accessible Pop-up Window Generator.* This tool, developed by Accessify, creates pop-up windows that are accessible and search engine-friendly through a very intuitive user interface. Figure 12.4 depicts the dialog window of this tool.
2. Accessible Table Builder.† This online tool, also developed by Accesify, guides users step by step to create an accessible table. Figure 12.5 depicts the first step of the table building activity.
3. CC for Flash, ccPlayer, and ccMP3Player.‡ The Carl and Ruth Shapiro Family National Center for Accessible Media (NCAM) developed a series of tools to make Flash more accessible. The tool can be used to display captions of Flash video and audio content. These captions are stored in external files written in the W3C's DFXP§ format which can be created with MAGpie, NCAM's free captioning application. CC for Flash can also display captions saved in Apple's QTtext format. To help Flash programming, NCAM also created two flexible players: ccPlayer that allows users to embed a Flash Video (FLV) player on the web page and ccMP3Player that plays back MP3 files in

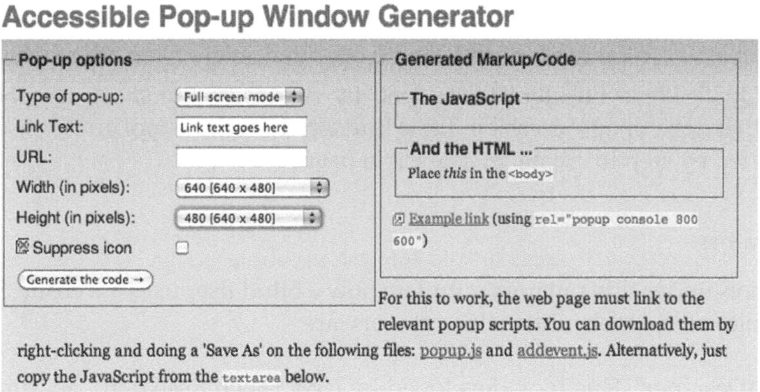

FIGURE 12.4
The Accessible Pop-up Generator.

---

* http://accessify.com/tools-and-wizards/accessibility-tools/pop-up-window-generator/
† http://accessify.com/tools-and-wizards/accessibility-tools/table-builder/
‡ http://ncam.wgbh.org/invent_build/web_multimedia/tools-guidelines/ccforflash
§ DFXP is an abstract document type of a profile of the Timed Text Markup Language intended to be used for interchange among distribution systems.

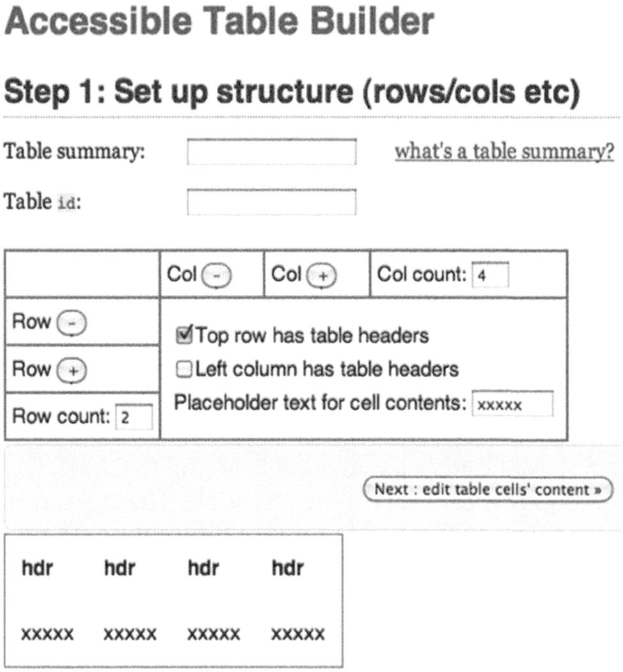

Accessible Table Builder

Step 1: Set up structure (rows/cols etc)

Table summary: [   ]   what's a table summary?

Table id: [   ]

	Col ⊖	Col ⊕	Col count: 4
Row ⊖	☑ Top row has table headers		
Row ⊕	☐ Left column has table headers		
Row count: 2	Placeholder text for cell contents: xxxxx		

(Next : edit table cells' content »)

hdr	**hdr**	**hdr**	**hdr**
xxxxx	xxxxx	xxxxx	xxxxx

FIGURE 12.5
The first step of creating an accessible table from Accessible Table Builder.

a web page with corresponding caption files. Both players are accessible to screen readers and can be operated solely from a keyboard.

4. Quick Form Builder.* Developed by Accessify, the same company that developed Accessible Table Builder, this online tool guides users step by step to create an accessible form.

Simulators

The tools under this category simulate how a blind user uses a website. Some examples of the tools under this category are

1. aDesigner.† This tool, developed by IBM Tokyo Research Lab, simulates a blind and low-vision web user. The tool looks at such elements as the degree of color contrast on the page, the ability of the user to change the font size, the appropriateness of alternate text for images, and the availability of links in the page to promote navigability. The tool also checks the page's compliance with various

---

* http://accessify.com/tools-and-wizards/accessibility-tools/quick-form-builder/
† http://www.trl.ibm.com/projects/acc_tech/adesigner_e.htm

accessibility guidelines, including Section 508, WCAG, and IBM Web Accessibility Checklist. The result of this analysis is a report with lists of problems. In addition, each page is given an overall score of general accessibility.

2. AnyBrowser.* While this website provides a variety of services, such as checking for compatibility with various browsers, tools relevant for accessibility include simulation of various screen sizes and viewing with images replaced by ALT text. It also provides HTML validation and link checking.

3. Fangs.† This Mozilla Firefox extension creates a textual representation of a web page similar to how the page would be read by a modern screen reader.

4. Lynx Viewer.‡ This online tool allows web authors to see what their pages will look like when viewed with Lynx, a text-mode web browser.

5. VIS.§ VIS stands for Visual Impairment Simulator for Microsoft Windows. Developed and hosted at Campus Information Technologies and Educational Services (CITES) and Disability Resources and Educational Services (DRES), University of Illinois at Urbana/ Champaign, VIS is a downloadable program that simulates what it is like to use Microsoft Windows with a visual impairment.

6. Web Anywhere.¶ Web Anywhere is a nonvisual interface to the web that requires no new software to be downloaded or installed. It allows the users to interact with the browser in a similar way users would interact with a screen reader, and therefore can be used to simulate how the webpage will be read by a screen reader for those developing websites for blind persons.

Repair Tools

Very few repair tools are available for public use, and many are packaged with checking tools. An example of these tools is:

1. HiSoftware Compliance Sheriff Accessibility Module.** This commercial module combines several applications: AccMonitor, AccRepair, and AccVerify. It verifies accessibility compliance with Section 508 and WCAG 1.0 and 2.0, repairs website content, and monitors all online portals across an enterprise for ongoing accessibility. It then

---

* http://www.anybrowser.com/
† http://www.standards-schmandards.com/projects/fangs/
‡ http://www.delorie.com/web/lynxview.html
§ http://vis.cita.uiuc.edu/
¶ http://webanywhere.cs.washington.edu/wa.php
** http://www.hisoftware.com/solutions/hisoftware-compliance-sheriff/accessibility-compliance.aspx

creates custom reports as requested. It deals with HTML, XHTML, SVG, XML, and any other text- or element-based content. Custom validation is supported for cascading style sheets (CSS), XSL, SVG, JavaScript, VBScript, and other text or element-based content.

Accessibility Checkers

The majority of the tools listed in the WAI website are automatic or semiautomatic accessibility checking tools. Because of the large variety of checking methods, the tools are further divided into the following subcategories:

Layout Checkers

Layout checkers include tools that check for the accessibility of layout elements, including tables, CSS, and so on. Examples of these checkers are as follows:

1. Complex Table Toolbar.* The toolbar is an add-on to FireFox and can be used to: reveal "headers" and "id" complex data table markup, create such markup either manually or automatically and create a linear version of the data table content. Complex data table markup is needed for screen reader users in order to make sense of a complex data table.

2. CSS Analyser.† This online tool checks the validity of an uploaded CSS against the W3C's validation service, along with a color contrast test, and a test to ensure that relevant sizes are specified in relative units of measurement.

3. Image Analyser.‡ This online tool was developed by the creator of CSS Analyser. It examines all images found on a web page to check for any accessibility issues. The width, height, alt, and longdesc attributes are examined for appropriate values.

4. Table Inspector.§ This tool is a Mozilla Firefox's extension that reveals the hidden accessibility features of data tables, such as summary, headers, axis, scope, and abbr.

5. Tablin.¶ Tablin is a filter program developed by the WAI Evaluation & Repair (ER) group that can linearize HTML tables and render them accordingly to preferences set by the presentation layer (e.g., the screen reader end-user). It is available as downloadable executables or Java codes as well as an online service.

---

* http://www.visionaustralia.org.au/info.aspx?page=1812
† http://juicystudio.com/services/csstest.php
‡ http://juicystudio.com/services/image.php
§ http://juicystudio.com/article/firefox-table-inspector.php
¶ http://www.w3.org/WAI/Resources/Tablin/

W3C CSS Validator results for http://www.cnn.com (CSS level 2.1)

Sorry! We found the following errors (20)	
URI : http://z.cdn.turner.com/cnn/tmpl_asset/static/mobile_phone/1387/css/lib-min.css	
1 body	Property overflow-x doesn't exist in CSS level 2.1 but exists in [css3] : hidden
1 body	Property -webkit-text-size-adjust doesn't exist : none
1 .redButtonsend, .redButton	Property -webkit-border-image doesn't exist : url("data:image/png;base64,iVBORw0KGgoAAAANSUhEUgAAADwAAAAWCAYAAACcy/8iAAAAC 0 5 0 5
2 .module_bgroup	Property -webkit-border-radius doesn't exist : 6px
2 #mixx	Property background-size doesn't exist in CSS level 2.1 but exists in [css3] : 20px 20px
3 #delicious	Property background-size doesn't exist in CSS level 2.1 but exists in [css3] : 20px 20px
3 #digg	Property background-size doesn't exist in CSS level 2.1 but exists in [css3] : 20px 20px
3 #facebook	Property background-size doesn't exist in CSS level 2.1 but exists in [css3] : 20px 20px
3 #friendfeed	Property background-size doesn't exist in CSS level 2.1 but exists in [css3] : 20px 20px
4 #stumbleupon	Property background-size doesn't exist in CSS level 2.1 but exists in [css3] : 20px 20px
4 #google	Property background-size doesn't exist in CSS level 2.1 but exists in [css3] : 20px 20px
5 #twitter	Property background-size doesn't exist in CSS level 2.1 but exists in [css3] : 20px 20px
5 #myspace	Property background-size doesn't exist in CSS level 2.1 but exists in [css3] : 20px 20px
5 #reddit	Property background-size doesn't exist in CSS level 2.1 but exists in [css3] : 20px 20px
7 .section_setwframe	Value Error : background Too many values or values are not recognized : none repeat scroll 0 0 rgba(

FIGURE 12.6
The report from W3C CSS Validator.

6. W3C CSS Validation Service.* W3C CSS Validation Service is a free
service that checks CSS in (X)HTML documents or standalone for
conformance to W3C recommendations. It can check a URL, an
uploaded file, or CSS text pasted into its textbox. It also allows users
to specify the CSS level and the medium that the website will be
rendered in (Figure 12.6 shows the error report based on CSS level
2.1 when the medium used is Braille).

Multilingual Checkers

While the majority of the tools hosted by the WAI website are for English
websites and only check against WCAG or Section 508, several tools check
against the regulations that are enforced outside the United States in addition to WCAG and Section 508. These tools are also able to check non-English
websites. The following are some of the examples of such tools:

1. Hera.† Hera was developed by Fundación Sidar, a group of experts in
new technologies and accessibility based in Spain. The name SIDAR
stands for Spanish words that translate into "Latin American
Foundation on Disability and Accessibility on the Web." It is an
online tool that performs some automated WCAG 1.0 testing, then

---

* http://jigsaw.w3.org/css-validator/
† http://www.sidar.org/hera/

guides the user through tests which need to be done or confirmed manually. Hera is multilingual (it currently supports 11 languages). The system is written in PHP and is available for adaptation under the GNU General Public License (GPL) open-source licensing.

2. daSilva.* daSilva is an online and downloadable tool that checks the accessibility of HTML/XHTML pages against WCAG 1.0 and e-GOV (Brazilian government accessibility rules for web) conformance. It is available in English, French, and Portuguese, although the information in English is limited.

3. Ocawa.† This online service in English and French runs accessibility tests based on the WCAG 1.0 using a built-in expert system. The Ocawa website offers free single or multiple page site audits with output reports indicating all inaccessible aspects of a page by highlighting the page's source code. For large clients and intranet facilities, an Ocawa Server can be installed for unlimited testing.

4. SortSite.‡ This downloadable tool is not free but the company offers a free trial. This tool checks for accessibility issues against Section 508, WCAG 1.0 and 2.0 as well as United Kingdom's DDA guidelines. It checks HTML, CSS, JavaScript, PDF, GIF, and Flash files.

5. TAW online.§ It is an online tool that checks against WCAG 1.0, WCAG 2.0 and mobileOK¶ guidelines. It is available in English, Spanish, Catalan, and Galician. It is complemented by TAW3,** the downloadable multiplatform version.

6. WDG HTML Validator.†† This bilingual (French and English) online tool validates against W3C HTML DTDs. It also provides its own DTDs to support nonstandard HTML features that can be added such as the EMBED element or the LEFTMARGIN attribute on BODY. This tool allows users to upload an HTML file, type in a URL, or paste the code, and also allows batch mode processing.‡‡

7. Web Accessibility Inspector.§§ This multiplatform (Mac and Windows OS) multilingual (English, Japanese, Chinese, and Korean) downloadable tool is provided by Fujitsu, and consequently, in addition to

---

* http://www.dasilva.org.br/?blogid=2
† http://www.ocawa.com/accueilEn.htm
‡ http://www.powermapper.com/products/sortsite/checks/accessibility-checks.htm
§ http://www.tawdis.net/
¶ mobileOK (http://www.w3.org/TR/mobileOK/) is a W3C scheme that allows content providers to promote their content as being suitable for use on very basic mobile devices.
** http://www.tawdis.net/ingles_downloadTaw.html
†† http://www.htmlhelp.com/tools/validator/
‡‡ http://www.htmlhelp.com/tools/validator/batch.html.en
§§ http://www.fujitsu.com/global/accessibility/assistance/wi/

checking accessibility issues against WCAG 1.0, it also checks against Fujitsu web accessibility guidelines.* Users can specify the file to be checked by its file name, folder. or URL.

Beyond Accessibility Checkers

Some tools check for problems with the web page or website beyond accessibility issues, such as interoperability, usability, and so on. Below are the examples of some of these tools:

1. Foxability.† Formerly called "Acc," it is a Firefox extension that is capable of evaluating and reporting some accessibility violations. It reports HTML coding flaws and it includes features such as visual layout extraction implementation, basic scalability test, testing deeply nested layout tables, Skip to Main Content link check, navigation consistency check, and scripted page evaluation. The last version developed in 2009 was for Firefox v.3 (as of September 29, 2011, the version of Mozilla's Firefox is 3.6.22).

2. Functional Accessibility Evaluator.‡ Developed and hosted by University of Illinois Urbana Champaign, this online tool analyzes web pages for markup that is consistent with the use of iCITA HTML Best Practices for the development of functionally accessible web resources that also support interoperability. The iCITA HTML Best Practices are a statement of techniques for implementation of the WCAG, Section 508, and the Illinois Information Technology Accessibility Act (IITAA). Although the URL above only allows evaluation of a single page, FTA provides multiple page evaluation after the user registers for a free account. The downloadable version in the form of Firefox add-on is also available.§

3. HTML Validator.¶ This downloadable tool is a Mozilla extension that adds HTML validation inside Firefox and Mozilla. The number of errors of a HTML page is represented as an icon in the status bar when browsing. The details of the errors are seen when looking at the HTML source of the page. This extension is based on Tidy and OpenSP. The tool also cleans up the codes from unnecessary syntax.

4. InFocus Suite.** The InFocus Suite is the heart of SSB BART Group's Accessibility Management Platform (AMP). InFocus is an integrated

---

* http://www.fujitsu.com/downloads/US/GND/web-accessibility-guide.pdf
† http://foxability.sourceforge.net/
‡ http://fae.cita.uiuc.edu/
§ http://firefox.cita.uiuc.edu
¶ http://users.skynet.be/mgueury/mozilla/
** https://www.ssbbartgroup.com/amp/infocus.php

solution that includes testing and analysis tools, a rules builder, a checking engine, and content spidering.

5. Site Valet.* This downloadable tool spiders sites checking validity, accessibility against WCAG 1.0, metadata and link integrity, saving results to an SQL database. It incorporates monitoring, change detection, and audit trail. It supports a wide range of reports: on the spot analysis, database queries, and historical, in detailed (developer) and executive summary (management) formats.

6. Total Validator.† It is a downloadable multiplatform (X)HTML validator, an accessibility validator (against WCAG 2.0 and Section 508), a spell checker, and a broken links checker all rolled into one tool allowing one-click validation of a page. For validation of the entire site and other more advanced features, the company offers Pro Tool.‡

General Checkers

There are too many tools that perform general accessibility checking, and therefore, the following list includes only the tools that provide extra services beyond a single page general accessibility checker.

1. Accessibility Wizard.§ This tool breaks down the WCAG version 1.0 checkpoints into individual tasks for each job role in a development team (e.g., interface designer, content writer, and information architect). Once the user chooses the desired job role, he or she is asked to choose the level of accessibility compliance required (A, AA, and AAA). Finally, the user is asked to choose the design elements that he or she would be working on (e.g., for an interface designer, the choice is either navigation or color). Upon choosing the design elements to work on, a set of guidelines will be displayed. A web client that supports the Flash 6 (or higher) plug-in is the minimum requirement to use the wizard. Figure 12.7 described the guidelines for a content manager requesting the AAA level of compliance for markup design elements.

2. EvalAccess.¶ This is one of a small number of online tools that evaluate multiple pages. It evaluates HTML markup and crawls for a site up to third level deep and up to 15 URLs. It then returns the report of the number of errors in each page (see Figure 12.8 for a sample report. Clicking the URL brings up the detailed error report).

---

* http://valet.webthing.com/2.0/
† http://www.totalvalidator.com/
‡ http://www.totalvalidator.com/tools/protool.html
§ http://www.binaryblue.com.au/access_wizard/
¶ http://sipt07.si.ehu.es/evalaccess2

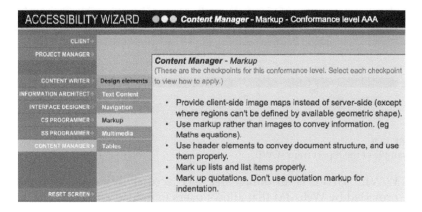

FIGURE 12.7
Accessibility Wizard.

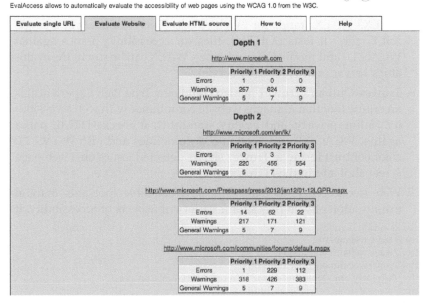

FIGURE 12.8
The report from EvalAccess.

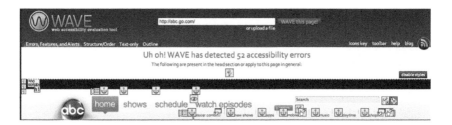

FIGURE 12.9
An example of the report from WAVE.

3. WAVE.* WAVE is an online free web accessibility evaluation tool provided by WebAIM that allows users to upload an HTML file, fill in a URL, or paste the HTML code. Rather than providing a complex technical report, WAVE shows the original web page with embedded icons and indicators that reveal the accessibility of that page as shown in Figure 12.9. WAVE is also available as Firefox toolbar† or Dreamweaver extension.‡

4. Accessibility Favelet.§ This is another tool developed by Accessify that consists of little pieces of JavaScript that can be saved as favorites in Internet Explorer, Mozilla, and Opera. It performs a variety of accessibility checking such as missing ALT tags and pairing ALT text to its corresponding image for easier cross-checking of whether the ALT text matches the image content. It also provides a function to disable a style sheet.

5. WAEX.¶ WAEX stands for "Web Accessibility Evaluator in a single XSLT** file." It tests (X)HTML files for accessibility issues against WCAG 1.0 and mobileOK guidelines. WAEX can be run in the evaluator's server or at W3C XSLT servlet.

6. Truwex Online.†† Truwex (which stands for True Web Experience) is an online tool that manages website compliance with web accessibility, online privacy, and quality standards. It checks HTML pages against WCAG 1.0 and Section 508 guidelines and also WCAG 2.0 color contrast formula. Truwex shows detected issues on a web page screenshot and in the HTML code.

7. Web Accessibility Toolbar. This downloadable tool aids manual examination of web pages for a variety of aspects of accessibility. It

---

* http://wave.webaim.org/
† http://wave.webaim.org/toolbar
‡ http://wave.webaim.org/dwextension
§ http://accessify.com/tools-and-wizards/accessibility-tools/favelets/
¶ http://www.it.uc3m.es/vlc/waex.html
** XSLT is a language for transforming XML documents into XHTML documents or to other XML documents.
†† http://checkwebsite.erigami.com/accessibility.html

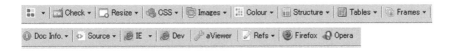

FIGURE 12.10
Web Accessibility Toolbar for Internet Explorer.

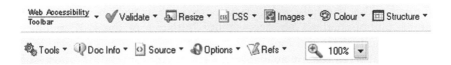

FIGURE 12.11
Web Accessibility Toolbar for Opera.

consists of a range of functions that identify components of a web page, provide access to alternate views of page content, and facilitate the use of third-party online applications. This work is licensed under a Creative Commons License.* It is available for Internet Explorer† or Opera‡ (the Opera version is not compatible with Opera 10 or newer). The screenshot for the IE version is depicted in Figure 12.10 while the Opera version is depicted in Figure 12.11.

8. Web Developer extension.§ The Web Developer extension adds various web developer tools to a browser. The extension is available for Firefox and Chrome, and will run on any platform that these browsers support, including Windows, Mac OS X, and Linux.

Conclusion

World Wide Web is said to bridge the information gap for people who are blind or visually impaired. It allows people who are blind to read newspapers on the day they are published, order groceries and know the prices before checking out, and find out what titles are on a CD before making a selection.¶

---

* Creative Commons licenses (http://creativecommons.org) are several copyright licenses that allow the distribution of copyrighted works that has been ported in 50 jurisdictions worldwide. The original set of licenses grant the "baseline rights," such as the right to distribute the copyrighted work worldwide, without changes, at no charge.
† http://www.paciellogroup.com/resources/wat-ie-about.html
‡ http://www.paciellogroup.com/resources/wat/opera
§ http://chrispederick.com/work/web-developer/
¶ http://www.afb.org/Section.asp?SectionID=57&TopicID=167

But the role of the web as an information bridge for those who are blind will only be effective if the web pages are designed with regard to accessibility.

It is possible that the lack of accessibility consideration for blind users is due to the small number of web designers who follow guidelines for accessibility. Or it could be due to the fact that only companies that have government contracts are mandated by Section 508 of the ADA to make their websites accessible. However, it is also possible that it is because of lack of readily available information that can help web designers make their website accessible. For example, although the Web Accessibility Initiative of the W3C publishes guidelines online, not everyone knows about them. Training for developers in this area is also not readily available in most places, especially because computer technology continues to progress and change at lightning speed.

This chapter aims at providing information for web designers, hosts, users, and researchers on the issues surrounding web accessibility for screen reader users at a conceptual level, which is hopefully less prone to technological changes. It starts by describing how blind persons usually access web-based information and some guidelines on how to design web pages in such a way that would make them more screen reader friendly. This chapter also lists a selection of tools that can improve web accessibility for blind users either through providing guidelines and wizard for web designers at the design and development stage, simulating how a website looks to a blind user, or automatically checking and correcting accessibility errors.

While all of these tools have been helpful in facilitating more blind-friendly web environment, many of these tools had not touched on the interaction between blind persons and Web 2.0. One of the most significant features of Web 2.0 that differentiates it with its predecessor is the dynamic visual content, such as tickers, calendar, and other time-sensitive changes without changing URL or refreshing the page. This can result in exciting experience for sighted users. However, unfortunately, most screen readers cannot handle dynamic content. To mediate this problem, W3C proposed ARIA markup for web developers to tag web pages to guide screen readers on reading the Web 2.0 content, but very few tools are able to fix Web 2.0 inaccessibility after the fact. The good news is the majority of web pages that provide pages in Web 2.0 also provide an alternative, and for that, the tools listed above can hopefully ameliorate the accessibility problems that blind users face when interacting with the web.

References

Brophy, P. and Cavern, J. 2007. Web accessibility. *Library Trends* 55: 950–972.

Chong, C. 2011. Making your web site accessible to the blind. National Federation for the Blind, http://www.nfb.org/nfb/Web_accessibility.asp?SnID=3873666.

Di Blas, N., Paolini, P., and Speroni, M. 2004. "Usable accessibility" to the web for blind users. *Proc. of 8th ERCIM Workshop: User Interfaces for All*, pp. 28–29. Berlin, Germany: Springer Verlag.

Richards, J.T. and Hanson, V.L. 2004. Web accessibility: A broader view. *Proc. of the 13th International Conference on World Wide Web (WWW '04)*, pp. 72–79. New York: ACM.

Royal National Institute for the Blind (RNIB). 2011. UK law for websites: Does the law require me to make my site accessible? http://www.rnib.org.uk/professionals/webaccessibility/lawsandstandards/Pages/uk_law.aspx.

Theofanos, M.F. and Redish, J.C. 2003 Guidelines for accessible and usable web sites: Observing users who work with screen readers. *Interactions* 10(6): 38–51.

World Wide Web Consortium's Web Accessibility Initiative (W3C WAI). 2006. Complete List of Web Accessibility Evaluation Tools, http://www.w3.org/WAI/ER/tools/complete.

13

Accessible DAISY Multimedia: Making Reading Easier for All

George Kerscher, Varju Luceno, and Lynn Leith

CONTENTS

What Is DAISY?

DAISY is the acronym for digital accessible information system. The DAISY/NISO Standard is the digital talking book (DTB) specification for accessible digital books. It is a multimedia standard which supports the traditional presentation of text and images, similar to what you would find in a printed book—but with the added features of navigation to points and audio content. In a DAISY publication, the text and audio are synchronized, allowing readers to navigate through the audio in a meaningful way. The current specification, DAISY 3, is based on extensible markup language (XML). DAISY is the basis for the National Instructional Materials Accessibility Standard (NIMAS) in the United States.

Publications produced in the DAISY format provide readers with flexible access to the digital content through enhanced navigation. In the same way that a sighted reader goes through a print publication, a reader with a print disability can skip past the front matter of a book, select and skip to chapter headings, go to a specific page, move to the required or desired part of the book as fast or faster than a sighted reader can, or read the book from cover to cover. It is even possible to search for a word in the text content and go directly to points in the publication where it occurs—all of this and more is possible with a DAISY DTB.

The current audience for DAISY books is large; however, the potential audience is enormous. When a DAISY book and player are brought into a classroom for a print-disabled student, all the students want them. The current and potential DAISY audiences include:

- Readers who may benefit from the multimedia features
- Readers who are blind or have low vision and who therefore are unable to read standard print publications
- Readers with dyslexia or other learning differences who have difficulty reading and understanding standard print content
- Language learners who may benefit from the audio and text synchronization and the navigability of DAISY DTBs
- Readers who may, for any number of reasons, benefit from the variety of ways to access the content of a book in DAISY format
- Educators who can create and provide their students with custom-made DAISY books tailored to their individual student and classroom setting needs

Short History of DAISY

In 1988, after recognizing the limitations of cassettes, TPB began the development of a new talking book format, a format that from its inception was known as DAISY. In 1991, TPB received a government grant to develop the "DAISY idea" into a working platform that could replace cassettes and revolutionize the way talking books were used, introducing document structuring that would provide readers with easy navigation through books. In 1994, the first prototype of the DAISY system was developed and later that year it was shown at the International Conference on Computers Helping People with Special

Needs (ICCHP) in Vienna. Interest in the DAISY project began to grow. At very early stages in the development of the DAISY Standard, talking book readers from many countries were surveyed regarding their reading requirements and their vision of a fully accessible audio book. Those who provided input made it very clear that analog recordings did not meet their reading and information needs. As the project evolved, the following list of requirements was added to the core concept of phrase-based navigation:

- Skimming of the text, phrase by phrase or section by section, where a section is a collection of phrases
- Searching for different parts in the text-based table of contents
- Searching for specific pages in the talking book and navigation by page
- Bookmarking which supports both placing and searching for bookmarks in the content of the book
- Functionality to underline and make notes in the talking book

In April 1995, 30 people from 11 countries, representing organizations of and/or for the blind, met in Toronto, Canada. The purpose of the meeting was to discuss digital technologies, future directions, and alternatives for talking books on cassette. TPB introduced DAISY to the participants. The outcome of that meeting was the formation of the worldwide DAISY Consortium in 1996. The primary purpose of the newly established consortium was to promote new and evolving DTB technologies. In 1997, the DAISY Consortium decided to adopt open standards based on file formats being developed for the Internet.

The first DAISY DTB specification was released in 1997. The consortium revised the early DAISY format to conform to several World Wide Web Consortium (W3C) multimedia standards in 1988. Version 2.0 combined the HTML and SMIL (synchronized multimedia integration language) standards, providing a more active, synchronized multimedia reading experience. Additional enhancements led to the development of the 2.01 and 2.02 specifications. For example, skippable and escapable structures were added to the DAISY 2.02 Standard.

The DAISY 2.02 specification which is based on XHTML, SMIL, audio, and images became the most widely implemented standard for talking book libraries and other organizations serving the print-disabled population. It has been the implementation standard since 2001 and many organizations around the world still create digital content that conforms to this specification.

The DAISY/NISO Z39.86-2005 Standard, first approved in 2002 as ANSI/NISO Z39.86, also known as DAISY 3,* is XML-based and supports further enhancements in DAISY DTBs. The DAISY Consortium is the designated

---

* How to Markup a Book with DAISY XML (DAISY 3 Structure Guidelines).

maintenance agency for the DAISY 3 (ANSI/NISO Z39.86) Standard. All DAISY Standards are open, international standards.

DAISY 3 *supports modular extensions.* For example, the MathML in DAISY extension supports access to mathematical notation such as complex equations. The MathML in DAISY specification requires that images and alternative text be "attached" to the MathML.

The NIMAS, which was incorporated in 2004 into the revised Individuals with Disabilities Education Act in the United States as the technical standard for all K–12 textbooks and related instructional materials, is an application of the set of elements in the DAISY/NISO Standard.

The National File Format Technical Panel unanimously agreed that adoption of the well-established and actively implemented DAISY Standard would increase the availability of high-quality alternate format materials— Braille, audio, digital text, and large print—for qualifying students with print disabilities in the United States.

Anatomy of a DAISY Book

The evolution of accessible information from analog audio tapes to DAISY multimedia is much like the evolution of the written word from papyrus scrolls to bound books. Like a scroll, an audiotape must be read in linear fashion, that is, from beginning to end. Disadvantages of print publications include the fact that the display of the words on the page cannot be altered, the contrast between the print and background cannot be changed, and there is no way for someone with a print disability to move easily from one part of the book to another. Print publications must be converted into an alternate format to meet the reading needs of all learners and readers.

A navigable DAISY book can provide a rich reading experience and can be explained as a set of digital files that may include

- One or more digital audio files containing the human narration or synthesized speech of part or all of the text content (WAV, MP3)
- A marked-up file containing some or all of the text (XML or XHTML)
- A synchronization file to associate markup in the text file with time points in the audio file/s (SMIL)
- A navigation control file which allows the user to move easily, quickly, and smoothly between files while synchronization between text and audio is maintained (NCX)

Image files (JPG, PNG) are also often present in a DAISY DTB.

DAISY books support formatting through both cascading style sheets (CSS) and extensible style sheet language (XSL) styling. The styling can be applied to the visual, audio, or Braille presentation of the publication's content.

The document type definition (DTD) defines a collection of allowed elements and attribute names and the relationship between them. For example, the DTBook 2005-2 DTD is at the center of the DAISY/NISO Z39.86-2005 Standard. It defines the markup for the textual content of a DAISY DTB and consists of a machine-readable list of allowable tags, the attributes that may be applied to them, and the rules stipulating where the tags may be used.

Within the XML text file, DAISY elements are classified as

- Structural
- Block
- Inline elements

Major structural elements include levels (<level1> through <level6>), <frontmatter>, <bodymatter>, and <rearmatter>.

In DAISY, level elements are the most fundamental. The following basic example of this element shows a top-level section of a textbook identified using <level1 class = "part">, which has two sections identified using <level 2 class = "chapter">.

These levels may contain other content elements, such as additional chapters, sidebars, block quotes, and so on.

```
<level1 class = "part">
<h1> Part 1 </h1>
<p> This is an introductory paragraph for Part 1. </p>
<level2 class = "chapter">
<h2> Chapter 1 </h2>
<p> This paragraph is within Chapter 1. </p>
</level2>
<level2 class = "chapter">
<h2> Chapter 2 </h2>
<p> This paragraph is within Chapter 2. </p>
</level2>
</level1>
```
DAISY DTBs also contain block elements such as <list>, <paragraph>, and <sidebar>, and inline elements such as <a>, <pagenum>, and <span>.

Books produced in the DAISY format are made up of multiple files in order to

- Support enhanced navigation
- Support synchronization of text and audio

The NCX file can contain information that

- Supports navigation by heading and by page
- Allows direct navigation to tables, figures, sidebars, and other content within the book

DAISY books may contain text content, audio content (with a structural text file), or a combination of both the full text of the book and the audio. DAISY reading systems (players) must provide synchronized playback of the text and audio content. This is done using information in the SMIL files which associates text with audio. Some DAISY reading devices provide the audio of the textual content using automatically generated synthesized speech.

A DAISY 3 full-audio, full-text book contains

- A DTB package file (OPF), which contains metadata and a list of the other files in the DTB
- A navigation control file (NCX)—similar to a table of contents
- A DTBook file (XML) which contains the textual content of the book
- A set of audio files (WAV, MP3)
- A set of SMIL files (to synchronize the text and audio)

The DTB structure created by the producer determines the degree of navigation available to the reader.

It is important that each document included within a DAISY DTB, including the XML content, be valid to the specification.

Three Types of DAISY Digital Talking Books

There are three types of DAISY DTBs: text only, audio with navigation, and full text plus full audio. All three types can be played with DAISY players that support text-to-speech (TTS). DAISY players which do not support TTS cannot be used with text-only DAISY books. A brief description of each type of DAISY books follows:

- *Text only*: Provides all the content of a DTB, including navigation and display options, but does not include any prerecorded audio. Text-only books are often rendered using TTS for audio playback. Example: DAISY Consortium member Bookshare provides its members with DAISY 3 text-only books.
- *Audio with navigation*: Audio books with DAISY navigation deliver the entire document as recorded audio plus the additional navigation features. For example, DAISY Consortium members RNIB and Learning Ally provide this type of DAISY book.

- *Full text plus full audio*: These are the richest form of DAISY books. They contain the entire text of a document synchronized with the recorded audio.

By synchronizing audio and text, DAISY multimedia books address the needs of all types of readers and learners. Full-text, full-audio DAISY books synchronize the audio playback with the text displayed on a computer screen, benefiting people who read most easily and learn most effectively with content that is visually rendered. The easy navigation provided in DAISY DTBs offers tactile/kinetic learners the opportunity to explore documents and interact with information in a way that holds their attention and improves their learning.

DAISY Book Production

People with print disabilities such as blindness or dyslexia have benefited from DAISY's synchronized multimedia for more than a decade. Thanks to the recent development of new open-source and commercial software tools for the production of DAISY multimedia, today everyone can have access to information in a way that best suits their personal reading and learning style. DAISY content production and delivery are at various stages in libraries for the blind and other organizations serving people who need information in accessible formats. Historically, the DAISY book production process began with the print book. This is now changing in some parts of the world as publisher files become more available.

Different types of workflows exist; some begin with the print publication, some with electronic text files, and some with prerecorded audio.

Open-Source Software

Over the last 5 years, the DAISY Consortium has developed a suite of open-source tools for production of DAISY multimedia content. These tools, including Tobi, Obi (structured audio production tool), and the DAISY Pipeline, are making information accessible to increasing numbers of readers with print disabilities.

Tobi: Digital Content Authoring Tool

Tobi is a free, open-source DAISY 3 multimedia production software designed to facilitate the process of synchronizing a text document with human narration. This tool provides a live recording workflow that is fully integrated with structured text. Tobi can also be used to import existing audio. The waveform editor supports audio-editing functions such as selection, delete, insert, cut/copy/paste, playback, and punch-in punch-out recording. Examples of possible uses for Tobi are

- Original full text and audio DTB production
- Podcast synchronization with a structured script
- Improving and/or upgrading an existing DAISY DTB

Although Tobi has basic text-editing functions, it is not an XML editor. External tools must be used to create the XML source document. Readily available tools such as Microsoft Word, Open-Office, or Libre Office can be used to produce a marked-up XML DTBook source document with their respective "Save as DAISY" add-ins.[*]

Tobi is the first accessible production tool that supports image description authoring workflow. Research carried out under the DIAGRAM project[†] will contribute to the development of a content model for descriptions for various kinds of graphical material. More information can be found on the Tobi Project page of the DAISY Consortium website.[‡]

Obi: Creating Accessible Audio Books Can Be Easy

Obi is a free DAISY software application used for audio recording to produce DAISY 3 DTBs with structure. It is simple to use and requires minimal training. By empowering mainstream users, Obi brings the benefits of DAISY technology to a broader range of consumers in situations where time and cost constraints limit the use of sophisticated synchronized multimedia production tools (e.g., a classroom environment or people and organizations in developing countries).

Obi 2.0 features and benefits include

- Users can produce DTBs conforming to both DAISY 3 and DAISY 2.02 standards.
- Full accessibility—supports keyboard navigation, magnification of text and graphics, and audio clues.
- Screen readers, including open-source screen readers, are supported.
- Bookmarking—any section or phrase can be bookmarked.
- Customizable keyboard shortcuts per user's individual preferences.
- Supports internationalization—can be easily localized into other languages.

---

[*] http://www.daisy.org/projects/save-as-daisy
[†] http://www.daisy.org/project/diagram
[‡] http://www.daisy.org/project/tobi

- Gentle learning curve—simple user interface makes Obi easy to learn.
- Recording process caters to the needs of both beginners and advanced users.
- Users can import projects ranging from full-text full-audio DAISY book files to navigable (audio-NCX) DAISY 3 books, DTBook XML and XHTML files, and WAV and MP3 files.
- Automated project recovery feature reduces the possibility of losing data.
- Supports undo and redo editing operations.
- Obi is open-source and is released under the LGPL license which means its source code is available for anyone to run, modify, and redistribute.

"We use Obi every day," said Greg Kearney of the Association for the Blind of Western Australia. "We use it to both create and convert books to DAISY format. We have found it to be easy to use and able to generate books that are of high quality."

More information can be found on the Obi Project page of the DAISY Consortium website.*

DAISY Pipeline: DTB-Related Document Transformations

To meet the growing need for digital content in various accessible formats, in 2005 the DAISY Consortium launched a development project to create the DAISY Pipeline,† a cross-platform, open-source transformation utility. This tool converts documents from a variety of file formats into accessible multimedia formats. It is designed to be used in both server-side and desktop environments. An accessible desktop–user interface is provided with full support for language localization.

As the DAISY Pipeline offers several content file transformation options, it can also help optimize the accessible publishing process. The Pipeline is a valuable tool in achieving the DAISY Consortium's vision of *a world where everyone has equal access to information and knowledge.*

The DAISY Pipeline efficiently and economically meets the changing needs for conversion and transformation utilities within the DAISY community. It provides a comprehensive solution for converting text documents into accessible formats for people with print disabilities. XML-based DTBook, which is a pivotal document format, is used to represent the book content prior to publishing. Documents in DTBook XML can be stored by

---

* http://www.daisy.org/project/obi
† http://www.daisy.org/project/pipeline

organizations, and a variety of output formats can be generated from it on demand.

Production using the DAISY Pipeline is an automated, noninteractive conversion of digital content into DAISY and other formats, possibly used in conjunction with manual editing environments. The publishing stage is the conversion of documents into various output formats. The current DAISY Pipeline supports multiple formats, including DAISY 2.02, DAISY/NISO Z39.86 2005, Open eBook, XHTML, RTF, and LaTeX. Manipulation of existing content includes functions such as audio encoding, DTBook repair, and format migration (e.g., from DAISY 2.02 to DAISY 3).

The collaborative nature of this project reduces duplication of effort and ensures maximum sharing of best practices within the community.

Organizations can reuse the Pipeline functionality in multiple deployment scenarios and they are free to contribute components in both for-profit and not-for-profit contexts. The current Pipeline core functionality is available in several "flavors" which can be chosen based on the deployment requirements:

- *The Command Line Interface:* This is the most minimalist Pipeline distribution. It is deployed as a compressed archive (ZIP), and allows users to run the Pipeline from a command line environment.

- *Desktop Application, the Pipeline GUI:* This is a stand-alone desktop application. It is usually deployed via an installer and provides the end user with a rich graphical user interface to create Pipeline jobs, execute transformations, and track the execution progress and messages.

- *Pipeline Lite:* This is a minimalist GUI for the Pipeline functionality consisting of a set of dialogs, from a simple progress dialog to a dynamic job configuration dialog. It is intended to be embedded in third-party software to provide some Pipeline functionality (e.g., "Save as DAISY" for Microsoft Word or Obi).

- *PipeOnline:* This is a web application for creating and executing Pipeline jobs over the Internet. It is a robust database-backed application with built-in execution queues, email notification, and usage statistics.

- *Remote Component, Pipeline WS:* This is a web service layer on top of the Pipeline functionality. It allows users to "drive" the Pipeline remotely in a platform-independent manner. This is useful for organizations that want to run an online Pipeline service or whose home environment is not directly compatible with the regular Pipeline Java API (e.g., in an MS.Net environment).

The DAISY Pipeline 2* is a project that is developing a next-generation framework for automated production of accessible materials for people with

---

* http://www.daisy.org/pipeline2/

print disabilities. Pipeline 2 is also intended to provide mainstream publishers with a framework for automated production of accessible materials. It is the follow-up and total redesign of the original DAISY Pipeline.

Commercial Production Tools

Software

Several commercial production tools have been developed for DAISY book production.

Dolphin Publisher,[*] for example, is a tool for creating professional DAISY DTBs with human narrated or synthetic voices. It is designed for alternative formats and DAISY specialists who want to create professional DAISY talking books. Dolphin Publisher is a production software solution for publishers of DAISY talking books, professional transcription services, DAISY talking book libraries, and specialist DAISY talking book producers in education. Producers can convert material to DAISY format from .html, .txt, .rtf, and .doc files; insert footnotes, page numbers, and pop-up pictures; add images and synchronize them with audio and text; mix human audio with synthetic speech; use synthesized speech or record human narration.

Another example of commercial DAISY book production software is the Book Wizard Producer,[†] which creates DAISY/NISO Z39.86-2002 DTBs.

Hardware

The PLEXTALK PTR2[‡] is well suited for structured audio-only recordings. Examples of how it may be used include people who wish to record lectures or seminars and organizations which use volunteer readers to record DAISY books. PLEXLATK PTR2 can also be used to play DAISY DTBs and music compact discs (CDs). It can be used to write DAISY DTBs or audio content to CD or to a memory card when it is connected to a computer. PLEXTALK Recording Software (PRS) is packaged with PTR2, providing DAISY book publishers with the necessary tools to quickly and easily record, edit, and finalize "audio and structure" DAISY 2.02 books.

Some portable DAISY reading devices can also produce DAISY books from prerecorded audio and also offer wireless features. Examples include PLEXTALK Pocket[§] and BookPort Plus.[¶]

---

[*] http://www.yourdolphin.com/productdetail.asp?id=12
[†] http://tech.aph.org/bwp_info.htm
[‡] http://www.plextalk.com/americas/top/products/ptr2/
[§] http://www.plextalk.com/americas/top/products/ptp1/
[¶] http://tech.aph.org/bt_info.htm

DAISY Reading Systems

Book lovers can listen to DAISY books on

- Computers using DAISY playback software
- Stand-alone DAISY players (desktop DAISY players or portable DAISY players)
- Mobile phones (Android and Symbian phones)
- MP3 players (will only provide limited navigation within the audio)
- Apple devices with a DAISY app: iPhone, iPod Touch, and iPad

A text-only DAISY book can be

- Read using a refreshable Braille display or screen reading software
- Printed as Braille book on paper
- Converted to a talking book using synthesized voice
- Printed on paper as a large print book
- Read as large print text on a computer screen

DAISY Playback Software (Features and Capabilities)

Typically, DAISY software players render the text, audio (human narration or synthetic speech), as well as embedded images (if present). Readers can make adjustments to the font size and color and also the background color and in most cases adjust the playback speed. Most software players feature variable playback speed and synchronized highlighting of text and audio as well as numerous other functions. Some DAISY software players have built-in synthetic TTS. These players therefore support playback of text-only DAISY DTBs.

AMIS is a free, open-source DAISY playback software developed by the DAISY Consortium. Highlights of AMIS include its self-voicing interface, playback rate control, text searching and bookmarking, reading options, and page style customization. AMIS is available in multiple languages.[*] It runs on Windows and supports DAISY 2.02 and DAISY 3 (formally ANSI/NISO Z3986-2005) books.

Emerson is a cross-platform audio DTB player. It does not support text-only DTBs; it supports only MP3-encoded DTBs. The DAISY formats supported are DAISY 2.02 and DAISY 3.

---

[*] http://www.daisy.org/amis/download/translations

Examples of commercial software DAISY players include ida-reader[*] and Book Wizard Reader.[†] New College Worcester in the United Kingdom has chosen Dolphin's EasyReader as their preferred DAISY software player.

Praise for Two DAISY Software Players

Jonathan Fogg[‡] stated that he liked the ease and straightforward interface on EasyReader. He believed that the students would: (1) find it easy to use and navigate and open the books and documents; (2) be able to quickly return to books they have used before; and (3) be able to jump between all of the headings, whether from one to the next, or between all the levels 2s or level 3s.

> Our students need, or even deserve the opportunity to have the best experience as they can get and as we can deliver. If DAISY is appropriate for some of our students, then we should be delivering DAISY documents to those students.
>
> Because EasyReader is able to play text files and html files and EPUB files it gives the students the flexibility to access materials that other people are producing.

ReadHear™ Mac is the other DAISY player. It is the first fully featured DTB player for the Mac. ReadHear Mac[§] provides excellent benefits to those who enjoy and appreciate learning and listening to DAISY books, math content, articles, and documents.

DAISY Hardware Players (Features and Capabilities)

DAISY hardware players, which are in some ways similar to CD players or MP3 players, can be of great assistance to print-disabled users as well as to auditory learners who benefit from audio playback, whether the audio is presented through a TTS feature or with human narration.

The reader's experience can vary widely depending on the type of book and the playback system being used. Some hardware DAISY reading systems such as Victor Reader Classic, Victor Reader Stratus,[¶] and PLEXTALK PTN 2[**] are desktop players with easy-to-locate large tactile buttons. All of these provide navigation features through voice guidance and allow users to adjust the playback speed (faster or slower). They also have built-in speakers and headphone jacks. Some models support placing multiple bookmarks.

---

[*] http://www.idareader.com/
[†] http://www.aph.org/products/bwr_bro.html
[‡] http://www.yourdolphin.com/productdetail.asp?id=9&act=show&csid=110&z=5
[§] http://www.gh-accessibility.com/software/readhear-mac-instant-download
[¶] http://www.humanware.com/en-usa/products/blindness/dtb_players/classic_models/
[**] http://www.plextalk.com/americas/top/products/ptn2/

Some hardware players such as HIMS BrailleSense Plus[*] incorporate a portable Braille display.

DAISY players can also be small and highly portable. Most portable DAISY players such as Milestone,[†] PLEXTALK Pocket, BookPort Plus, BookSense XT,[‡] and Victor Reader Stream[§] can also play music and other file formats. These players come with high-speed USB and higher-capacity SD card support.

The BookSense DS[¶] is a portable DAISY player with an OLED screen. Users can check the status of playback or view their file list on the OLED screen.

Another DAISY player for students with dyslexia or other learning difficulties is the ClassMate Reader.[**] It plays the audio and simultaneously displays and highlights the corresponding text on its full-color screen. Its simple, flexible interface can be configured to the user's specific needs. ClassMate Reader also includes helpful study tools such as bookmarks, voice recording, highlighting function, and a speaking dictionary to enhance learning. With built-in TTS, it also plays e-text and NIMAS files.

Students can download and store their curriculum directly on an SD card for easy access anytime, anywhere. The ClassMate Reader provides a solution for people who want to have access to their newspapers, articles, emails, and books wherever they are. Its full-color screen can be configured to change font type, text size, color, line spacing, and so on. The user can also adjust text scrolling speed and move text to be viewed above or below the passage read.

Using a fingertip or the stylus, readers can interact with the text on the touch screen and its simple, user-friendly interface. The ClassMate uses a proven multisensory multimodal approach, which consists of stimulating both sight and hearing by the simultaneous use of text and audio (the fundamental principle underlying the DAISY Standards). A number of studies have shown that multimodal approaches improve comprehension and understanding.

Praise for One of the DAISY Hardware Players

Educator Marie Kouthoofd[††] stated that the VR Stream and the rich reading experience DAISY books provide allows her to authentically proclaim to her students each and every semester that she would never assign any reading that she has not read.

---

[*] http://www.hims-inc.com/products/braille-sense-plus

[†] http://www.bones.ch/bones/pages/eng/products/milestone312.html

[‡] http://www.hims-inc.com/products/booksense-xt

[§] http://www.humanware.com/en-usa/products/blindness/dtb_players/compact_model

[¶] http://www.hims-inc.com/products/booksense-ds

[**] http://www.humanware.com/en-usa/products/learning_disabilities/_details/id_107/classmate_reader_audio_book_player.html

[††] http://www.daisy.org/stories/marie-kouthoofd

The DAISY Consortium maintains a list of DAISY players and production tools developed by the DAISY Consortium members (Friends) on the DAISY Consortium website.[*]

There are many different types of DAISY hardware and software players available (including DAISY apps for iPhone, iPod Touch, iPad, and Android). However, some of these systems have not been tested with or approved for Learning Ally, National Library Service for the Blind and Physically Handicapped (NLS, USA), Bookshare, or any other DAISY member organizations' digital content. Readers who want to acquire a DAISY hardware player should research the options carefully, and if needed, contact these organizations to find out which players support their DTBs and if it is necessary to authorize their players for the organization's books.

DAISY Book Distribution

The NLS talking book program was first established by an Act of the U.S. Congress in 1931—80 years ago, to serve blind adults. Originally, there were 19 libraries—today the NLS network includes more than 100 libraries across the nation and in the U.S. territories. These libraries distribute reading materials to a readership of more than 900,000. The Talking Book and Braille Program is a collaborative arrangement between federal, state, and local libraries. NLS provides free players to its patrons and uses the extension of the 2002 DAISY/NISO Standard, DTB_2002_NLS.[†] An online service, called BARD,[‡] is also available.

Learning Ally[§] (formerly RFB&D) was established in 1948 to provide recorded textbooks to veterans who where blinded in World War II. This organization has been an educational resource for more than 50 years allowing people with print disabilities gain access to new opportunities, education, and careers. More than 70% of the people served by RFB&D (now Learning Ally) are identified as having learning disabilities. The population of students with learning differences is growing rapidly as serious learning disabilities are better diagnosed.

Learning Ally provide its members with downloadable DAISY books as well as DAISY books on CDs. Both offer the same variable speed, bookmarking, and navigational features. Learning Ally audio books with DAISY navigation deliver the entire document as human-narrated recorded audio with the additional navigation features. Learning Ally also has an Audio App[¶]

---

[*] http://www.daisy.org/tools-services/
[†] http://www.digitalpreservation.gov/formats/fdd/fdd000256.shtml
[‡] https://nlsbard.loc.gov/ApplicationInstructions.html
[§] http://www.learningally.org/
[¶] http://www.learningally.org/apple/

available for members to get their downloadable DAISY titles on iOS devices like the iPad, iPhone, and iPod touch.

Just like NLS and Learning Ally, Bookshare,[*] an online library of digital books for people with print disabilities operates under an exception to U.S. copyright law[†] which allows copyrighted digital books to be made available to people with qualifying disabilities. In addition, many publishers and authors have volunteered to provide Bookshare with access to their publications.

Bookshare members download books, textbooks, and newspapers in a compressed, encrypted DAISY 3 or electronic Braille file. They then read the material using adaptive technology, typically software that reads the book aloud (TTS) and/or displays the text of the book on a computer screen, or Braille access devices, such as refreshable Braille displays. Bookshare books are also available on Apple devices via their Read2Go[‡] application.

An extensive list of DAISY content providers around the globe[§] is available on the DAISY Consortium website.

CDs, Portable and Mobile Media

Books that once had to be stored on multiple audiotapes can now be distributed on a single CD, flash drive, cartridge, memory card, and/or even stored in the cloud.

A portable media unit may contain more than one DAISY book. On the other hand, extremely large DAISY books may need to be stored on more than one media unit—content of a very large DTB can be processed to span more than one media unit without loss of navigation throughout the book. DAISY content can also be made available as a download, streamed, or read from a web browser over the Internet (examples are Dorina DAISY Reader[¶] and AnyDAISY[**]).

Mobile technologies increasingly provide benefits to persons with disabilities and the aging population by improving safety, offering accessible interfaces such as voice recognition or TTS, as well as various messaging functions. As a result, more individuals can access the information they want and need and ultimately fully participate in society.

As an example, DAISY2Go[††] is a part of the Nuance Accessibility Suite. It has been optimized for Nuance TALKS, to allow easy alternation between audio and textual content. It is free for users who own a license for TALKS&ZOOMS Premium Edition. DAISY2Go is a Mobile player/viewer for

---

[*] http://www.bookshare.org
[†] http://www.bookshare.org/_/aboutUs/legal/chafeeAmendment
[‡] http://itunes.apple.com/us/app/read2go/id425585903?mt=8
[§] http://www.daisy.org/multimedia
[¶] http://www.caracol.com.br/agora/doc.cfm?id_doc=1982&lang=en
[**] https://launchpad.net/daisyextension
[††] http://www.nuance.com/for-individuals/by-solution/talks-zooms/daisy/index.htm

books conforming to the DAISY 2.02 and DAISY 3 specifications, for Symbian phones utilizing S60 3rd Edition or 5th Edition.

Dolphin EasyReader Express is a fairly new, web-based subscription service which allows DAISY talking book providers to include an Express version of EasyReader to their DAISY talking books.

Olav Indergaard[*] explains the benefits that the Norwegian Library of Talking Books and Braille (NLB) have experienced in adding EasyReader Express to their DAISY talking books:

> NLB (The Norwegian Library of Talking Books and Braille) has been a provider of DAISY-content for several years. One of our challenges as a DAISY-content provider has been to ensure that our users have access to DAISY-playback systems in order to fully utilize the DAISY-format. NLB therefore decided to provide DAISY-player software to all our users by including a DAISY-player in all our books. EasyReader Express was the software of choice.

Like many DAISY talking book libraries, NLB had an existing catalog of a large number of DAISY talking books. In NLB's case, this was over 14,000 DAISY talking book titles. Dolphin worked with NLB to make sure that EasyReader Express could be added to all of their DAISY talking books with the minimal effort.

DAISY Online Distribution

The DAISY Online Delivery Protocol (DOP)[†] is a web service API that facilitates the delivery of digital resources from service providers to end users. The protocol features a core set of operations that can be configured to enable a variety of different download models, making it a flexible and lightweight solution to the growing need for online delivery of published content.

The simplest use case for this protocol is the nontechnical user who receives content directly to a DOP-enabled DAISY player through automatic book selection by the library computer, based on a stored profile of the user's reading interests. In this case, the DOP will simply push content from the library server to the user's player as soon as the user releases content he or she has already read.

During the development of the specification, it was decided that DOP would not address the security of the content. The proposed solution to any security requirement is the *Specification for DAISY Protected Digital Talking Book*[‡] *(PDTB2)*. This specification, already in use in France and United States (NLS), is based on industry standards like AES and RSA technologies that are used in e-commerce and online banking.

---

[*] http://www.yourdolphin.co.uk/productdetail.asp?id=33&act=show&csid=123&z=5
[†] http://www.daisy.org/project/daisy-online-delivery
[‡] http://www.daisy.org/project/protected-dtb

Other libraries producing DAISY content, such as those in Sweden and Denmark, are using watermarking which hides a digital signature of the person who downloaded it within the books themselves. Watermarking has no negative impact on playback systems or usability of DAISY DTBs. DOP provides a mechanism for service providers to implement controlled lending of content as described in the *Lending model* section of the protocol.

The protocol, in and of itself, must not be seen as a full-proof security mechanism. PDTB2 support in the DAISY Online Protocol is the recommended way to protect content being distributed through the DOP system.

It was decided by the DAISY Consortium working group, during the development of the DOP, that streaming content would not be part of the protocol itself, but simply a possible way for players to operate. A library cannot force a player to operate in a streaming mode using the DAISY Online Delivery Specification.

Example of DAISY Content Online Distribution

Flemish organizations built a common online distribution platform[*] for all accessible reading material in Flanders. The platform hosts daily newspapers; soon magazines as well as books will be added. At that point, all accessible reading material in Flanders will be available from the same place.

In order to support as many readers as possible, the platform allows access in various ways, including online network DAISY players, web browsers, and podcasting. Both downloading and streaming are available (The DAISY Planet: September 2011[†]).

How Does It Work?

Content providers publish new titles on the online platform. When titles are requested they become available in the clients' online bookshelves. From the bookshelf it is possible to begin reading or downloading DAISY books. In a typical scenario, users can download a title via podcast to their mobile DAISY players and read it on the way to work. During lunch break they can continue reading on their computers using a web browser-based DAISY player. Back home, users can finish reading on an online network DAISY player like the Plextalk PTX1 Pro[‡] (the world's first DAISY Online Delivery standard compatible player).

When streaming with the online service on a DAISY player, navigating within a DAISY book is even faster than it is when using a CD. For content

---

[*] http://www.anderslezen.be
[†] http://www.daisy.org/planet-2011-09#a2
[‡] http://www.daisy.org/tools/578#t162

providers, online distribution is easier and less expensive than preparing and distributing physical media such as CDs.

Although CDs will not disappear for a few years, online reading of DAISY titles is here now, with benefits for both producers and readers. Approximately 61% of European households have a broadband Internet connection and that number is growing yearly by 5%—online reading will be possible for everyone in the near future. The goal of the Online DAISY platform is to improve the availability of accessible reading material and contributing to the principle of "information access for all."

DAISY Is the Future

EPUB 2.0.1* was approved as a Recommended Specification in May, 2010. It is defined by three open standard specifications, the first of which is the Open Publication Structure (OPS)†:

> DTBook is an XML vocabulary defined in the DAISY/NISO standard, formally, the ANSI/NISO Z39.86-2005 Standard. This vocabulary is specifically designed for eBook content...It is strongly recommended that Content Providers select this XML Preferred Vocabulary for their educational publications and for content that is highly structured.

DAISY XML (or DTBook) is thus part of the EPUB 2 standard. From a pure accessibility perspective, EPUB borrows heavily from the DAISY Standards and W3C and Web Accessibility Initiative (WAI) specifications. The text must be present for presentation through synthetic speech, refreshable Braille displays, and enlarged character display.

All of the features we are beginning to see in EPUB reading systems have been part of DAISY reader systems for more than a decade. Accessibility features are working their way into the mainstream.

All of the major features targeted for the new DAISY Standard, the Authoring and Interchange Framework (DAISY AI), which are based on the gathered and approved requirements, have been adopted by EPUB and are incorporated into the new EPUB 3 standard. EPUB 3 is a blend of what DAISY has done and what the commercial market wants and needs.

It will be possible to transform all existing DAISY 2.02 and DAISY 3 content to EPUB 3. DAISY AI XML will remain the standard for accessible content source file authoring, content preservation, and archiving. The semantics (the relationship between a document's content and its structure) in DAISY

---

* http://idpf.org/epub/201
† http://idpf.org/epub/20/spec/OPS_2.0.1_draft.htm#Section2.4

AI authored documents will be preserved in distributed EPUB 3 digital content.

The next DAISY Standard, DAISY AI,* will support Braille production. In EPUB-based publications, rendering with refreshable Braille is supported. The harmonization of the accessible DAISY Standard with the EPUB specification is designed to ensure that EPUB-based publications can be fully capable of supporting the accessibility requirements that are the foundation of DAISY.

Simultaneously, this blending of the two specifications supports the needs of the DAISY Consortium to attend to the accessibility challenges that digital materials can create if not addressed at the development and production stage. EPUB 3 incorporates sophisticated support for TTS (computer-generated synthetic speech), as well as Math Markup Language (MathML) for effectively rendering mathematics in an accessible manner. It also includes support for Scaled Vector Graphics (SVG) which can be used to create layered and navigable versions of images with embedded text equivalents, offering a significant boost to the production of tactile graphics.

The DAISY Consortium anticipates adopting EPUB 3 as the distribution format for its members. EPUB 3 reached the Recommendation Specification† status on October 11, 2011.

No longer a mixture of e-book and DTB technologies, the new revision of EPUB actually has the DTB accessibility components more fully integrated into the specification:

- The Navigation Control Center (NCC) for XML applications (NCX) has been reformulated as an XHTML document to simplify its processing and rendering as well as improve its international language capabilities.

- The subset of SMIL used for synchronization of audio and text content, now called Media Overlay document, lives outside the content markup. The provision of audio and text synchronization has generated interest from mainstream publishers.

- The integrated support for TTS markup allows digital content producers to enhance the content with pronunciation and prosody instructions.

The incorporation of the DAISY accessibility requirements into the new EPUB 3 standard holds significant promise for the increased availability of commercial products that are useable, out of the box, by a wide range of consumers—those with disabilities and those without. EPUB supports

---

* http://www.daisy.org/zw/ZedAI_UserPortal#Recent_Events
† http://idpf.org/epub/30

reflowable content, which means that it can be deployed on multiple devices, and it efficiently supports in-house publisher workflows as well as commercial product distribution and digital rights management (DRM). EPUB is steadily emerging as the format of choice for eBook development and distribution.

EPUB 3 supports interactive content—support for W3C ARIA markup has been integrated to improve the accessibility of dynamic content. Further, EPUB 3 adds native support for new types of content such as MathML and SVG, and it also adds support for correct representation of many new scripts (such as Arabic, Chinese, and Japanese) by integrating, for example, W3C Ruby Annotation[*] and vertical writing[†] support.

Through EPUB 3, which will be the recommended distribution format for DAISY content, the accessibility and enhanced navigation features of DAISY will be experienced by many more people everywhere. Even more significant than this is the fact that when an EPUB 3 book is published, *it can be accessible from the point of publication—content available to mainstream readers will be available and accessible for everyone, everywhere.*

However, not all EPUB 3 books, distribution portals and Reading Systems will be created the same, and may therefore not fulfill all expectations in terms of accessibility. There is a very important role for the DAISY community to play, including providing input and advice to content and tool developers and providers, and ensuring that end users have access to consolidated information which will allow them to navigate this emerging new landscape with ease and take full advantage of the benefits that EPUB 3 will bring.

Accessible publishing has existed for many years in the form of narrated audio, large print, and Braille. However, only recently have mainstream reading technologies begun to make it possible to achieve equal access to published content for people of all ages and disabilities. Mainstream digital content producers are beginning to recognize and embrace new opportunities and extend the potential audience and market for their publications—but there is still a very long way to go.

In addition, life expectancy is increasing, with current projections suggesting that the number of people over 80 years of age will more than double within the next 10 years. Currently, 21% of people over 50 experience severe vision, hearing, or dexterity problems, and that likelihood only increases with age. Publishers need to be ready to meet the needs of this growing group of readers.

---

[*] http://www.w3.org/TR/ruby/
[†] http://idpf.org/epub/30/spec/epub30-overview-20111011.html#sec-gls-css

The digital revolution in publishing is causing all publishers and organizations providing digital content to rethink their business models, their way of doing business and workflows.

O'Reilly Media, in collaboration with the IDPF, has released a white paper "What Is EPUB 3? An Introduction to the EPUB Specification for Multimedia Publishing" by Matt Garrish. It can be downloaded at no cost from the O'Reilly Media website* (registration required).

---

* http://shop.oreilly.com/product/0636920022442.do

14

Math and the Blind

Arthur I. Karshmer, Yonatan G. Breiter, and Cristian Bernareggi

CONTENTS

Introduction

Mathematics has often been called "The Mother of All Science," but for most students of the subject this description carries little weight. Math is viewed by many students to be a hurdle that must be cleared in their educational experience. Clearing this hurdle is a prerequisite to entering any of the so-called traditional STEM* careers. In reality, the need for math skills goes well beyond the traditional view of science to include the social and behavioral sciences, economics, and many others. The message is clear: without knowledge of some advanced level of mathematics, entry into a growing number of professional fields is difficult, if not impossible. Not only does the problem have a negative impact on career choice and earning power, but it also affects national competitiveness and decreases the scientific capabilities of our society. For students with visual impairment, the problem is even more profound. What we call "The Mother of All Science" is viewed as "The Bane of the Blind."

Much of the problem is based on the techniques traditionally used to present information to the blind. Louis Braille, a blind Frenchman, in the early nineteenth century, invented the almost universal system for textual and numeric presentation to the blind. Interestingly, the concept was devised as an aid to the French military, which desired a tactile method of presenting important information to soldiers at night.

The Braille system uses a 3 × 2 matrix of raised and/or not raised dots (see Figure 14.1) to represent both characters and numeric digits. For a variety of reasons, the Braille system has been criticized over the years; yet it still remains the universal system of information transfer for the blind. Whether Braille is presented embossed on special paper, or presented via electronic means, Braille is still the standard.

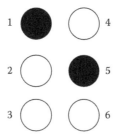

FIGURE 14.1
The Braille representation of the letter "e" with dot numbers (not to scale).

---

* STEM is an acronym for the words science, technology, engineering, and mathematics. This term was coined by the U.S. National Science Foundation in 2002.

Unfortunately, a system such as Braille has some inherent problems. As Braille is a matrix of six dots, in which any dot can be raised or not, the limit on character set is restrictive. Indeed Braille can only represent 2^6 or 64 unique characters. Using the English alphabet as an example, the problem becomes clear. The minimal English character set requires 26 lowercase letters, 26 uppercase letters, and 10 digits. The basic set requires 62 of the possible 64 characters representable by Braille.

Unfortunately, teaching math to the blind requires many more special characters than required by literary Braille. To solve this problem, special forms of the traditional 6-dot and 8-dot Braille have been developed to present mathematics. More on this subject is presented later in this chapter. Given these, and other reasons, teaching mathematics to the blind is a daunting challenge. There can be no doubt that mathematics is "the bane of the blind."

Problem in Historical Perspective

Early History of Education for the Blind

To better understand the technical issues associated with teaching mathematics to the blind, it is first helpful to get a historical overview of the place of the blind in society. The creation of the first school for the blind, which took place in Paris in 1785 by Valentine Hauy, was an important landmark in an earlier period in which the blind were effectively ostracized from the seeing world. In an interesting paper (Lowenfeld 1956), the author characterizes the history of the blind in society as developing through three different phases. Briefly stated, these periods included:

The primitive society: During this period, the blind were considered unable to survive and consequently were doomed to die with no support by the rest of the society.

Great religions come of age: Along with the development of large religious movements came an important turning point in the treatment of the blind in society. Rather than a policy of abandonment, the blind became the beneficiaries of a more humanitarian view of their situation in society. This new approach yielded unexpected consequences that would go a long way in their behalf in the future. As a result of this new attitude, many blind individuals thrived, accomplished impressive achievements, and demonstrated that the blind could, indeed, be functional and valued members of society.

Societal inclusion: By the strength of their own achievements, the blind demonstrated their ability to survive and more importantly to thrive in, and contribute to, society in general. At this point, society was in a position to consider the concept of special education for the blind. The process would be carried out in schools separated from the seeing with curricula different from that offered to the seeing, and finally offered only in residential schools.

The residential model of educating the blind began in France in the late eighteenth century and then became the norm on the continent. By the third decade of the nineteenth century, it arrived in the United States. For all but a few instances, the basic model of educating the blind changed little for the next century. Yes, this was advancement for the blind, but by its very form, morphed into a system of questionable value.

In an unexpected, but understandable, twist of fate, the residential school for the blind became a veritable prison for its students. The curriculum was based more on the practical rather than the abstract, and stressed providing work for the student—not any work, but rather work that could easily be carried out by the students attending the closed world of the residential school. Students, upon completion of their basic studies, worked in what came to be called the "sheltered workshop," creating simple items that were readily sold to the outside world, profiting both the student and the school.*

Louis Braille and Major Changes in Education of the Blind

Amid major changes in the American educational system for the blind, Braille perfected his literary Braille code, which had, and still has, a key role in educating the blind. In the period between 1829 and 1834, the American scene was poised to make major changes to the education of the blind. In addition to Braille's major contribution, three now famous schools for the blind were founded. In 1829, the New England Asylum for the Blind (now the Perkins School for the Blind) was founded; in 1831, the New York Institution for the Education of the Blind (now known as the New York Institute for Special Education) was incorporated; and in 1832, the Pennsylvania Institution for the Instruction of the Blind (now known as the Overbrook School for the Blind) was established. The events of this period became the foundation for modern instruction of the blind.

While the residential school was a major improvement in the education of the blind, it fostered the concept that the blind and the sighted were intended to be separated. Over time, however, the situation changed, as more and more blind students were able to transition into the sighted society. The twentieth century witnessed a major change in the blind person's place in society, and with this change also came a new view of their education in the regular classroom. While change came slowly, it was clear that a new era had

---

* The fear of the sheltered workshop continues today. There are jobs available to the blind as telephone agents or operators that become almost totally populated by other blind individuals and form the modern sheltered workshop (see Chapter 17).

arrived for the blind student. A time when they could become full-time educational partners with the sighted, a change dubbed "mainstreaming." This
change in no way meant the end of the residential school, but did portend
the decline of many of their number. In general, mainstreaming has been a
success. In certain educational domains, however, new issues have surfaced.
One of these problem domains relates directly to the subject of this work:
science, and more specifically, math and the blind.

The teaching of mathematics has been, from the earliest days to today, one of
the most difficult endeavors in the educational process of the blind. Whether
in the residential school or the mainstreamed classroom of today's public
schools, teaching math to the blind is an arduous, and often unsuccessful, task.

The residential schools have been considerably more successful in this
task. These schools have developed tools to help in this process, and have
developed curricula and applied best practices learned in their long history
of teaching this difficult subject. And, indeed, many of them continue on
today. While the number of the residential schools have continually declined
over the recent past, the ones still in operation do an excellent job. Highly
trained teachers, experience-based techniques, and deep commitment to the
work make them the best at this task. One needs to look no further than
institutions such as the Perkins School, the Overbrook School for the Blind,
and the Texas School for the Blind and Visually Impaired to see how far they
have progressed over the years.

But times have changed. Students that would, in the past, been in residential
schools are now mainstreamed into the general educational system. A system
without the experienced and well-trained special education teachers is now
forced to deal with classes of a variety of students exhibiting a variety of special
needs. These teachers are looking toward technological innovations to help
make the task more feasible. In the remainder of this work, the various reasons
for this difficulty are presented and emerging technologies are discussed.

But first, it is important to make the following comment on developing
tools and methods to help the blind master mathematics. Simply stated,
every blind student trying to learn mathematics is actually only 1/3 of the
group involved in this difficult learning process. The other two members of
this team are their teachers and their parents. Later in this work, new technologies are described that include the other 2/3 of the group in the process.
This is an important insight rarely discussed in this domain.

Difficulties of Braille in the Domain of Mathematics

Why Does Literary Braille Fail in the World of Mathematics?

Literary Braille is a powerful tool. It allows the blind to read text accurately
and speedily. It is generally easy to produce and there are numerous electronic

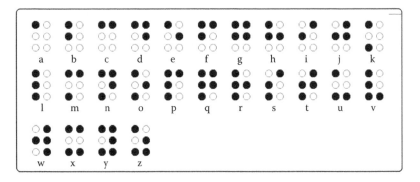

FIGURE 14.2
The lowercase alphabet in Braille.

devices that can present and modify Braille output in real time. While these devices, normally called "refreshable Braille," are expensive, they are readily available in the developed world. The refreshable Braille device is normally a 40–80 character linear display of 6-dot Braille characters along with a variety of other control buttons. Figure 14.2 shows the American Braille cells that form the lowercase letters of the alphabet (not to scale).

Note that there are no Braille characters to indicate the digits from 0 to 9, or the uppercase alphabet. In the case of numbers, a special character to indicate that they now represent digits, not letters, prefixes the letters "a" through "j." The number "31987" would then be represented in Braille as shown in Figure 14.3. The representation of the five digits is composed of six Braille characters. The leading character is the special breakout character that indicates that all following lowercase letters between "a" and "j" represent the 10 digits used in numerical representations. In a similar manner the method to indicate an uppercase letter is to precede the lowercase letter by a special breakout character (see Figure 14.4).

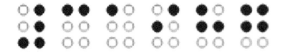

FIGURE 14.3
The number "31987" in Braille shown as the appropriate letters preceded by the special breakout character for numbers (not to scale).

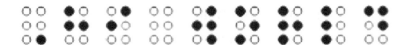

FIGURE 14.4
The use of capitalization in Braille of the characters "Hi world" (not to scale).

To make literary Braille reading faster, several special characters have been added. These special characters represent letter sequences commonly used in English, or the common sequences used in a particular national language. In the English Braille code, there are special characters for the letter sequence "ing" and others. Other national Braille codes would have similar notation common to their language. In fact, there are several grades of literary Braille that offer even more contractions to speed the reading process. The higher the level of contractions, the more difficult the character set is to learn.

While the majority of the blind community uses literary Braille, it is of little value in the representation of mathematics. Given the maximum character set in literary Braille (64 characters), it became clear that a change was needed for mathematics. One of the new ideas to expand the Braille's range of characters in a dramatic way was the 8-dot code proposal. Instead of the two columns and three-row characters, the proponents of the 8-dot system suggested characters of two columns and four rows.

The resulting set of characters would allow a character set of 2^8 or 256 unique characters. The 8-dot system, while improving the size of the Braille alphabet, has posed several problems that have made it unattractive (several of the 8-dot systems are described later in this chapter.)

- The millions of 6-dot Braille users around the world are not anxious to learn a new system.
- Many of the users of the 6-dot systems are older Braille users reporting that their sense of touch had deteriorated over time.
- The cost of such a change is prohibitive.

Historically, engineering a better system does not necessarily make the new system more attractive than its predecessor. A perfect example of this phenomenon is the keyboard layout used on effectively all systems using the Roman character set. Called the "QWERTY" keyboard, it actually represents a deoptimization of the original typewriter keyboard. This action was required on early typing machines as most of the typists could easily type at a speed that would jam the machine. In recent years, several new and more efficient keyboard layouts have been suggested, with the most famous being the Dovorak (1936) keyboard. Due to the rejection of the new keyboards by the vast number of people who type, the QWERTY keyboard is still dominant.

Birth of a New 6-Dot System for Mathematics

Louis Braille's development of the first system of tactile character representations became a boon for the blind. Suddenly, the blind could read and write. But Braille also represented a key to many more doors for the blind. Braille users were now able to consider using the code for other endeavors beyond literature. Blind students considered having Braille-like codes for music, science, and mathematics. But these studies needed a more robust code to express the much more complex structure and larger alphabet of mathematics.

Enter Abraham Nemeth. Born blind in 1918 on the Lower East Side of Manhattan. As a child, Dr. Nemeth had a love for mathematics and perused his studies at several educational institutions in the New York City area attaining his undergraduate and master's degrees in psychology. With discouragement from his advisor and encouragement from his wife, Nemeth decided to continue his studies in mathematics.

Nemeth quickly realized that literary Braille was not adequate for advanced studies in math and science. To achieve his educational goal, Dr. Nemeth created a system of Braille-like codes for the reading and writing of math and science. His system was completed in 1952 and subsequently became the standard system used in the United States and other countries.

While math codes have been developed in a number of countries (Britain, Germany, Italy, France, Spain, and others), they all suffer from the same problem. Briefly stated, literary Braille and Braille-like math codes can only represent information in a linear format. For literary purposes, this is not a major issue, but for mathematics it is. This point can be made clear with a few very simple examples.

In our first example, we will use a simple equation: $a = b + c$. Here, there is no need for anything more than a linear presentation. Unfortunately, the study of math rapidly involves much more complex equations. For example, consider the following simple equation: $a = b - cd$. It is still quite simple, but clearly two-dimensional in nature. While two-dimensional, this simple equation can be presented in two different linear ways, one of which is prone to error and the other is not.

- *Prone to error*: $a = b - c$ over d. This linear representation does not capture the fact that this equation contains a complex fraction.
- *Not prone to error*: $a = (b - c)$ over d. While still linear, there is no ambiguity in this representation. Indeed, any equation, regardless of its complexity, can be presented in a linear format using enough parentheses. Unfortunately, using this approach can cause the reader to become lost—trying to differentiate the forest from the trees.

The first rendering of our equation is clearly ambiguous—a feature not acceptable in mathematics. The second rendering is totally unambiguous. Next, we examine a bit more complex equation. Known worldwide as the Pythagorean theorem, it is simply stated in the following way: $c = \sqrt{a^2 + b^2}$. This simple equation, to be linear and unambiguous, could be expressed as c = square root of (a squared + b squared). The rendering is correct, but is also a bit clumsy.

Dr. Nemeth recognized the difficulties and subsequently devised a scheme to present even the most complex mathematics in a linear form. In 1952, the Nemeth code was officially recognized by the Braille Authority of North

America (BANA) as the standard representation of mathematics. While offering a partial solution to the linearity problem, Nemeth code does present other difficulties: (1) due to the minimal character set available in 6-dot Braille and the extensive alphabetic demands of math, many new break-out sequences were needed; and (2) to make the code more compact, certain characters have meaning defined by their placement in an equation, making contextual information become a vital feature of the code.

Nemeth code, and other national mathematics codes, fall into a category of languages know as "context-sensitive"[*] languages. The classification by language theorists indicates that there will be cases in which context-sensitive languages cannot be mechanically translated to a context-free language.

The process of translating from Nemeth code to a context-free language is commonly known as "back translation." For many years, this process was considered unsolvable. Work by Reddy et al. (2005) proposed the use of techniques of programming language semantics and logic programming to achieve back translation. Other attempts at back translation include (1) the Labradoor project (Miesenberger et al. 1998), (2) the MAVIS project (Karshmer et al. 1998), (3) the Insight project (Karshmer et al. 1998; Annamalai et al. 2003; Gopal et al. 2007), and (4) the Multi-Language Mathematical Braille Translator (Archambault et al. 2005).

Several Math Braille Formats

The goal of the various standardized national math codes is to present all printed math in a linear form—for refreshable Braille presentation devices. While currently available refreshable Braille devices can only present a line of 40 or 80 6-dot Braille characters,[†] the future will bring large-scale refreshable presentation devices with resolutions of 1000 by 1000 refreshable points. In this format, math codes will be presentable in a two-dimensional form. Some devices of considerably smaller resolution (Handy Tech) have come to the market (see Figure 14.5), but with two major drawbacks: (1) relatively low resolution, and (2) extremely high price. New technologies to solve these problems are currently in the research phase.

The previous simple equation, $a = (b - c/d)$ and the representation of it as "the quantity of $b - c$ over d" would be expressed in Nemeth as ?$b - c/d$# where the "?" symbol represents the beginning of a fraction and the "#" character represents the end of a fraction. It should be noted that codes such

---

[*] Given: X, a1, and a2 are strings in a language, then if the meaning of X in the expression a1 X a2 remains the same regardless of the values of a1 and/or a2, we say that the expression is context free. Otherwise the expression is context sensitive.

[†] The resolution of these devices is either 80 by 3 or 160 by 3 refreshable Braille points.

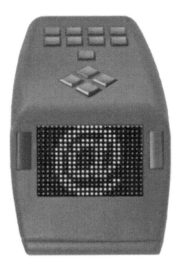

FIGURE 14.5
The Handy Tech Graphic Window professional. (Courtesy of Handy Tech Gmbh, Germany.)

as Nemeth apply different symbols to the various parts of an equation in order to make a linear presentation. Each different grouping signal indicates what sort of mathematical structure is about to begin. If common parenthesis were used, the reader would have to wait until the first instance of a "/" to recognize what has already been read is the numerator of a fraction. The cognitive value of this approach is the grouping of already known information in the reader's memory while not yet being aware of what is to come.

The Nemeth code, while being difficult to parse, does offer some cognitive advantages to the reader. However, it can make machine translation to another math code extremely difficult, and often impossible. The difficulty increases when we realize that there are numerous different math codes in use around world. At a small meeting of math code experts held in Lakeland, Florida, the decision was made to attempt to build tools to translate various popular math codes to each other (Karshmer et al. 2002, 2004). The meeting led to the development of the Universal Mathematics Access project. See Archambault et al. (2004, 2005) and Archambault and Moço (2006) for illustrations of these encodings.

The problem of representing math to the blind is clearly complex. The needs associated with reading linear math representations by the blind dictate the use of a complex set of context-sensitive markers. The math codes developed in a number of countries use context sensitivity to alleviate the problem. Representation of equations in context-free languages, while solving the translation problems, does in turn create representations that are extremely complex, and more difficult for the visually impaired reader.

Braille itself has become a target of deep criticism. The structure of Braille makes it an easy target for dramatic overhaul or replacement. The 6-dot Braille cell, while being adequate for literary purposes, falls well short of serving the scientific community. The technique of using cells with different meaning depending on their location puts math codes into the world of context-sensitive languages (Hopcroft et al. 2000), and the problems associated with them.

Making Braille More Useful in the Domain of Mathematics

Tactile feedback is currently the foundation for transmitting information to the blind. Given this status, and the ubiquity of tactile Braille systems, it would seem obvious that the best fix would come from expanding the number of tactile dots in each cell. Adding only two extra dots to the Braille cell expands its alphabet by a factor of four. Such a system was suggested by Schweikhardt in 1985. Other approaches to creating an 8-dot system (Schweikhardt 1998, 2000) have been reported, but have shown only marginal acceptance in the world of the blind. Two systems of note were developed primarily for mathematics, and are the work of the LAMBDA Group (Schweikhardt et al. 2006) and DotsPlus (Gardner 2002, 2003, 2005).

LAMBDA Project

The European LAMBDA system offers a linear representation of information much like the manner that mathematical information is presented in the markup language* known as MathML. The goal is to convert math code to a context-free markup language as opposed to the context-sensitive nature of other math codes. Achieving this goal eliminates many of the problems with math codes described earlier. Essentially, LAMBDA is a markup language. Using this approach, the LAMBDA team was able to use a common language as the foundation of other tools available in LAMBDA. The key to LAMBDA's approach was the development of an 8-dot Braille system.

While the 8-dot Braille cell can represent 256 unique characters, there is still need for more Braille characters. To make 8-dot systems easier to use, the LAMBDA team defined the breakout sequences in a logical way, to simplify interpretation, and increase the use of recognition, rather than recall by the

---

* A markup language is a special computer language used to encapsulate and describe data and their attributes. A markup language embeds processing instructions (tags) in electronic documents so they are accurately presented regardless of the hardware and software used. They are also able to include additional descriptive information (metadata) about the encapsulated data. Some examples of markup languages include: Extensible Markup Language (XML), Hypertext Markup Language (HTML), Math Markup Language (MathML), Scalable Vector Graphics (SVG, a subset of XML, is a tool for drawing complex objects, such as equations, from other markup languages), and VoiceXML.

user.* To accomplish this, they created prefixes that do not simply redefine the next character, but rather act as identifiers of a class to which following characters belong.

Finally, the LAMBDA team has designed and implemented an advanced editing system for creation of code by the user, which offers a simple method of using the hierarchical elements of equations and smoothly manages the various elements of the equation.

DotsPlus System

The DotsPlus system, like the LAMBDA system, relies on 8-dot Braille cells. Through a clever design, the majority of the multiple Braille cell breakout encodings of 6-dot Braille are eliminated. The use of the two extra dots allows a very powerful set of tools for identifying special characters. For example, DotsPlus would represent the uppercase "C" as the 6-dot definition of the basic letter "c," plus the use of one of the other dots in the last row of the cell. This approach eliminates the breakout character denoting upper-case in the traditional 6-dot system. Using this technique, DotsPlus is able to minimize the use of breakout characters in a large number of cases.

The result of this design achieves important goals. First, due to the graphi-cal notation and the reduction of breakout sequences, the language is consid-erably easier to learn and remember. Second, the basic goal of this 8-dot system is to represent the majority of special symbols as tactile graphical characters. Once again, the general disdain of changing from 6-dot to 8-dot Braille has had a negative effect on its broad acceptance.

In reality, both LAMBDA and DotsPlus represent interesting and useful concepts to make the representation of math easier to learn and use, and should be considered in any future efforts in this domain. However, both of these systems are still bound to linear representation of complex information.

Other systems developed in the recent past aim directly at solving the lin-earity problem. Four systems of interest deserve note: View+, the Handy Tech system, the AutOMathic Blocks (Karshmer et al. 2007) system, and, finally, the HyperBraille† system.

View+ System

The View+ system offers two-dimensional information in a static environ-ment. Through the use of two products from the parent company, the Tiger‡ printer and the Iveo touch pad can present quite elegant tactile representations

---

* A basic principal of human–machine interface design is to make use of tools a matter of rec-ognition rather than recall. In HCI, recognition represents "instant" identification while recall requires intermediate thought.
† http://www.hyperbraille.de
‡ http://www.viewplus.com/products

on special paper. The system can also present maps, graphs, and other information. For presenting math, the problem is printed on the Tiger device, and its output is then placed on the Iveo touch pad. A computer with a custom program is used in the system to supply information concerning the problems presented. In this manner, students are able to read their exercises tactilely, and have tutoring from the attached computer.

The system is quite useful in representing math in a multidimensional manner. However, each new problem, or set of problems, requires teacher creation on the Tiger printer. Only after this step can the Tiger printer output be made available for student usage. An additional problem with this approach is that it requires expensive equipment, a Tiger printer, and an Iveo touch pad to present static information. The system costs several thousand dollars, making it affordable only by schools and generally out of the price range of individuals.

Handy Tech System

The Handy Tech system[*] is one of the first two-dimensional refreshable dot systems capable of presenting complex objects and math. With a low resolution of 24 by 16 and a price tag of almost $11,000, the system is more of a research tool than a system usable in the average school. The system has software to present numerous refreshable images useful in the process of teaching math. Its low resolution and high price make it an expensive partial solution in the math domain.

AutOMathic Blocks System

The AutOMathic Blocks (Karshmer et al. 2007) system is a tactile system designed to help young blind students master arithmetic and beginning algebra (see Figure 14.6). The key element in all the systems described above was their ability to present two-dimensional representation of the educational material that can be read and "visualized" tactilely. While the View+ and the Handy Tech systems are able to accomplish this task, they fall short in their abilities to do so in a dynamic way at a reasonable price. The AutOMathic Blocks system was designed to deal with these issues and then go several steps further with the following features: (1) it provides a tactile two-dimensional representations of problem sets; (2) it allows for concurrent use of a refreshable Braille device; (3) it has a price below $500; and (4) it allows the student, teacher, and parent to create their own problem sets and to obtain real-time tutoring from any laptop or desktop computer.

The system employs the concept of teaching sighted and blind students using technologies from the early twentieth century along with inexpensive electronic devices. The base technology of the past is the wooden blocks

---

[*] http://www.handytech.de

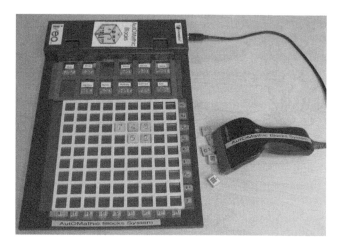

FIGURE 14.6
The AutOMathic Blocks system prototype.

containing letters of the alphabet and the digits from "0" to "9." The student (the child) was then free to manipulate these blocks by hand to solve simple spelling and arithmetic exercises. The parent or teacher then evaluated the correctness of the student's solution.

The AutOMathic Blocks system offers a similar approach. Small blocks (1.6 × 1.6 × 0.5 cm) are used with visible digits on one side along with their Braille representation, while the reverse side of the block contains the barcode for the number. Students are able to choose blocks from an organized block reservoir, read their barcode, and then place the blocks on the touchpad. At the end of the selection and placement phase, the problem exists in two-dimensional form on the touch pad along with an internal model of the touchpad. When ready, the student presses the Braille button marked "Solve" and the computer–student interaction begins. The student is now free to read the problem in two-dimensional space with his/her fingertips and receive a more realistic view than the traditional linear view.

HyperBraille System

The HyperBraille system is a step into the ultimate refreshable tactile system to present a very large range of problems and solutions in tactile format (Figure 14.7). The initial prototype system has a resolution of 120 by 60 pins that can be controlled by a computer in real time. Its resolution is approaching high-quality presentation of complex mathematics.

The current model has two drawbacks, one being its weight (over 20 pounds) and the other its price ($90,000). The system is based on an array of 7200 piezoelectric pins. While not ready for general use, it does represent progress in large-scale refreshable tactile devices.

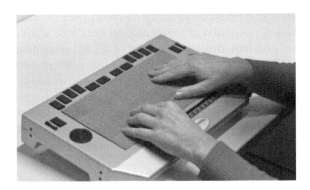

FIGURE 14.7
The HyperBraille tablet. (Courtesy of Metec Ingenieur AG, Germany.)

Broader View of the Problem

The display of math code as a series of equations to be solved is only half of the goal of allowing the blind to become practitioners in the world of STEM. If we are to provide superior tools to allow the blind meaningful access to mathematics, it is critical to realize that the entire document must be accessible, not only the equations. All equations of a proof, along with the embedded textual materials, must be seen as a single document. In this regard, the following sections present the notions of static and dynamic presentations (National Library of Service 2000; Pontelli and Palmer 2004) in relation to their ability to present math and text in a meaningful manner.

Static View

The static approach basically translates mathematical content into a form usable by a variety of assistive technologies. This group of devices has the ability to present the equations on Braille embossing printers, refreshable Braille presentation tools, as well as high-resolution pin displays. The presentation of the material is nothing more than an inactive presentation much like a page of a book.

Dynamic View

In the dynamic approach, the mathematical content is presented in a somewhat different way than used in the static view. The material is presented with tools that aid in the understanding of the content both in a static fashion and as a structure that can help uncover the innermost structure of equations.

Without the dynamic presentation of an equation, the presentation can easily become a confusing potpourri of mathematical notation. Math codes attempt to alleviate this problem through the use of context-sensitive presentation tools. While these approaches are certainly an improvement over a strictly linear presentation, they do not allow the user to navigate in and out of the deepest corners of an equation. Finally, dynamic systems must also provide a tool to permit the user to enter information into a document via interactive techniques. Again, while this tool is of great importance, writing in Braille code, especially math-based codes, leaves the teacher and parents out of the loop.

Holistic View

The static and dynamic views assumed that math for the blind could only be delivered in some linear fashion, and that special tools are needed to make this linear view more useful to the reader. However, tools offering a dynamic view allow the reader to navigate in a mental model of the math to build internal models of the equation. The user is then required to use the smaller "visualizations" to build a model of the entire equation.

What current presentations of math lack is a method of displaying the entire equation in a two-dimensional tactile model that can yield the intricacies of the mathematics in a tactilely equivalent manner to what the sighted student sees. While this can be accomplished with full-page embossed renderings of equations, the static nature of the output is a deterrent to interactive learning. The best model of the holistic view would be a high-resolution refreshable pin display device. Such devices are emerging on the market, and in the future will become the foundation of the effective teaching of math to the blind using tactile input. Short of any dramatic breakthrough in the domain of transferring information directly to the brain, high-resolution pin displays would appear to be the future of teaching and manipulating of mathematics by the blind.

Examples of Dynamic Approaches

The elements associated with a dynamic view of mathematics are based on understanding of the structure of math, the way in which math is manipulated by the user, techniques that are effective tools for highlighting the "road surface" of the equation, and a set of tools to travel this complex roadway.

Understanding the Way People Interact with Mathematics

While several designs for assistive technologies for the blind have come to the market in recent years, the notion of extensive usability testing and cognitive evaluation have been lacking. As part of the MAVIS project (Karshmer et al. 1998) and its ensuing MathGenie equation browser, a team of cognitive scientists was employed to gain understanding of how sighted individuals read and understand mathematics. The results of the study (Barraza et al. 2004; Karshmer and Gillan 2003) were intended to aid in the design of the MathGenie system's aural interaction with the user. Three basic studies were carried out in order to gain a better understanding of the processes used by the sighted in reading equations. The three studies focused on different areas essential to the understanding of mathematics:

- How people verbalize equations
- The effect of isolating (called chunking) parts of the equation:
- The initial scan of the equation:

Interestingly, the results mapped very closely with the guidelines outlined by Nemeth in his MathSpeak (Nemeth 1972) protocol (see Barraza et al. 2004 for further details).

Overview of Some of the Systems That Are Considered Dynamic

MathGenie Equation Browser

The MathGenie system was designed as a tool to help blind mathematicians, at all levels, to understand equations through the use of a highly flexible browser. The input to the MathGenie is the presentation level of MathML, which can be generated by a variety of equation editing systems from a commercial copy of MathType* to free editors available on the Internet.

The equation editor permits the teacher to create well-formed equations to be printed for the sighted and sent electronically to the blind users. Once the MathML file is loaded, the user is given a number of options on navigation styles from simply reading the entire equation to much finer-grained evaluation (see Figure 14.8). In all cases, navigation techniques are selected by pressing the various function keys and navigation controlled via use of the arrow keys. The MathML input is also converted via SVG and placed in a prominent place on the display device. In this way, the teacher can follow the student in a visual way.

The insertion of words such as "begin fraction" and "end fraction" are attractive due to their ability to inform the reader of structural elements of the equation. Without these lexical indicators, the aural presentation would include levels of ambiguity that are unacceptable to the reader. A simple example of this problem would be presenting the equation shown in Figure 14.8 without the lexical indicators:

a equals *b* minus *c* over *d*

---

* http://www.dessci.com/en/products/mathplayer/

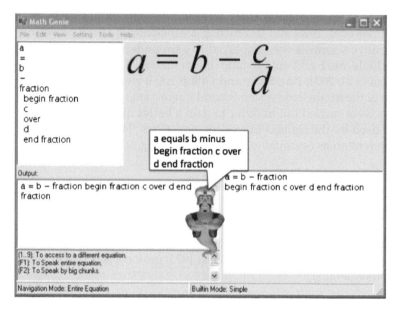

FIGURE 14.8
The MathGenie screen.

The ambiguity here is clear. Does the equation mean

$$a = b - \frac{c}{d} \quad (1) \quad \text{or} \quad a = \frac{b-c}{d} \quad (2)?$$

By using lexical indicators, all ambiguity is avoided. Using "begin fraction" and "end fraction," the meaning becomes clear. The following are two unambiguous statements that avoid any misunderstanding.

Equation 1 would be read as
　a equals *b* minus begin fraction *c* over *d* end fraction
while Equation 2 would be read as
　a equals begin fraction *b* minus *c* over *d* end fraction.

The use of lexical indicators was clearly indicated in the work of Chang (1983) as well as the work done by Barraza et al. (2004), and the MathSpeak language suggested by Nemeth. The use of lexical indicators, when properly applied, is a simple way of avoiding ambiguity. The MathGenie architecture includes other features useful to blind, visually impaired, and dyslexic users.

AsTeR System

AsTeR or audio system for technical readings, developed by Raman (1994), was designed to convert LaTeX documents to a format that could be used as

TABLE 14.1

Representation of the Pythagorean Theorem in Nemeth, MathML, and LaTeX

The equation	$c = \sqrt{a^2 + b^2}$
MathML representation	\<mrow\> \<mi\>c\</mi\>\<mo\>=\</mo\>\<msqrt\> \<mrow\> \<mi\>a\</mi\> \<mn\>2\</mn\> \<msup\> \<mo\>+\</mo\>\<msup\> \<mi\>b\</mi\> \<mn\>2\</mn\> \</msup\> \</mrow\> \</msqrt\> \</mrow\>
LaTeX representation	\[c = \sqrt {{a^2} + {b^2}} \]
Nemeth representation	C.k > a^2″ + b^2″]

audio documents. The audio documents can then be used to speak both textual and technical text. In his PhD thesis abstract, Raman states: "Visual communication is characterized by the eye's ability to actively access parts of a two-dimensional display. The reader is active, while the display is passive. This active-passive role is reversed by the temporal nature of oral communication: information flows actively past a passive listener. This prohibits multiple views—it is impossible to first obtain a high-level view and then 'look' at details. These shortcomings become severe when presenting complex mathematics orally."

The AsTeR system is based on a document representation model, which is used to expose the logical structure of the document. Mathematical material is then enhanced through the inclusion of "visual specifiers" such as "radical symbol," "subscript," and so on, which aid in the delivery of semantic information to the user. AsTeR offers active browsing and mathematical information, which can be navigated as a tree structure.

Table 14.1 illustrates a sample of representation in three of the most popular tools used in the world of mathematics: Nemeth, MathML, and LaTeX. The equation is the famous Pythagorean theorem which is an ideal candidate to demonstrate the tools associated with math and the blind.

Browsing Mathematics by Telephone (VoiceXML)

In an attempt to bring equation browsing to a broader community, Reddy et al. (2005) suggested using VoiceXML as the foundation of a telephone-based equation browser. As VoiceXML is a context-free markup language, documents in MathML can be readily translated to it. While VoiceXML was originally developed for the purpose of voice-based information telephony, it was not designed to handle and manipulate complex queries. Through the use of voice anchors, the user can interactively attach speech labels to subexpressions in the equation and then navigate via these labels. Any telephone, stationary or mobile, can then be used as a math browser.

MATHS System

The MATHS (Mathematical Access for Technology and Science) was one of the first of the crop of math browsing software developed in recent years. The system (Stevens et al. 1997; Weber and Stevens 1996) became the model of sophisticated math browsing for the blind and many of its innovations are still in use today. MATHS used an interesting combination of both speech and nonspeech audio to form the basis for transmitting useful information to the user. Two of the most interesting nonspeech features of this system are (1) the use of standardized prosody for describing different aspects of the content of the equation being read (see also Fitzpatrick 2002, 2006), and (2) the "Audio Glance" which is used to obtain an overall visualization of the form of the equation at hand.

The MATHS system was also dependent on special hardware in the form of what was called the "MATHS Workstation," which did not come to fruition. Finally, MATHS was able to generate both English and Stuttgart Braille and included an integrated editing system.

Other Browser-Based Systems to Teach Mathematics

While we have covered a number of well-known browser-based (dynamic) systems, there are others worth mentioning in this category. All of these systems have offered different approaches to solving the same problem—a problem not yet resolved. Some interesting projects in this domain include (1) the MathSpeak project (gh LLC 2006), (2) the MathTalk Project (McClellan 2007), and (3) MathEx (Gaura 2002).

Holistic Systems Available Now or in the Foreseeable Future

Among the numerous assistive technologies covered in this chapter, only three stand out as currently or potentially holistic. The system that is currently holistic is the AutOMathic Blocks System, while the HyperBraille system has the ability to be in this category. The Handy Tech system is in the same category as the HyperBraille but with a dramatically smaller resolution. These three systems have been described in an earlier part of this chapter.

Other Destinations for, and Sources of, Information

Learning math is a two-way street. The works covered to this point have dealt with the presentation of mathematics to the blind student. But, there is more than just reading in the educational process. At some point, information must be prepared for review by the teacher. In most cases, a teacher that does not read literary Braille will also not read math codes.

Another aspect of this issue is the techniques needed to collect mathematical content from non-electronic sources and to prepare it for presentation by the browser. The systems examined to this point have the advantage of receiving digital input in a format that could easily be converted to their internal representations.

Input from Printed Page: Infty Project

For many years, groups wrestled with the task of scanning printed math documents for conversion to a format usable in assistive technologies for the blind. The problem was considered one of the most difficult tasks in processing textual information that could be used in a digital form. Electronic publications offered a bit easier task, but the conversion of scanned text and equations from a paper document poses a great hurdle.

Even today, student services for the blind on most university campuses are only able to scan a textbook to extract the literary portion of the textual material. With the advent of electronic texts, most of the mathematical content is still only offered as an image.

The Infty project in Japan (Suzuki et al. 2004) has developed the InftyReader OCR application, which can accurately recognize scientific documents scanned from paper or from PDF formatted documents. The software can recognize complicated math expressions, tables, graphs, and other technical notations and then convert them to accessible formats. As these formats are all context-free languages, the translation of them to any other context-free or context-sensitive language is routine.

The complete Infty package contains (1) the Infty reader described above (Fukuda et al. 2000), (2) the Infty editor via ChattyInfty (Suzuki et al. 2004), and (3) ChattyInfty browser and editor (Suzuki 2005).

The Infty project has given us an important set of tools to build accessible technologies for the blind that are more usable. The software requires no expensive or sophisticated document-scanning technology and works well from most inexpensive desktop scanners.

Input from Student to Teacher

Yet another problem area for teachers of the blind is evaluating work submitted by the student. Braille embossed documents are of little to no value depending on the teacher's Braille skills. The problem becomes even more difficult when the subject matter is mathematics and the homework is submitted in a national code for math.

Solving this problem presents unique and difficult challenges in converting a math code document into either the actual equation or a verbalization of the homework. The actual Braille cells are susceptible to damage simply through normal handling. While a trained human reader can read such content with the help of context, it is a difficult task for an OCR program. The software is thus used to make its best approximation of the meaning of the Braille and the teacher must then examine and edit the output.

One of the first software tools of this type is the Winsight System (Gopal et al. 2007). The system takes hard copy input in the form of embossed pages of Braille, scans them, and then performs image recognition and finally analyzes these data to generate an ASCII version of the Braille being scanned. The system then separates the Nemeth coded equations and the Braille text, and converts it to LaTeX. From this point, the LaTeX can be easily printed for the teacher's perusal.

Input from Internet

Design Science Inc. is a company best known for its MathType equation editor. It is a powerful editing and document preparation tool that can generate MathML as its output. The system, called MathPlayer (Soifer 2005), enables Microsoft Internet Explorer to display mathematical content in web pages.

MathPlayer interfaces with the user's screen reader to deliver control and speech output. Simple equations are simply read left to right, while the user can also choose to navigate complex equations with tools somewhat similar to those used in the MathGenie system. The system also contains authoring tools to allow teachers to present math content to both their sighted and blind students.

Summary

In this chapter, we have discussed the issues associated with teaching math to the blind. From the earliest days of residential schools for the blind to today's mainstreamed students, learning math is one of the most difficult components of a broad-based education. And, without strong math skills, blind students are precluded from having careers in any of the hard sciences as well as social and behavior sciences.

In some sense, the movement of blind students into the mainstream of K-12 education was a step backward in the quest to learn math. The residential schools are staffed by teachers having extensive experience in teaching a variety of subjects, including math. Using this experience, these schools offer superior help for the young blind student.

Unfortunately, many U.S. K-12 schools are not prepared to supply the help that is required to effectively teach technical subjects to the blind. One solution to this problem is to send the blind students to special schools for the blind to receive their technical education and return them to the public school for their other classes. Unfortunately, this system, while being attractive, does have a major problem—there are not enough special schools in the United States to work in cooperation with the public school systems.

Given the realities of the special school working in concert with the public schools, there have been numerous projects to offer expert teaching to the blind. The current work has described the issues associated with the problem as well as many of the most interesting efforts to make mathematics accessible to the blind. While many of the projects break ground in their approach to the problem, none of them offers a comprehensive solution. The projects that come the closest to a broad solution suffer from extremely high pricing.

What is needed is a more general approach. Each of the projects described herein are focused on limited aspects of the problem without having a generalized understanding of all the issues associated with a comprehensive solution. This situation is partially due to the lack of a comprehensive understanding of the problem. Designers and developers of assistive technologies for the blind normally approach their work with a narrow focus, therefore seeing only a small part of the overall problem.

To be fair, many of the assistive technologies being developed are truly interesting and useful. For example, the Infty project has developed tools that are very useful, but the final output of the project is still a method to cast mathematics in a linear view based on math codes (Braille-like). The same is true in other interesting, but narrowly focused, projects. What has been done solves small pieces of the complex puzzle without enough consideration of the totality of the problem.

One of the most promising tools on the horizon is the HyperBraille system and its successors. Currently, and for at least the near future, the system is out of the financial reach of virtually all potential customers. Equally as important, the HyperBraille system simply takes Braille to a higher level through the use of high-resolution pin displays. It does not break new ground in the understanding of the nature of the problem and therefore it keeps us in the domain of Braille and other Braille-like codes used for mathematics.

What is needed is research that uncovers the entire process of reading, visualizing, understanding, and solving problems in mathematical notion. Accomplishing this goal requires truly interdisciplinary teams of scientists to gain a general understanding of the problem. Such teams would naturally require the participation of psychologists, cognitive scientists, neurophysiologists, computer experts, as well as experts in the domain of HCI (human–computer interaction).

Surprisingly, there is a paucity of research which explains how sighted people read and understand mathematics, no less explaining how best to present mathematics to the blind. With the exception of a small number of projects, the vast majority of the work in this domain is done based on the designer's hypotheses, but with no testing or verification of these hypotheses.

But the problem cannot be totally explained by the lack of science used by the developers. The problem is broader and the main problem is one of public policy and the support of the assistive technology industry.

References

Annamalai, A., Gopal, D., Gupta, G., Guo, H., and Karshmer, A. I. 2003. INSIGHT: A comprehensive system for converting Braille based mathematical documents to LaTeX. In *Universal Access in HCI: Inclusive Design in the Information Society, Volume 4 of the Proceedings of the 10th International Conference on Human-Computer Interaction (HCI International 2003)*. Crete, Greece.

Archambault, D., Batusic, M., Berger, F. et al. 2005. The Universal Maths Conversion Library: An attempt to build an open software library to convert mathematical contents in various formats. In *Human-Computer Interfaces: Concepts, New Ideas, Better Usability, and Applications, Volume 3 of the Proceedings of the 11th International Conference on Human-Computer Interaction (HCI International 2005)*. Las Vegas, Nevada.

Archambault, D., Fitzpatrick, D., Gupta, G., Karshmer, A. I., Miesenberger, K., and Pontelli, E. 2004. Towards a universal maths conversion library. In *Proceedings of the 9th International Conference on Computers Helping People with Special Needs (ICCHP 2004)*. Paris.

Archambault, D. and Moço, V. 2006. Canonical MathML to simplify conversion of MathML to Braille mathematical notations. In *Proceedings of the 10th International Conference on Computers Helping People with Special Needs (ICCHP 2006)*. Linz, Austria.

Barraza, P., Gillan, D. J., Karshmer, A. I., and Pazuchanics, S. 2004. A cognitive analysis of equation reading applied to the development of assistive technology for visually-impaired students. In *Proceedings of the Human Factors and Ergonomics Society 48th Annual Meeting (HFES 2004)*. Denver, Colorado.

Chang, L. A. 1983. *Handbook for Spoken Mathematics (Larry's Speakeasy)*. Lawrence Livermore Laboratory, The Regents of the University of California.

Dvorak, A., Merrick, N., Dealey, W., and Ford, G. 1936. *Typewriting Behavior*, New York: American Book Company.

Fitzpatrick, D. 2002. Speaking technical documents: Using prosody to convey textual and mathematical material. In *Proceedings of the 8th International Conference on Computers Helping People with Special Needs (ICCHP 2002)*. Linz, Austria.

Fitzpatrick, D. 2006. Mathematics: How and what to speak. In *Proceedings of the 10th International Conference on Computers Helping People with Special Needs (ICCHP 2006)*. Linz, Austria.

Fukuda, R., Ohtake, N., and Suzuki, M. 2000. Optical recognition and Braille transcription of mathematical documents. In *Proceedings of the 7th International Conference on Computers Helping People with Special Needs (ICCHP 2000)*. Linz, Austria.

Gardner, J. 2002. Access by blind students and professionals to mainstream math and science. In *Proceedings of the 2002 International Conference on Computers Helping People with Special Needs (ICCHP 2002)*. Linz, Austria.

Gardner, J. 2003. DotsPlus Braille tutorial: Simplifying communication between sighted and blind people. In *Proceedings of the 2003 CSUN International Conference on Technology and Persons with Disabilities (CSUN 2003)*. Los Angeles, California.

Gardner, J. 2005. *Introduction to DotsPlus® Braille.* http://dots.physics.orst.edu/dotsplus.html.

Gaura, P. 2002. REMathEx: Reader and editor of the mathematical expressions for blind students. In *Proceedings of the 8th International Conference on Computers Helping People with Special Needs (ICCHP 2002)*. Linz, Austria.

gh LLC 2006. *Welcome to the MathSpeak Initiative.* http://www.gh-mathspeak.com.

Gopal, D., Wang, Q., Gupta, G., Cnitnis, S., Guo, H., and Karshmer, A. I. 2007. Towards completely automatic backtranslation of Nemeth Braille Code. In *Universal Access in Human-Computer Interaction. Applications and Services, Proceedings of the 4th International Conference on Universal Access in Human-Computer Interaction, Volume 7 of the Combined Proceedings of HCI International 2007*. Beijing, China.

Hopcroft, J. E., Motwani, R., and Ullman, J. D. 2000. *Introduction to Automata Theory, Languages, and Computation.* Boston: Addison Wesley.

Karshmer, A. I. and Gillan, D. 2003. How well can we read equations to blind mathematics students: Some answers from psychology. In *Universal Access in HCI: Inclusive Design in the Information Society, Volume 4 of the Proceedings of the 10th International Conference on Human-Computer Interaction (HCI International 2003)*. Crete, Greece.

Karshmer, A. I., Gupta, G., Geiger, S., and Weaver, C. 1998. Reading and writing mathematics: e MAVIS project. In *Proceedings of the Third International ACM Conference on Assistive Technologies (ASSETS 1998)*. Marina del Rey, California.

Karshmer, A. I., Gupta, G., and Gillan, D. J. 2002. Architecting an auditory browser for navigating mathematical expressions. In *Proceedings of the 8th International Conference on Computers Helping People with Special Needs (ICCHP 2002)*. Linz, Austria.

Karshmer, A. I., Gupta, G., Pontelli, E. et al. 2004. UMA: A system for universal mathematics accessibility. In *Proceedings of the 6th International ACM SIGACCESS Conference on Computers and Accessibility (ASSETS 2004)*. Atlanta, Georgia.

Karshmer, A.I., Daultani, P., and McCaffrey, M. 2007. AutOMathic Blocks: An automated systems to teach math to K-12 children with severe visual impairment allowing both physical and haptic interaction with an automated tutor. In *Proceedings of the Learning with Disabilities Conference*, Dayton, Ohio.

Lowenfeld, B. 1956. History and development of specialized education for the blind. *Exceptional Children*, 23:53–57.

McClellan, N. 2007. The MathTalk System. http://www. metroplexvoice.com/tech_notes.htm.

Miesenberger, K., Batusic, M., and Stöger, B. 1998. Labradoor: A contribution to making mathematics accessible for the blind. In *Proceedings of the 6th International*

Conference on Computers Helping People with Special Needs (ICCHP 1998). Vienna and Budapest.

National Library of Service 2000. *Braille: Into the Next Millennium*. Library of Congress.

Nemeth, A. 1972. *The Nemeth Braille Code for Mathematics and Science Notation*. Louisville, Kentucky: American Printing House for the Blind.

Pontelli, E. and Palmer, B. 2004. Translating between formats for mathematics: Current approach and an agenda for future developments. In *Proceedings of the 9th International Conference on Computers Helping People with Special Needs (ICCHP 2004)*. Paris.

Raman, T. V. 1994. *Audio Systems for Technical Reading*. PhD dissertation, Cornell University, Ithaca, NY.

Reddy, H., Gupta, G., and Karshmer, A. I. 2005. Dynamic aural browsing of MathML documents with VoiceXML. In *The Management of Information: E-Business, the Web, and Mobile Computing, Volume 2 of the Proceedings of the 11th International Conference on Human-Computer Interaction (HCI International 2005)*. Las Vegas, Nevada.

Schweikhardt, W. 1998. *Stuttgartermathematikschrifürblinde*. Universität Stuttgart, Institut für Informatik.

Schweikhardt, W. 2000. Requirements on a mathematical notation for the blind. In *Proceedings of the 7th International Conference on Computers Helping People with Special Needs (ICCHP 2000)*. Karlsruhe, Germany.

Schweikhardt, W., Bernareggi, C., Jessel, N., Encelle, B., and Gut, M. 2006. LAMBDA: A European system to access mathematics with Braille and audio synthesis. In *Proceedings of the 10th International Conference on Computers Helping People with Special Needs (ICCHP 2006)*. Linz, Austria.

Soifer, N. 2005. Advances in accessible web-based mathematics. In *Proceedings of the 2005 CSUN International Conference on Technology and Persons with Disabilities (CSUN 2005)*. Los Angeles, California.

Stevens, R. D., Edwards, A. D. N., and Harling, P. A. 1997. Access to mathematics for visually disabled students through multi-modal interaction. *Human-Computer Interaction* 12:47–92.

Suzuki, M. 2005. *Infty Project: About ChattyInfty*. http://www.inftyproject.org/download/AboutChattyftInyE.txt.

Suzuki, M., Kanahori, T., Ohtake, N., and Yamaguchi, K. 2004. An integrated OCR software for mathematical document and its output with accessibility. In *Proceedings of the 9th International Conference on Computers Helping People with Special Needs (ICCHP 2004)*. Paris.

Weber, G. and Stevens, R. D. 1996. Integration of speech and Braille in the MATHS workstation. In *Proceedings of the 5th International Conference on Computers Helping People with Special Needs (ICCHP 1996)*. Linz, Austria.

15

Video Games for Users with Visual Impairments

Eelke Folmer

CONTENTS

Introduction

Over the last three decades, video games have evolved from an obscure pastime into a force of change that is transforming the way people perceive, learn about, and interact with the world around them. According to the NPD Group, currently more than 100 million consoles are present in U.S. households,* and an estimated 63% of the US population plays video games with 51% of players playing games on at least a weekly basis (ESA 2008). Beyond pure entertainment, video games are increasingly used for more serious applications such as education, health, and rehabilitation.

---

* http://www.npd.com/press/releases/press_090520.html

Games have been identified to be powerful motivators—especially for children (Blumberg 1998; Squire 2005; Shaffer and Gee 2006)—and consequently video games are increasingly used in academic contexts as education tools. For example, many K12 schools incorporate video games in their curricula (Odenweller et al. 1998). Though video games have been identified as a contributing factor to children's increasingly sedentary behavior and associated higher levels of obesity (Trost et al. 2001; Wack and Tantleff-Dunn 2009), a new genre of video games, called *exergames*, has the potential to turn couch potatoes into jumping beans (Ni Mhurchu et al. 2008). Exercise games are video games that use upper and/or lower body gestures, such as steps, punches, and kicks to provide their players with an immersive experience that engages them into physical activity and gross motor skill development (Lieberman 2007; Mueller et al. 2008; Adams et al. 2009). Studies with exergames, such as Nintendo Wii, show that they stimulate greater energy expenditure than when playing sedentary video games (Lanningham-Foster et al. 2006; Graves et al. 2007; Leatherdale et al. 2010). Games have also been developed for various rehabilitation purposes. For example, an interface for the popular Guitar Hero game has been developed that allows upper extremity amputees to train the dexterous control of upper-extremity neuroprostheses (Armiger and Vogelstein 2008).

Despite this increased interest in using video games for more serious applications, a significant number of people encounter barriers when playing games, due to a disability (Grammenos 2008; Yuan et al. 2010). It could be argued that the social, educational, and health opportunities offered by games could potentially benefit users with disabilities the most. For example, users with disabilities are often isolated and lonely (Stuart et al. 2006) and games and virtual worlds could offer new opportunities for socialization. There is considerable evidence that the overweight and obesity rates are higher among persons with disabilities than among the general population (Cooper et al. 1999; Rimmer and Braddock 2002; Rimmer 2005). Exercise games such as Nintendo Wii, could offer new opportunities for individuals with disabilities to participate in physical activity. In certain circumstances, such as when games are used in the classroom for educational purposes, there is a legal obligation to make them accessible. Section 508 of the US Rehabilitation Act (U.S. Government 1998) states that schools and universities that rely on federal funding must make their electronic and information technologies accessible.

Video game accessibility is an emerging field of research within human computer interaction (Yuan et al. 2010). This chapter surveys existing work in the area of video game accessibility for users with visual impairments. It starts by discussing visual impairments and the benefits of users with visual impairments being able to play games. It then discusses the specific barriers that users with visual impairments encounter when trying to play a video game based on a generic interaction model for games. A number of games developed for different types of visual impairments are surveyed, along with several strategies to make video games accessible to users with visual impairments. The last section of this chapter envisions the future of visually impaired gaming.

Visual Impairments

The US has an estimated 1.3 million individuals who are legally blind* and 6.8 million individuals who have a visual impairment. Individuals with visual impairments have reduced mobility and as a result they participate in fewer social activities, have more difficulty attending school and using educational resources.

Visual impairments are strongly related to the current obesity epidemic in the US. Obese individuals are twice as likely to lose their sight (Johnson 2005; Habot-Wilner and Belkin 2005; Cheung and Wong 2007) due to an increased chance of developing cataracts. Loss of sight has further identified to significantly reduce remaining years—and quality of life (Karpa et al. 2009; Chadha and Subramanian 2010; Crewe et al. 2010).

Benefits of Access to Video Games

Access to video games could offer new socialization, education, employment, and health opportunities for individuals with visual impairments:

- *Socialization*: Video games and virtual worlds offer social communities for users *with* disabilities. For example, the Heron Sanctuary (Talamasca 2008) is a meeting place in Second Life for individuals suffering from disabilities such as multiple sclerosis and muscular dystrophy. Naughty Auties is a virtual resource center and meeting place within Second Life for those with autism.[†] Visually impaired individuals are currently excluded from participating in such communities. Social interaction offered by virtual worlds could benefit the visually impaired as the severity of their disability may make them feel socially and physically isolated within their geographic communities (Talamasca 2008).

- *Education*: Virtual worlds such as Second Life have successfully drawn academic interest as a viable environment for learning due to its high degree of customization (Robbins 2007). Many educational institutions use Second Life as a virtual classroom.[‡] Second Life has also been adopted for foreign language training.[§] A high school

---

* http://www.afb.org/info_document_view.asp?documentid=1367
[†] http://www.cnn.com/2008/HEALTH/conditions/03/28/sl.autism.irpt/index.html
[‡] http://slusage.com/chemistry.asp
[§] http://www.languagelab.com/en

opened up in 2010 that only uses video games in their curricula to teach children about STEM.[*] Accessibility to video games and virtual worlds could open up new education opportunities for individuals with visual impairments, especially considering that they can easily facilitate distance learning (Dickey).

- *Employment*: Only 11.9% of individuals with visual impairments have a bachelors or higher degree and only 25% of 16–65-years-old individuals with visual impairments are employed. Virtual worlds have thriving economies where people make a living out of selling virtual content. Second Life is also successfully used as a collaborative workspace in industrial[†] environments. Games and virtual worlds could offer new employment opportunities for individuals with visual impairments.

- *Health*: Compared to children and adolescents in other disability groups, those with visual impairments have been identified to be the most inactive, with 39% classified as sedentary and only 27% classified as active (Longmuir and Bar-Or 2000). Children with visual impairments have limited access to physical education, recreation, and athletic programs because of: (1) *limited social opportunities*, such as lack of exercise partners or sighted guides with whom to exercise (Ponchillia et al. 2002; Shapiro et al. 2005); (2) *fear of injury* while exercising (Lieberman, Houston-Wilson, and Kozub 2002) and safety concerns of parents and teachers (Lieberman and Lepore 1998; Nixon 1988); and (3) *self barriers*, such as fear of being made fun of while exercising (Nikolaraizi and De Reybekiel 2001), and a general lack of exercise opportunities (Lieberman et al. 2002). Although schools are mandated by law to have adapted physical education programs, few children with visual impairments participate in them (Stuart et al. 2006; Houwen et al. 2007). Psychosocial factors, such as parents' lack of understanding of their child's ability to be physically active, often lead to overprotective behaviors in an attempt to assist the children (Lieberman and Lepore 1998; Longmuir 1998). Exergames have been successfully used for engaging adults with cerebral palsy into physical activity (Hurkmans et al. 2010). When compared with regular physical activities, exergames have some attractive properties for individuals with visual impairments because: (1) exergames can be played independently and do not require an exercise partner or sighted guide to be present; (2) exergames are performed in place, which significantly minimizes the risk of injury; and (3) the ability to play the same games as their peers, either alone or with their peers

---

[*] http://www.popsci.com/entertainment-amp-gaming/article/2009-12/new-school-teaches-students-through-videogames

[†] http://secondlife.reuters.com/stories/2006/11/09/ibm-accelerates-push-into-3-D-virtual-worlds

and family, may increase socialization opportunities, which is important as users with visual impairments are often isolated and lonely (Stuart et al. 2006).

Barriers to Access

Users with visual impairments encounter various barriers when trying to play video games.

Game Interaction Model

Yuan et al. (2010) presents the following game interaction model (Figure 15.1) that illustrates how players interact with video games and which also allows for identifying how users with disabilities face barriers to play video games. This model was derived by analyzing how a player interacts with a game for a number of different game genres and finding commonalities between the steps that are performed when playing a game. The game interaction model consists of three steps:

1. *Receive stimuli.* Games provide stimuli in three different forms: visual, auditory, and haptic. Depending on the type of game, stimuli can be further divided into two categories:

   a. *Primary* stimuli must be perceivable by the player in order to play the game. Almost all games use visuals as primary stimuli. For

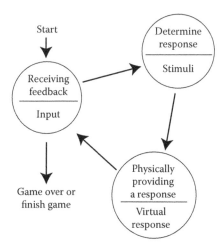

FIGURE 15.1
Game interaction model expressed as a finite state machine.

example in a First Person Shooter (FPS) game, visuals are used as a primary stimulus and without visual feedback the game cannot be played. Though sound and haptic feedback may be provided, this typically does not provide sufficient information to be able to play the game. For example, the player may hear or feel the presence of an enemy but may not be able to determine the enemy's location. Though a game typically has only one primary stimulus, some games such as dance/music games rely upon music to such an extent that visuals and audio are both primary stimuli.

    b. *Secondary* stimuli are provided as a supplement to a primary stimulus. Being able to play a game does not depend upon being able to perceive a secondary stimulus. In an FPS without sound or haptic feedback, the player can still play the game to a large extent, but the player may suffer from a reduced gaming experience.

2. *Determine response.* Based on the specific set of stimuli that the game provides, the player must cognitively determine which in-game response(s) to provide from the set of available game actions. These actions are specific to the game and are typically defined by the game's genre. For example, an FPS may allow the player to navigate his or her character, whereas an RTS game may allow the player to group units together. The player either chooses a combination of one or more actions or may decide to not provide an action at all.

3. *Provide input.* After deciding which in-game response(s) to provide, the player must physically issue the chosen action(s) through the input device used to interact with the game. Typically, games require the player to actuate a physical device such as keyboard, mouse, controller, or a steering wheel.

After successfully performing these three steps, the internal state of the game may change and new stimuli may be provided. The subsequent steps rely on each other, for example, if a user cannot receive stimuli, it will impair their ability to successfully determine what response to provide. The steps are repeated until the player wins, loses, or quits the game.

Barriers for Players with Visual Impairments

A visual impairment primarily affects Step 1 of the interaction model. The barrier players with visual impairments encounter is that they are unable to or limited to perceive primary stimuli. Without this feedback it may be impossible to determine what in-game response and what physical input to provide and when, though these players are cognitively and physically able to perform such tasks. For example, a first person shooter provides primarily visual cues that indicate what to do and when. If an enemy appears this indicates to the player to determine a response and to provide an input. Players who are unable to see are unable to perceive these primary cues and cannot proceed with steps 2 and 3 and are hence unable to play the game. Although games do provide audio and occasionally haptic feedback, these are typically provided as secondary stimulus as they do not contain information on what to do and when. For example, if the player hears footsteps this could be the footsteps of an enemy or of a friend (in case of multiplayer cooperative games).

The accessibility barrier varies with the type of impairment. Someone with no vision is unable play video games that only provide visual cues. Individuals with minor visual impairments such as color blindness—for most games—only suffer from a reduced gaming experience (e.g., not being able to read a red text on a green background in a first person shooter) though for some games they may encounter barriers that prevent them from being able to play the game at all.

Games Accessible to Visually Impaired Players

We now survey a number of video games that have been specifically developed to accommodate the abilities of users with visual impairments.

Low Vision Games

Individuals with low vision may find it difficult or impossible to receive feedback from games because visuals are typically used as a primary stimulus. Features, such as high-contrast color schemes accommodating color blindness, scalable fonts, or the ability to zoom in, are recommended by accessibility guidelines for software and the web* and can be found in a number of commercial games. For example, many games allow for increasing the font size. A number of puzzle games allow for using different color schemes when a player is color blind (Schiesel 2009), and many first person shooter and real time strategy games may allow for customizing the colors of the units of the enemy. Figure 15.2 shows solutions for low vision offered by a strategy and a puzzle game.

Individuals with severe visual impairments, for example, legally or totally blind, are excluded from playing video games that rely upon visual stimuli. Primary visual cues must be substituted with nonvisual cues to allow a player who is blind to play video games (Yuan and Folmer 2008). Sensory substitution is challenging due to the limited spatial and temporal resolutions of audio and tactile modalities (Bach-y Rita and Kercel 2003).

---

* http://www.w3.org/TR/WCAG10

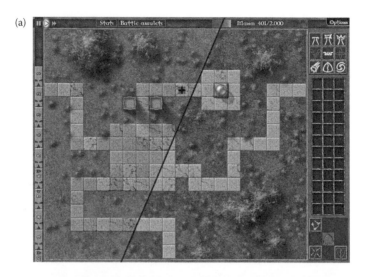

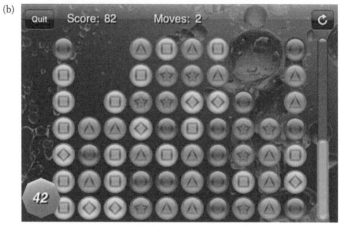

FIGURE 15.2
(a) Screenshot from the strategy game Gem Craft that offers a high-contrast mode. (b) Puzzle game that in addition to color also uses symbols to distinguish individual objects.

Patterns for encoding information tactually generally include intensity, duration, temporal patterns, and spatial locations (Van Erp 2002). Within the domain of video games primarily audio has been explored for making games accessible to users who are blind. These games are commonly referred to as *audio games*.

Audio Games

Many audio games have been developed for the blind (Friberg and Gärdenfors 2004; Roden and Parberry 2005). An extensive list of audio games is maintained on the website (http://www.audiogames.net). Some of these games were created for research purposes but many are developed by independent game developers. A number of games have been selected that cover a broad range of game genres as well as all the different strategies that are used to make the game accessible to blind gamers.

- *Mach 1 Car Racing* (Kitchen 2008) is a remake of the classic racing game *Pole Position*. Audio cues, such as the echo of your engine, are used to indicate which direction to turn. The game uses self-voicing with an adjustable rate of speech. Players control their car using the arrow keys.

- *Shades of Doom,*[*] *AudioQuake* (Atkinson et al. 2006), *Terraformers* (?) are first person shooter games. These three games use different strategies for accessibility. Shades of Doom uses audio cues such as footsteps to help find one's way through the levels. A navigation tool provides synthetic speech about the player's surrounding. AudioQuake uses "earcons" which are structured sounds that obey musical conventions (Brewster et al. 1995). These alert the player to an object or event. Terraformers uses a sound compass where different tones are used to indicate the direction the player is pointing. It also offers a sound radar that can be used to identify what is in front of the player. By using a "ping," it is possible to tell how far objects are in front of the character. Using a key on the keyboard, it is also possible to tell what type of object is in front of the character, using a voice playback system. All games use stereo sound to convey spatial information. These games have the same controls as regular FPS games.

- *The Last Crusade* (Dwyer and VanLund 2008) is a role-playing RPG game that uses self-voicing to read out the events of the game. A player uses keyboard for basic control including spacebar for stats reporting and instructions and arrow keys for navigation.

- *AudioBattleShip* (Sánchez et al. 2003) is a turn-based strategy game (Figure 15.2a) that was initially designed to be used for cognitive development purposes with blind children. A wacom tablet is used as an input device. A grid system is built over the tablet in order to represent the matrix of the battlefield and some additional help buttons for triggering actions. Audio cues are provided to inform about a specific spatial location on the board or the occurrence of certain actions such as the sound of a bomb dropping over certain cells in the battle grid. Though the wacom tablet does not provide haptic feedback, because it is a constrained input device, it allows for better mental mapping of the battlefield.

---

[*] http://www.gmagames.com/sod.html

- *GMA Tank Commander* (GMAGames 2008) is an audio-only version of the classic game *Tank Commander*. The type of enemy is indicated using audio cues and its location through surround sound. The player controls their tank using their keyboard.

- *Speed Sonic Across the Span* (Oren 2007) is a platform game. Audio cues are used to indicate objects and obstacles. The sound is consecutive with the platform panning to the right–left throughout the game. Players control their characters using a controller.

- *Metris* (InspiredCode 2008) is a musical version of the puzzle game *Tetris* that works with a screen reader. Audio cues such as tone and beats determine what input the player must provide.

- *Powerup* (Trewin et al. 2009) is a multiplayer educational 3-D game developed by IBM where players explore environments and solve various quests. This game supports various accessibility features for visual, motor, and cognitive impairments. Visually impaired users can play this game using built-in self-voicing. Audio cues such as footsteps provide additional guidance. Four different islands are available with four different challenges to complete. Visually impaired users have the same options as sighted players and can issue a number of commands such as "look left" activated by key presses to get information about their environment.

- *Finger Dance* (Miller et al. 2007) is a pattern matching dance/rhythm games. Finger dance is a modification of *Dance Dance Revolution* (DDR). Music games provide visual feedback based on the music that is played, indicating which inputs to provide on specific input devices such as a dance mat or a guitar controller. Finger Dance changes the original game play of the DDR game significantly because it replaces the original music with audio cues that indicate which keys the player must provide.

- *AudiOdyssey* (Glinert and Wyse 2007) is a gesture-based music game (Figure 15.3b). AudiOdyssey uses speech instructions to indicate to the player what gesture needs to be provided with a motion-sensing controller. A specific gesture reveals an instrument and players must perform a sequence of this gesture that matches the beat of the song as indicated using an audio cue to activate the instrument. After activating the instrument, a new gesture is taught that conveys a new instrument as to iteratively fill in the song.

Haptic Games

In recent years new types of video games have emerged that put constraints on the use of audio for sensory substitution. Examples of such game genres are exergames and music games. Exergames and music games are often

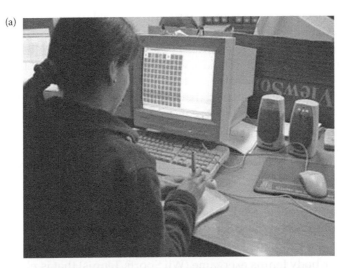

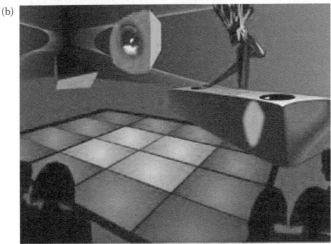

FIGURE 15.3
(a) Blind player playing AudioBattleShip using a wacom tablet. (b) Screenshot from AudiOdyssey.

played in social contexts (Mueller et al. 2003; Bianchi-Berthouze et al. 2007; Sinclair et al. 2007) and feature music (Hoysniemi 2006; Parker and Heerema 2007; Stanley and Calvo 2009) as the input the player needs to provide is matched with the rhythm and beats of the songs. Extra audio feedback may interfere with being able to socialize and layering audio over music may be overstimulating and detrimental to the player's experience (Yuan and Folmer 2008). Instead of audio cues several accessible implementations of these games have been implemented that explore the use of haptic feedback.

- *Blind Hero* (Yuan and Folmer 2008) is an accessible version of the pattern matching music game Guitar Hero* in which players play rock music using a guitar-shaped controller (see Figure 15.4). Due to the presence of music, Blind Hero provides vibrotactile cues provided with a haptic glove that indicate what input to provide and when. User studies with three blind players showed they could successfully play the game and they could memorize input sequences using vibrotactile feedback.

- *Rock Vibe* (Allman et al. 2009) is an accessible version of the Rock Band† pattern matching music game. Players with visual impairments can play the drumming part by providing users with vibrations on upper and lower arms to represent the drumhead cues and on ankle to represent the kick drum cue. Auditory information is used to provide feedback on correct and timely hit (with various drumming sounds) or errors (with a click sound).

- *VI Tennis* (Morelli et al. 2010) implements the gameplay of a popular upper-body tennis exergame (Wii Sports Tennis) that is played with a motion-sensing controller called a Wii remote (see Figure 15.4c). Wii Sports Tennis only involves a temporal challenge, for example, when the ball gets close, the player has a few seconds to provide the upper-body gesture (swing their Wii remote from back to forward like a tennis racket) to return the ball. There is no spatial challenge as the computer automatically moves each player to the location of the ball. The sensitivity and timing of gestures in VI Tennis are based on Wii Sports Tennis, which is relatively forgiving to appeal to a mass audience.

- *VI Bowling* (Morelli et al. 2010) implements the gameplay of an upper-body bowling exergame (Wii Sports) that is played with a Wii remote. Because bowling is self-paced, it consists predominantly of a spatial challenge, for example, throwing the ball at the pins. Wii Sports Bowling implements the gestures used in bowling, however, players aim their ball by adjusting a visual marker using the arrow keys on their controller that indicates the direction in which their ball will be thrown. The direction of the ball can be adjusted by twisting the Wii remote while throwing, though the direction in which the gesture is performed is not taken into account. VI Bowling implements the same gestures and audio feedback as Wii Sports Bowling, but the spatial challenge is performed using a technique where users scan their environment with the controller and a vibrotactile cue indicates whether the controller is pointed at the direction of the pins.

- *Pet-n-Punch* (Morelli et al. 2011) is a whack-a-mole like exergame that can be played using two Wii remotes. Players are asked to help a

* http://www.guitarhero.com
† www.rockband.com.

farmer rid his farm of rodents by smacking them on the head with their hammer(s). Pet-N-Punch provides audio and tactile cues as to indicate what motions to provide and when. Players need to hit the rodents with a certain intensity. In order to avoid players simply swinging wildly, cats are also present within the playing field and

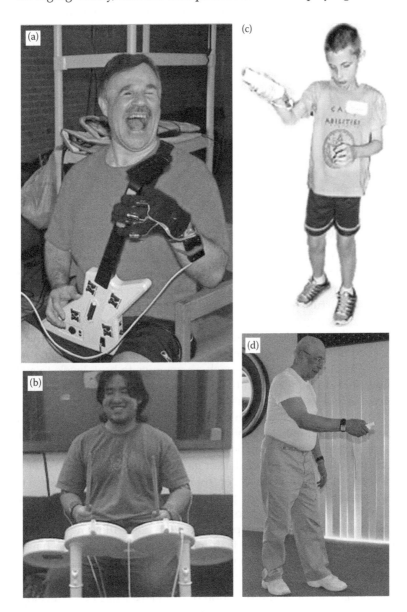

FIGURE 15.4
(a) Guitar Hero. (b) Rock Vibe. (c) VI Tennis. (d) VI Bowling.

players are penalized if cats were hit on the head. The idea of using two arms to play this game as opposed to one (as is common with most Wii-based exergames) is to stimulate larger physical activity.

- *Real Time Sensory Substitution* (Morelli and Folmer 2011) is a generic solution for making gesture-based controllerless video games accessible. Real-time sensory substitution has been implemented for the Kinect Sports hurdles game. Kinect is a camera-based gaming device used for gesture-based input. Kinect does not have a controller which makes it difficult to provide haptic feedback in sensory substitution. Real-time sensory substitution uses real-time video analysis to detect visual cues that require a gestural response from the player which are then provided to the user using haptic feedback using a Wii remote.

Video games and virtual worlds share the same interaction mechanisms and therefore we also review accessible virtual world interfaces for users with visual impairments.

Accessible Virtual World Interfaces

The immersive graphics, large amount of user-generated content, and social interaction opportunities offered by popular virtual worlds, such as Second Life, could eventually make for a more interactive and informative World Wide Web. Unfortunately, virtual worlds are currently not accessible to users who are visually impaired. Two different types of virtual worlds can be distinguished: (1) Game-like virtual worlds such as World of Warcraft or Star Wars Galaxies are modeled after role playing games with all the typical elements found in most games—such as: enemies to beat, levels to attain, a story line, goals to achieve, and the possibility for the avatar to die; (2) Non-game-like virtual worlds, such as Second Life, There and Active Worlds are characterized by the lack of such elements. A main difference between current game- and non-game-like virtual words is that non-game-like virtual worlds are entirely created, owned, and maintained by their users. Though such virtual worlds are modeled after games in terms of their use of three-dimensional graphics and basic control features, they allow for a variety of different usages varying from playing games, visiting museums, taking classes, or socializing with others in numerous communities.

The Second Life viewer was open-sourced in 2007, allowing developers to enhance the viewer with new features. Several modifications have been developed that allow users with visual impairments to access them.

- *Haptic navigation.* A modification of the viewer has been developed that allows users who are visually impaired to navigate their avatar using force feedback (Pascale et al. 2008). Different object types are distinguished through different vibration frequencies. However, this approach is limited to a few object categories as the user has to memorize the vibration frequencies of these categories.

- *Max the virtual guide dog.* The guide dog project* developed by the Virtual Ability Group† offers a virtual guide dog object that can be "worn" by a user's avatar (Figure 15.5a). The guide dog provides a number of functions such as navigation and querying the environment through a chat-like interface. Feedback is provided using synthetic speech. Because it is integrated into the Second Life viewer, this solution allows for hearing in-game audio, but it may also

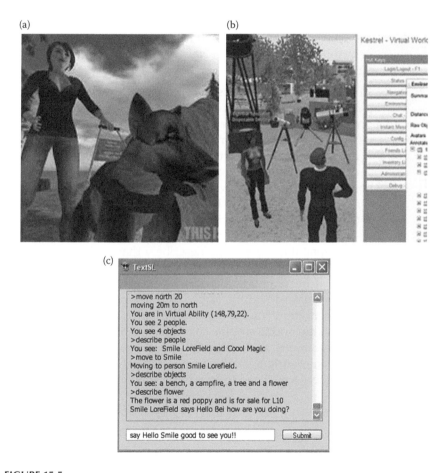

FIGURE 15.5
(a) Max the virtual guide dog. (b) IBM Alphaworks client. (c) TextSL client.

---

* http://virtualguide dog.org
† http://virtualability.org

require a sighted user to initially set up the guide dog object. Built-in speech synthesis typically does not allow for the same customizations as external screen readers.

- *Alphaworks.* IBM's Human Ability and Accessibility Center developed a Web-based interface for Second Life* that can be accessed with a screen reader (Figure 15.5b). This client provides basic navigation, communication, and perception functions using various hot keys. A hot key-based interface is limited in supporting a large number of different actions on large numbers of objects and avatars. A notable feature of this client is that it also provides a plug-in for the Second Life viewer, which allows users to add names to objects in Second Life, as such data is often missing. These names are stored in an external database and the IBM's client can retrieve such object descriptions when a user encounters an object with missing meta-information.

- *TextSL* offers screen reader access to Second Life using a command line interface (CLI) (Figure 15.5c). Shells and early text-based adventure games such as Zork are examples of command line interfaces that are very accessible to screenreaders as they provide textual output and users iteratively interact with them using commands. We implemented a command line interface (TextSL) on top of Second Life whose output can be read with a screen reader. TextSL accepts commands from the user allowing the user to move their avatar around ("move north"), interact with other avatars ("say") and objects ("sit on chair"), and get information on their environment using simple spatial queries (e.g., "describe") that can be parametrized (e.g., "describe chair"). This command line interface is turned into a simple natural language interface by mapping common verbs ("go," "walk," "proceed") to the same internal command ("move"). This allows users to interact using natural language which avoids users having to memorize specific commands. A interpreter allows for using propositions and conjuctions, for example, "sit on the chair." When answering spatial queries a simple form of pruning and iterative queries are used to avoid overwhelming the user with feedback.

Video Game Accessibility Strategies

Table 15.1 shows an overview of all games and accessible virtual world interfaces surveyed in this chapter. We now list a set of strategies for making

---

* http://services.alphaworks.ibm.com/virtualworlds

TABLE 15.1

Blind-Accessible Games and Strategies Used

Name of Game	Genre	Adaptation	Feedback	Input
Mach 1 car racing	Racing	Yes	Audio cues	Keyboard
Shades of doom	FPS	Yes	Audio cues, speech	Keyboard
Audio quake		Yes	Sonification, speech	
Terraformers		No	Sonification, speech	
The last crusade	RPG	No	Speech	Keyboard
AudioBattleShip	RTS	Yes	Audio cues	Tablet
GMA tank comm.	Arcade	Yes	Audio cues	Keyboard
Speed sonic	Platform	No	Audio cues	Controller
Metris	Puzzle	Yes	Sonification	Keyboard
Powerup	Educational	No	Audio cues	Keyboard
AudiOdyssey	Music	No	Audio cues	Wiimote
Blind hero		Yes	Haptic	Guitar controller
Finger dance		Yes	Audio cues	Keyboard
VI Tennis	Exergame	Yes	Haptic + audio cues	Wii remote
VI Bowling		Yes		
Pet-n-punch		No		
Haptic navigation	Virtual world	Yes	Haptic cues	Joystick
Max the guide dog	Virtual world	Yes	Speech synthesis	Keyboard
Alphaworks	Virtual world	Yes	Speech synthesis	Hot keys
TextSL	Virtual world	Yes	Screenreader	Natural language

video games and virtual worlds accessible to users with visual impairments based on the games we surveyed.

Low Vision Strategies

- *Enhance visual feedback.* Players with low vision can be supported by modifying visual stimuli using:
- *High-contrast color schemes.* By reducing the amount of colors and using colors that are visually very dissimilar it becomes easier for user with visual impairments to see what is rendered on the screen.
- *Scalable fonts.* Being able to increase fonts size increases readability. Often this functionality is available through hot keys.
- *Zoom options.* Users can zoom in on particular parts of the screen to see what is rendered.
- *Customizable color schemes.* Users can customize the colors of certain game units to increase their visibility.
- *Color blind mode.* A built-in mode that avoids certain color combinations (e.g., red–green) depending on the type of color blindness.

No Vision Strategies: Sensory Substitution

Sensory substitution is required for players that have no vision. It basically means converting visual feedback into audio or haptic modalities. Sensory substitution is challenging due to the limited spatial and temporal resolutions of audio and tactile modalities (Bach-y Rita and Kercel 2003) and often trade offs are required to not represent all visual feedback but only what is relevant to be able to play the game.

- *Replace visuals with AUDIO feedback.* This strategy is most commonly used as most computers feature speakers and no extra hardware is required. A drawback of using audio is that it may interfere with existing audio in the game.
- *Speech* can be provided either by a screen reader when text is provided or using self-voicing. Screen readers have the benefit that they are more customizable and users with visual impairments often already have them customized to their specific preferences and abilities.
- *Audio cues* use real world sounds such as the sound of wind or footsteps to provide information or hints to the player. Using binaural audio 3-D sound effects can be simulated using headphones.
- *Sonification* uses nonspeech audio to convey information using changes in pitch, amplitude, or tempo (Barrass and Kramer 1999). A number of specific sonification techniques can be used:
  - *Auditory icons*: real life sounds indicating different objects or actions.
  - *Earcons*: structured sounds (non-real-life) that obey musical conventions (Brewster et al. 1995) that can indicate different objects or actions.
  - *Sonar*: a sonar-like mechanism conveys spatial information on the locations of objects in front of the player.
- *Replace visuals with HAPTIC feedback.* When audio is difficult to provide such as with music games, haptic feedback may be considered. The drawback of this approach is that a gaming device is required that provides haptic feedback such as a Wii remote. A benefit of using haptic feedback is that it does not interfere with audio already present in the game.
- *Haptic cues* can be used to indicate a particular input to provide. Haptic cues can vary in length, pattern, and frequency. Multiple vibrotactors can be used to provide feedback at different parts of the human body.
- *Haptification*, or modulation of a continuous representation of a haptic cue (frequency, intensity, or a pattern), can be used to indicate spatial information such as the distance to or the location of an object in front of the player.

- *Replace visuals with AUDIO AND HAPTIC feedback.* In some cases visual cues can be encoded in haptic as well as audio. This has the benefit that multimodal cues presented simultaneously can be detected at lower thresholds, faster and more accurately than when presented separately in each modality (Miller 1982), which could lead to higher gaming performances and fewer errors.

Envisioning the Future

What will the future hold for visually impaired gamers? We outline three promising areas.

- *Mobile audio games.* Mobile games have transformed the landscape of video games. Apple's iPhone has become the number one mobile gaming device with thousands of games available. Recently an interesting audio game called Papa Sangre* was developed for the iOS platform. Papa Sangre is an audio game with no graphics and uses binaural audio to create 3-D stereo sound. The goal in each level is to acquire certain objects without disturbing a monster. You have no visual sight of anything, so you have to walk toward sounds using the on-screen footstep pads and a compass for changing direction. Though this game is completely accessible to users who are blind, it is actually marketed to a mainstream market. Its success has the potential to propel audio games from a niche to a mainstream market as several audio-only games for mobile devices are currently in development†.

- *Social gaming.* Social networks have also transformed the gaming space as many games are now being played with friends through social networks like Facebook. Popular titles include Mafia Wars and Farmville. Though major social networks such as Facebook and Twitter are to some extent accessible to users with visual impairments, a social network has been developed for users who are blind called BlinkNation http://www.blinknation.com/ which can be accessed with a screenreader. This network already allows for playing games, but it could be expanded to allow users who are blind to play games against each other. Such a game network could allow for creating gaming competitions and game-specific leaderboards that could offer challenges to blind users as well as new opportunities for socialization.

---

* http://www.papasangre.com
† http://toucharcade.com/2011/04/14/papa-sangre-2-and-the-nightjar-in-the-works

- *Collaborative paired gaming.* A study of gamers with disabilities in the popular World of Warcraft game (Theodore Lim 2011) shows that gamers with disabilities often pair up with nondisabled players to play the game. This can either be a disabled and a nondisabled player controlling one character or each controlling a character where the nondisabled person performs the task that is difficult or impossible to perform for the player who is disabled. For example, a sighted player can play a warrior that keeps an eye out for enemies and indicates to a blind wizard where to shoot fireballs. This type of symbiotic relationship between players or characters in a game is something that game designers could explore in the design of games. For example, particular characters could be given a handicap (e.g., no visuals feedback or limited navigation possibilities) and in return would be made more powerful to accommodate this handicap.

References

Adams, M. A., S. J. Marshall, L. Dillon, S. Caparosa, E. Ramirez, J. Phillips, and G. J. Norman. 2009. A theory-based framework for evaluating exergames as persuasive technology. In *Persuasive '09: Proceedings of the 4th International Conference on Persuasive Technology*, New York, NY, USA, pp. 1–8.

Allman, T., R. K. Dhillon, M. A. Landau, and S. H. Kurniawan. 2009. Rock vibe: Rock band® computer games for people with no or limited vision. In *Assets '09: Proceedings of the 11th international ACM SIGACCESS conference on Computers and accessibility*, New York, NY, USA, pp. 51–58. ACM.

Armiger, R. S. and R. J. Vogelstein. 2008. Air-guitar hero: A real-time video game interface for training and evaluation of dexterous upper-extremity neuroprosthetic control algorithms. In *Biomedical Circuits and Systems Conference, 2008. BioCAS 2008*, Baltimore, MD; Huddersfield, UK. *IEEE*, pp. 121–124.

Atkinson, M. T., S. Gucukoglu, C. H. C. Machin, and A. E. Lawrence. 2006. Making the mainstream accessible: Redefining the game. In *sandbox '06: Proceedings of the 2006 ACM SIGGRAPH Symposium on Videogames*, New York, NY, USA, pp. 21–28. ACM.

Bach-y Rita, P. and S. W Kercel. 2003. Sensory substitution and the human-machine interface. *Trends in Cognitive Sciences* 7(12), 541–546.

Barrass, S. and G. Kramer. 1999. Using sonification. *Multimedia Systems* 7, 23–31.

Bianchi-Berthouze, N., W. W. Kim, and D. Patel. 2007. Does body movement engage you more in digital game play? and why? In *ACII '07: Proceedings of the 2nd International Conference on Affective Computing and Intelligent Interaction*, Berlin, Heidelberg, pp. 102–113. Springer-Verlag.

Blumberg, F. C. 1998. Developmental differences at play: Children's selective attention and performance in video games. *Journal of Applied Developmental Psychology* 19(4), 615–624.

Brewster, S., P. Wright, and A. Edwards. 1995. Experimentally derived guidelines for the creation of earcons. In *Adjunct Proceedings of HCI*, Volume 95, pp. 155–159. Citeseer.

Chadha, R. K. and A. Subramanian. 2010, Sep. The effect of visual impairment on quality of life of children aged 3–16 years. *British Journal of Ophthalmology* 95(5), 642–645.

Cheung, N. and T. Y. Wong. 2007. Obesity and eye diseases. *Survey of Ophthalmology* 52(2), 180–195.

Cooper, R. A., L. A. Quatrano, P. W. Axelson, W. Harlan, M. Stineman, B. Franklin, J. S. Krause et al. 1999, Apr. Research on physical activity and health among people with disabilities: A consensus statement. *Journal of Rehabilitation Research and Development* 36(2), 142–154.

Crewe, J. M., N. Morlet, W. H. Morgan, K. Spilsbury, A. Mukhtar, A. Clark, J. Q. Ng, M. Crowley, and J. B. Semmens. 2010, Nov. Quality of life of the most severely vision impaired. *Clinical and Experimental Ophthalmology* 39(4), 336–343.

Dickey, M. 2005. Three-dimensional virtual worlds and distance learning: Two case studies of active worlds as a medium for distance education. *British Journal of Educational Technology* 36(3), 439–451.

Dwyer, P. and P. VanLund. 2008. The last crusade: http://www.cs.unc.edu/research/assist/et/projects/rpg/index.html.

ESA. 2008. Entertainment software association http://www.theesa.com/facts/game-player.asp.

Friberg, J. and D. Gärdenfors. 2004. Audio games: New perspectives on game audio. In *ACE '04: Proceedings of the 2004 ACM SIGCHI International Conference on Advances in Computer Entertainment Technology*, New York, NY, USA, pp. 148–154. ACM.

Glinert, E. and L. Wyse. 2007. Audiodyssey: An accessible video game for both sighted and non-sighted gamers. In *Future Play '07: Proceedings of the 2007 Conference*, New York, NY, USA, pp. 251–252. ACM.

GMAGames. 2008. Tank commander: http://www.gmagames.com/gtc1.shtml.

Grammenos, D. 2008. Game over: Learning by dying. In *CHI '08: Proceeding of the Twenty-Sixth Annual SIGCHI Conference on Human Factors in Computing Systems*, New York, NY, USA, pp. 1443–1452. ACM.

Graves, L., G. Stratton, N. D. Ridgers, and N. T. Cable. 2007. Comparison of energy expenditure in adolescents when playing new generation and sedentary computer games: Cross sectional study. *BMJ* 335(7633), 1282–1284.

Habot-Wilner, Z. and M. Belkin. 2005. Obesity is a risk factor for eye diseases. *Harefuah* 144(11), 805–809, 821.

Houwen, S., C. Visscher, E. Hartman, and K. A. P. M. Lemmink. 2007. Gross motor skills and sports participation of children with visual impairments. *Research Quarterly for Exercise & Sport* 78(2), 16–23.

Hoysniemi, J. 2006. International survey on the dance dance revolution game. *Computers in Entertainment* 4(2), 8.

Hurkmans, H. L., R. J. van den Berg-Emons, and H. J. Stam. 2010. Energy expenditure in adults with cerebral palsy playing wii sports. *Archives of Physical Medicine and Rehabilitation* 91(10), 1577–1581.

InspiredCode. 2008. Music tetris: http://www.inspiredcode.net/metris.htm.

Johnson, E. J. 2005. Obesity, lutein metabolism, and age-related macular degeneration: A web of connections. *Nutrition Reviews* 63(1), 9–15.

Karpa, M. J., P. Mitchell, K. Beath, E. Rochtchina, R. G. Cumming, and J. J. Wang. 2009. Blue mountains eye study: Direct and indirect effects of visual impairment on mortality risk in older persons. *Archives of Ophthalmology* 127(10), 1347–1353.

Kitchen, J. 2008. Mach 1 car racing: http://www.kitchensinc.net/.

Lanningham-Foster, L., T. B. Jensen, R. C. Foster, A. B. Redmond, B. A. Walker, D. Heinz, and J. A. Levine. 2006. Energy expenditure of sedentary screen time compared with active screen time for children. *Pediatrics* 118(6), e1831–e1835.

Leatherdale, S. T., S. J. Woodruff, and S. R. Manske. 2010. Energy expenditure while playing active and inactive video games. *American Journal of Health Behavior* 34(1), 31–35.

Lieberman, D. 2007. Dance games and other exergames: What the research says. http://www.comm.ucsb.edu/faculty/lieberman/exergames.htm.

Lieberman, L. J., C. Houston-Wilson, and F. Kozub. 2002. Perceived barriers to including students with visual impairments in general physical education. *Adapted Physical Activity Quarterly* 19(3), 364–377.

Lieberman, L. J. and M. Lepore. 1998. Camp abilities: A developmental sports camp for children who are blind and deafblind. *Palaestra* 14(1), 46–48.

Longmuir, P. 1998. Considerations for fitness appraisal, programming, and counselling of individuals with sensory impairments. *Canadian Journal of Applied Physiology* 23(2), 166–184.

Longmuir, P. E. and O. Bar-Or. 2000. Factors influencing the physical activity levels of youths with physical and sensory disabilities. *Adapted Physical Activity Quarterly* 17, 40–53.

Miller, J. 1982. Divided attention: Evidence for coactivation with redundant signals. *Cognitive Psychology* 14(2), 247–79.

Miller, D., A. Parecki, and S. A. Douglas. 2007. Finger dance: A sound game for blind people. In *Assets '07: Proceedings of the 9th International ACM SIGACCESS Conference on Computers and Accessibility*, New York, NY, USA, pp. 253–254. ACM.

Morelli, T., J. Foley, L. Columna, L. Lieberman, and E. Folmer. 2010. VI-Tennis: A vibrotactile/audio exergame for players who are visually impaired. In *Proceedings of Foundations of Digital Interactive Games (FDG'10)*, Monterey, California.

Morelli, T., J. Foley, and E. Folmer. 2010. VI-Bowling: A tactile spatial exergame for individuals with visual impairments. In *Proceedings of the 12th International ACM SIGACCESS Conference on Computers and Accessibility*, ASSETS '10, New York, NY, USA, pp. 179–186. ACM.

Morelli, T., J. Foley, L. Lieberman, and E. Folmer. 2011. Pet-n-punch: Upper body tactile/audio exergame to engage children with visual impairments into physical activity. In *Proceedings of Graphics Interface 2011*, GI '11, St. John's, Newfoundland, Canada, pp. 223–230. Canadian Human-Computer Communications Society.

Morelli, T. and E. Folmer. 2011. Real-time sensory substitution to enable players who are blind to play gesture based videogames. In *Proceedings Foundations of Digital Interactive Games 2011*, Bordeaux, France, pp. 147–153.

Mueller, F., S. Agamanolis, and R. Picard 2003. Exertion interfaces: Sports over a distance for social bonding and fun. In *CHI '03: Proceedings of the SIGCHI Conference on Human Factors in Computing Systems*, New York, NY, USA, pp. 561–568. ACM.

Mueller, F. F., M. R. Gibbs, and F. Vetere. 2008. Taxonomy of exertion games. In *OZCHI '08: Proceedings of the 20th Australasian Conference on Computer-Human Interaction*, New York, NY, USA, pp. 263–266. ACM.

Ni Mhurchu, C., R. Maddison, Y. Jiang, A. Jull, H. Prapavessis, and A. Rodgers. 2008. Couch potatoes to jumping beans: A pilot study of the effect of active video games on physical activity in children. *The International Journal of Behavioral Nutrition and Physical Activity* 5, 8.

Nikolaraizi, M. and N. De Reybekiel. 2001. A comparative study of children's attitudes towards deaf children, children in wheelchairs and blind children in Greece and in the UK. *European Journal of Special Needs Education* 16(2), 167–182.

Nixon, H. 1988. Reassessing support groups for parents of visually impaired children. *Journal of Visual Impairment & Blindness* 82, 271–278.

Odenweller, C. M., C. T. Hsu, and S. E. DiCarlo. 1998. Educational card games for understanding gastrointestinal physiology. *The American Journal of Physiology* 275(6 Pt 2), 78–84.

Oren, M. A. 2007. Speed sonic across the span: Building a platform audio game. In *CHI '07: CHI '07 Extended Abstracts on Human Factors in Computing Systems*, New York, NY, USA, pp. 2231–2236. ACM.

Parker, J. R. and J. Heerema. 2007. Musical interaction in computer games. In *Future Play '07: Proceedings of the 2007 Conference on Future Play*, New York, NY, USA, pp. 217–220. ACM.

Pascale, M., S. Mulatto, and D. Prattichizzo. 2008. Bringing haptics to second life for visually impaired people. In *EuroHaptics '08: Proceedings of the 6th International Conference on Haptics*, Berlin, Heidelberg, pp. 896–905. Springer-Verlag.

Ponchillia, P. E., S. V. Ponchillia, and B. Strause. 2002. Athletes with visual impairments: Attributes and sports participation. *Journal of Visual Impairment & Blindness* 96(4), 267–272.

Rimmer, J. H. 2005. Exercise and physical activity in persons aging with a physical disability. *Physical Medicine & Rehabilitation Clinics of North America* 16(1), 41–56.

Rimmer, J. H. and D. Braddock. 2002. Health promotion for people with physical, cognitive, and sensory disabilities: An emerging national priority. *American Journal of Health Promotion* 16, 220–224.

Robbins, S. S. 2007. Immersion and engagement in a virtual classroom: Using second life for higher education. In *EDUCAUSE Learning Initiative Spring 2007 Focus Session*, Muncie, Indiana.

Roden, T. and I. Parberry. 2005. Designing a narrative-based audio only 3-D game engine. In *ACE '05: Proceedings of the 2005 ACM SIGCHI International Conference on Advances in Computer Entertainment Technology*, New York, NY, USA, pp. 274–277. ACM.

Sánchez, J., N. Baloian, T. Hassler, and U. Hoppe. 2003. Audiobattleship: Blind learners collaboration through sound. In *CHI '03: CHI '03 Extended Abstracts on Human Factors in Computing Systems*, New York, NY, USA, pp. 798–799. ACM.

Schiesel, S. 2009. P.E. Classes turn to video game that works legs, not thumbs, *NY Times*, http://www.nytimes.com/2007/04/30/health/30exer.html.

Shaffer, D. W. and J. P. Gee. 2006. *How Computer Games Help Children Learn*. New York, NY, USA, Palgrave Macmillan.

Shapiro, D. R., A. Moffett, L. Lieberman, and G. M. Dummer. 2005. Perceived competence of children with visual impairments. *Journal of Visual Impairment & Blindness* 99(1), 15–25.

Sinclair, J., P. Hingston, and M. Masek. 2007. Considerations for the design of exergames. In *GRAPHITE '07: Proceedings of the 5th International Conference on*

Assistive Technology for Blindness and Low Vision

Computer Graphics and Interactive Techniques in Australia and Southeast Asia, New York, NY, USA, pp. 289–295. ACM.

Squire, K. 2005. Changing the game: What happens when video games enter the classroom? *Innovate: Journal of Online Education* 1(6).

Stanley, T. D. and D. Calvo. 2009. Rhythm learning with electronic simulation. In *SIGITE '09: Proceedings of the 10th ACM Conference on SIG-Information Technology Education*, New York, NY, USA, pp. 24–28. ACM.

Stuart, M., L. Lieberman, and K. Hand. 2006. Beliefs about physical activity among children who are visually impaired and their parents. *Journal of Visual Impairment and Blindness* 100(4), 223–234.

Talamasca, A. 2008. The heron sanctuary helps the disabled find a second. http://eurekadejavu.blogspot.com/2008/01/story-of-heron-sanctuary.html.

Theodore Lim, B. N. 2011. A study of raiders with disabilities in world of warcraft. In *Foundations of Digital Interactive Games 2011*.

Trewin, S., M. Laff, V. Hanson, and A. Cavender. 2009. Exploring visual and motor accessibility in navigating a virtual world. *ACM Transactions on Accessible Computing* 2(2), 1–35.

Trost, S. G., L. M. Kerr, D. S. Ward, and R. R. Pate. 2001. Physical activity and determinants of physical activity in obese and non-obese children. *International Journal of Obesity and Related Metabolic Disorders* 25(6), 822–829.

U.S. Government. 1998. 1998 amendment to Section 508 of the rehabilitation act. *SEC. 508. Electronic and information Technology*. http://www.section508.gov/.

Van Erp, J. 2002. Guidelines for the use of vibro-tactile displays in human computer interaction. In *Proceedings of EuroHaptics*, Edinburgh, UK, pp. 18–22.

Wack, E. and S. Tantleff-Dunn. 2009. Relationships between electronic game play, obesity, and psychosocial functioning in young men. *Cyberpsychology & Behavior* 12(2), 241–244.

Yuan, B. and E. Folmer. 2008. Blind hero: Enabling guitar hero for the visually impaired. In *Assets '08: Proceedings of the 10th International ACM SIGACCESS Conference on Computers and Accessibility*, New York, NY, USA, pp. 169–176. ACM.

Yuan, B., E. Folmer, and F. C. Harris. 2011. Game accessibility; a survey. *Universal Access in the Information Society* 10(1), 81–100.

16

Descriptive Video Services

Claude Chapdelaine

CONTENTS

Introduction

Description video (DV) is the art of enhancing audio-visual content by inserting verbal descriptions where circumstances permit, for example, between dialogues. These inserted descriptions translate relevant visual information so that an individual who is blind or has low vision can access, enjoy and understand audio-visual entertainment as much as a sighted person. It can be used for television programming, a theater play, a feature film, an opera, or any audio-visual content available on DVDs or through the Web. In 2006, a UK study established that close to 87% of blind and low vision people regularly listened to TV and videos or DVDs (Douglas et al., 2006). For them, the broadcast media provide important access to news, information and entertainment. We can infer that the proportion in North America is similar. So, the need for access to all these productions is widespread.

In writing this text, our hope is that readers will realize that producing accessible audio-visual content is as much an art as it is a technical challenge. We will cover the state of DV in North America. We will explain how DV is produced, its inherent difficulties, and the long production time necessary to reach the intended audience. We will review research done to understand this specific form of translation from visual cues to text and to find ways to assist the describers in making more effective DV. Finally, we will look toward the future and the work being done to assist in more cost-efficient production of DV. We will present in detail the work done at CRIM in the past 6 years where our efforts were along two axes: (1) automating and assisting the production of DV to reduce production time and cost and (2) building an accessible player based on the needs of the blind and low vision population, as identified by end-user studies. Producing DV is a challenge worth tackling since it is a means to access culture and no degree of visual impairment should exclude anyone from society or from understanding the world we live in.

State of DV Descriptive Video

The story of DV is a tale of many people, organizations, and countries. We will not be able to tell it all, but we will give an overview of what has been done in the United States, in Canada, and, to a lesser extent, in Europe. For a good review of what is being done in Europe, we recommend following the work of EBU (2006). A few facts are worth mentioning in regard to Europe: DV has been available in UK for 10 years, and in cinemas for 4 years so that about 40% of British cinemas are equipped with special transmitters that renders DV (Sonali, 2011); in theaters, DV has been available for 15 years with 14 theaters providing DV since 1990. The UK is also the European country offering the most DV on television with 8% coverage (representing about 10 h per week). However, this is not the standard in Europe as a whole. For example, the broadcast coverage by DV in Germany is 0.7%, in Italy it is 6 h per week, in Portugal one film per week, and in France, one film per month (Sonali, 2011). Improvement can surely be made. But, wherever the story comes from, it tells of courage, generosity, and determination on the part of the people and organizations determined to provide accessible culture to people with disabilities.

DV in the United States

In the United States, the history of DV originates in Hollywood. In the 1970s, Gregory Frazier, at the School of Creative Arts, San Francisco State University, found his idea after describing a movie to his blind students while they were watching television (Thomas Jr., 1996, Audio Description Coalition, 2010). Frazier, amazed by the experience, went to his Dean who just happened to be August Coppola, the brother of Francis Ford Coppola. An academic program was created and in 1988, the film Tucker was presented with DV. In the 1980s in Washington, DC, many DV events were created such as live theater performances, radio programs in collaboration with PBS, and audio cassettes for museum exhibitions, opera, and so on (Audio Description Coalition, 2010).

An essential player in DV proliferation is the WGBH Educational Foundation. In 1985, they started a multichannel television sound standard known as the Secondary Audio Program (SAP) that allowed the broadcasting of DV.[*] Descriptive Video Services (DVS®) was founded in 1990, with the purpose of providing DV to blind and low vision television viewers. They now provide this service to all of the American PBS stations and some programming for private television networks (CBS, FOX, etc.) as well as for feature films, IMAX films and DVDs. Since 2009, the American Council of the Blind (ACB) initiated the Audio Description Project (ADP) to increase the production of DV.[†] The accessibility of DV is also a story of laws and regulation. In 1990, the Americans with Disabilities Act (ADA) encouraged a strong mandate to eliminate discrimination in many aspects of life and public services. In 2000, the FCC (Federal Communications Commission) established rules to provide a certain amount of DV coverage of broadcasts. This ruling was later vacated by a federal court. In 2011, Congress passed the Twenty-First Century Communications and Video Accessibility Act, enabling the FCC to reinstate DV ratios for broadcasters and this should be implemented by July 1, 2012.[‡] This is a major step forward for blind and low vision people since it could amount to at least 50 h of DV broadcast coverage per week by all the major networks. The ruling targets mostly children's and prime time programming.[§]

DV in Canada

In Canada, the Charter of Rights and Freedoms included in the Canadian constitution ensures equal protection under the law for people with

---

[*] http://main.wgbh.org/wgbh/pages/mag/about/
[†] http://www.acb.org/adp/
[‡] http://www.broadcastlawblog.com/2011/08/articles/digital-television/fcc-releases-order-reinstating-television-video-description-rules/
[§] http://www.rnib.org.uk/livingwithsightloss/tvradiofilm/tvradiofilmnews/Pages/more_international_ad.aspx

disabilities. Even though Canadian government policies are committed to promote independence, employment, and accessibility for people with disabilities, the Government has not yet passed a law comparable to the Americans with Disabilities Act that would extend more strongly the rights of people with disabilities. Nonetheless, some regulations are in place. Established in 1968, the CRTC regulates all matters related to broadcasting in Canada.* The 1991 Canadian Broadcasting Act requires that accessible programming be provided by Canadian broadcasters. In 1995, the CRTC issued a public note that made accessibility a requirement for license renewals, which was applied at the time to closed captioning (Canadian Association of Broadcasters, 2004). Since September 2009, broadcasting licenses are renewed only if there is a commitment to broadcast a certain number of hours of DV per week, currently about 2 h per week (CRTC, 2009a). In 2009, the CRTC licensed TACtv which offers closed-captioned and accessible DV on a channel available 24 h with no special equipment or settings required. Furthermore, more than 2000 television providers are required to include this channel in their basic service (CRTC, 2009b). There is as yet no such channel available to the blind and low vision French Canadian population.

DV Production

Based on meetings with describers, we found that producing DV requires many steps and it is generally carried out as a postproduction activity.† Typically, describers would listen to the audio-video content to be described in order to identify the main characters, reviewing the script if available; to evaluate the gaps where DV could be inserted or not; and to document potential difficulties and list the key visual elements. This could require more than one viewing. The first work on the content would be to delimit with time codes the gaps where DV could be inserted (see Figure 16.1). Then the describing text has to be composed, carefully timing it to the length of the available gap, usually by reading the text aloud while playing the associated part of the video. This is where all the major constraints come into play, which we will describe in more detail later. The next step is quality control, usually done by an experienced describer or, in the best cases, by a blind or low vision evaluator.

Finally, the DV is recorded by a voice talent and synchronized with the sound track. The sound track is transferred to the desired format to be mixed with the video format of the content. This whole process is lengthy and

---

* http://www.crtc.gc.ca/eng/backgrnd/brochures/b19903.htm
† http://e-inclusion.crim.ca/

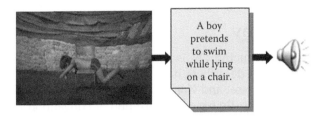

FIGURE 16.1
Process of translating a visual cue into a text and producing an audio file.

entails highly variable production costs depending on the difficulties encountered and the length of the audio-video content. In the ITC Standards, formerly Ofcom (UK), examples are provided such as a 2-h film, which would require 60 h of work to produce its DV version (giving a time ratio of 1:30) and a soap opera episode of 30 min, which took 1.5 h of work (giving a ratio of 1:3). Generally speaking, it is estimated that it takes an average of one working week to produce 1.5–2 h worth of DV (Foucher et al., 2007).

As we mentioned before, when the describing text is composed, stringent constraints have to be respected. There are many considerations to be taken into account (ITC, 2000; Foucher et al., 2007): finding the relevant information needed to understand the story such as the place of action, identifying the character doing the action, and identifying where the action takes place (not just the location but also the time in the case of flash-backs and dreams). Also, descriptions should not run over significant sound effects (although VD could also be used to give an explanation that clearly distinguishes a sound). There are also considerations about the nature of the language used: using the present tense is desirable, as are clear and simple descriptions, adapting the language to the tone of the content, and identifying characters in a consistent way that avoids confusion.

There are also important rules that have to be followed. Typically, the recommendation is to describe what you see and avoid interpretation, introduce a character as early as possible so that the character can subsequently be recognized by his voice, avoid overlapping of the description with the dialogue, leave some music and sound effects so as not to override the atmosphere of the content, and avoid repetition so as not to create monotony. All of these are subject to the biggest constraint of all, namely to render the description in the gap available. This is not always possible: some descriptions may have to be abandoned or shortened. In order to achieve this, the describer may have to rewrite or adapt his text, more than once. There is also the production time constraint that will impact on the cost of the production. More often than not, this constraint is stressed by postproduction companies and by broadcasters who regard DV as an imposed added cost needed to comply with government regulations (Gerzymisch-Arbogast, 2007) rather than as an essential service to their audience.

Research Done on DV

As we discussed, producing DV is a complex task since it involves many editorial decisions and describers have at their disposal only a few guidelines (Orero, 2005; Morisset and Gonant, 2008; ADS, 2009; Szarkowska, 2011). These guidelines are mostly based on intuition or convention without clear indications of the effectiveness of one strategy over another (Braun, 2008). Thus, DV producers could benefit greatly from research aimed at better understanding what is required, based on user-oriented feedback. The literature on this subject can be divided into two broad categories: (1) information value for indexing and classification and (2) linguistic content of DV.

On the information value side, Turner proposed a DV typology to enrich film indexing and, potentially, to automate DV production (Turner and Mathieu, 2008). From his study of 11 different audio-visual contents, he classified information to establish the most frequent types observed in DV. The types formed a typology of DV that includes action/movement, character identification, description of the surroundings, expressions of emotion, and textual information seen in the image. Piety (2004) did a textual analysis in which he also suggested a functional framework for describing/analyzing DV. His approach offers a classification of seven types of information: appearance, action, position, reading, indexical (indication of who is speaking), viewpoint, and state.

On the linguistic side, research aims to understand the specific linguistic nature of DV and how visual cues can be translated into words for blind and low vision people. In the previously mentioned study of Piety (2004), the author demonstrated how constraints such as available time free of speech (gap duration), choice of words, and choice of relevant information render DV production difficult. He found that DV required a distinctive language usage that has its own form and function. He analyzed not only the visual cues chosen by the describers for translation into DV, but also how they were described. He also stated that these choices had an impact on the cognitive load of blind and low vision people. Benecke (2007) found the linguistic aspect of DV so peculiar that he suggested the need for specialized terms such as "character fixation" in order to avoid describing a character by his role in one instance and then by his name in another. Salway (2007) showed a relation between the frequency of words used in DV and the frequency of occurrence of the characters, the actions, and the scenes. He found that the observable degree of regularity of words in the DV corpus might facilitate the automatic production of VD. Peli et al. (1996), Pettit et al. (1996), Schmeidler and Kirchner (2001), and Ely et al. (2006) reported on evaluations done with blind and low vision people on the value and importance of DV. These studies and many others provided valuable insights for designing guidelines. Unfortunately, they were rarely used by software developers who provide tools for the describers engaged in this complex task. After all, the production of DV is a small market, but as regulators demand greater DV coverage, more efficient tools will be needed.

Existing DV Tools and Research

To our knowledge, no standard exists to support the development of software tools currently used by describers in the postproduction industry. Most of these tools provide a video player window coupled to an editing window with a function to synchronize the time codes of the video with the associated piece of description. Mostly, these are the same tools as the ones used for captioning since postproduction companies are often engaged in both activities. In these cases, the captions serve to perform speech detection and the zones without captions indicate to the describer potential gaps to enter DV. These tools offer little automatic assistance, often just a shot detection. However, specific DV tools do exist and are available on the market. Some incorporate the recording process within the editing such as Swift Adept by Softel[*] while others, such as the Magpie by NCAM at WGBH, are designed both for DV and captioning.[†]

In the research community, some tools are being designed and tested to assist the describers more efficiently. Salway et al. (2007) used semantic-based indexing of video content in order to match events with actors. His approach involved algorithms based on shot detection and a classifier for speech, music, silence, and other sounds. Lakritz and Salway (2006) investigated the possibility of using an available script or screenplay to produce a first automatic draft of DV based on their analysis that such texts may contain up to 60% of the needed information for DV. The AVAC project in France proposes the use of speech processing to generate transcriptions of the audio content that would later assist annotation of visual cues (Champin et al., 2010). The involvement of CRIM in the E-Inclusion network initiated our project in DV. Two objectives were identified: (1) to provide a tool to assist DV production based on some automatic algorithms of image and speech processing to reduce production time and (2) to develop an accessible player design based on the results of usability studies to offer an enriched DV experience to blind and low vision people.

DV at CRIM

In the design of both the DV production tool and the DV player, our approach was to define specifications based on consultation, interviews, and testing

---

[*] http://www.softelgroup.com/Downloads/Swift-ADePT-page/Swift-ADePT-Datasheet.pdf
[†] http://ncam.wgbh.org/invent_build/web_multimedia/tools-guidelines/magpie

with the intended end-users. For the production tool, we consulted and tested our prototype with describers from the industry. The tool is named VDManager since in Canada the DV is known as video description (VD). Together with our collaborator, the University of Montreal, we consulted with blind and low vision people to query their needs by presenting them with existing DV productions (Mathieu and Turner, 2007) and with our initial DV productions (Chapdelaine and Gagnon, 2009). Each consultation gave us insights into how to improve the VDManager and to design an enriched accessible player.

Consultations with End-Users

We will briefly summarize the findings from these consultations and the analysis of existing DV done by the University of Montreal. From the describers, we found that the time needed to produce DV could be highly variable, depending not only on duration and type of the content but also on their knowledge of what is being described. Repeated episodes of television series would be considered easier and would be faster to do, as opposed to the first episode of a new series or a film, which would be considered a more complex task. The latter may require many viewings to assess the name and role of the characters, the evaluation of the number of gaps in speech and relevant sounds and their duration. Production involved the time coding of the beginning and the end of the gaps as well as selection of the visual cues to be described and editing of the associated text. The time needed to render the text would then be evaluated manually and, depending on the result, the text may need to be edited again (Gagnon et al., 2009). Based on the feedback from the blind and low vision people who participated, we found that priority should be given to identifying the principal characters as soon as possible, then presenting the action and the place. Participants disliked getting interpretation instead of description or added information not present in the image. Above all, we discovered that the quantity of DV needed could vary a lot from one individual to another. From the analysis of existing DV, it was observed that most of the description currently provided by producers is about action, movement of the characters, occupation/roles of the characters, decor, facial/corporal expressions, textual information included in the image, and attitude of characters (Mathieu and Turner, 2007).

Description of the VDManager

All of these inputs were considered in the design of a production tool that would assist the describers. However, automating all the visual cues identified from our consultation as being of interest was far beyond the current state of the art in computer vision and speech processing. We had to reach a trade-off between technical feasibility of automatic vision and speech algorithms and what would be most efficient for the describers. Thus, we implemented algorithms for shot transition detection, key-place recognition, speech/non-speech segmentation, text zone detection, and facial recognition of actors.

These algorithms are a combination of parametric and training paradigms and they can be seen as a collection of specialized filters that extract relevant audiovisual cues to assist in the creation of DV. We know that none of them can attain 100% detection accuracy when processing a highly uncontrolled environment like films. Nonetheless, we based our design on the actual performance of the algorithms while compensating for their deficiencies with efficient GUI interaction mechanisms. The algorithms used and their outcomes were documented at length in Gagnon et al. (2009) and Gagnon et al. (2010) where we also gave a complete description of the VDManager (Figure 16.2) and its functionalities.

We will concentrate on how VDManager deals with the deficiencies of the algorithms and how these deficiencies affect the task of DV description. The algorithms are run prior to the production work in order to detect the speech/nonspeech segments, the key-places, the faces, and the text. Shot detection is used to circumscribe the scope of the other algorithms. All the results of the algorithms are shown on an interactive timeline that can be controlled by keyboard shortcuts (see Figure 16.3). Typically, the describer has to validate the starting and ending boundaries of the nonspeech segments. The performance of this detection on four productions indicated that on the 533 nonspeech segments detected, 72% were correct and did not necessitate any modification by the describer while 13% were missed segments that needed to be added by the describers. The algorithm performance has, on average, a precision of 72% and a recall of 85%. The validation of boundaries is actually faster than what we observed since the describers have to wait for a caption

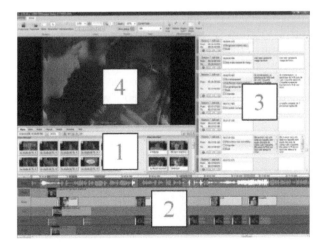

FIGURE 16.2
Overview of the VDManager GUI. The working areas are (1) resulting outputs of the automatic algorithm for validation, (2) interactive timeline, (3) VD editor, (4) embedded video player.

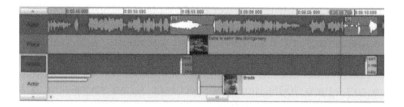

FIGURE 16.3
Screen shot of interactive timeline with items validated.

to be completed in order to take advantage of it. If a caption is not available, describers need only enter the first and last words of the caption line to create the boundaries.

When working with the key-places detector, the describers had to assign a name to the key places. If many key-places are related by being different points of view of the same environment, the describers can aggregate these key-places to form a scene (see Figure 16.4). Later on, if another key-place is already associated with the same cluster as one that has previously been encountered, then the interface would propose the same name to the describer. He or she would either accept the name or, in case of error, would select another name or enter a new name. As this validation proceeds, fewer and fewer key-places have to be named manually. At the end, this gives the describers a consistent identification of all of the scenes and of the number of different scenes to be named in the description scripts. A performance rating on this algorithm was run with three productions. It established that the describers did not need to identify the key-places 65% of the time, while for 35% of the time key-places had to be either named or given a name different from the one that had been proposed.

The next step is to identify and validate the principal actors in the film. Again, as the naming of the characters or the validation of the known characters proceeds, the probability of correctly recognizing characters later in the film (see Figure 16.5) increases. Performance on four productions indicated that for all the 1167 faces detected, close to 80% where properly identified by the algorithm while the describer had to manually validate or add 43% of the

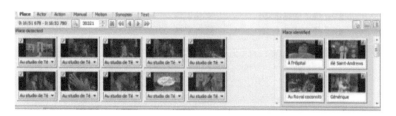

FIGURE 16.4
Example of key place validation showing on the left side the key places automatically associated with already named places, on the right side, identified places.

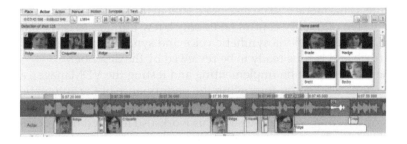

FIGURE 16.5
Example of face validation with the detected characters on the upper left side, the validated characters on the upper right side, and the appearance of the characters on the timeline at the bottom.

total faces. This also provides a consistent naming mechanism for the characters, the cue for their first appearance, and the frequency of appearance.

The describer needs to add all of the descriptions related to actions manually since no algorithm is provided for this item. Each action component is also rendered on the timeline. All the items validated in the timeline are then made available to the describers and are automatically imported into an editing window for the final scripting (see Figure 16.6). As the describer proceeds through the script, the software automatically flags the words in red if the number of characters does not approximately fit in the duration of the associated nonspeech segment. Furthermore, since we are using synthetic voice rendering, the describer can listen to the DV to validate his work. If some DV is too long for the duration of a given nonspeech segment, the describer can tag this as information to be used in an extended mode of DV

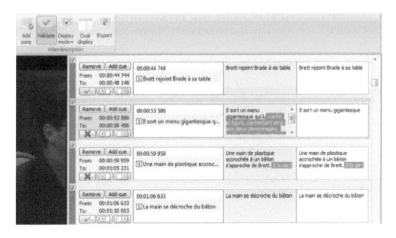

FIGURE 16.6
Screen shots of the editing window with items validated in available gaps and the finalized text with red warning to indicate that the text is too long for the gap.

rendering. (This mode will be discussed later in the section on the DV player.) The final step of quality control takes only a few minutes to carry out since all the DV is rendered via synthetic voice and synchronized with the video sound track and is thus ready to be reviewed by the describer.

In the 6 years spent on implementing and testing the VDManager, a team of 10 persons worked on improving the performance of the automatic algorithms, the development and design of the GUI, the production of a DV collection, and testing with end-users. This work also inspired us to develop an accessible DV player. In our study with end-users, we used this player to evaluate 104 DV productions made during this period and we evaluated the player itself.

Toward an Accessible and Innovative DV Player

From our first testing, we found that our DV production was widely accepted by the blind and low vision participants in our study, which was carried out with our new DV player. This player offers some innovative features which enabled participants in the study to choose between a standard mode which would give DV in the available speech gaps as it is rendered in real-time, or an extended mode that would automatically stop the video, render more DV, and automatically start the video again (Figure 16.7). The player had another feature that allowed the participant to personalize his or her experience by choosing to hear only the name of actors, or the identification of places, or the identification of actions or the text. As reported in Chapdelaine and Gagnon (2009), the possibility to choose the degree of DV was greatly appreciated but the personalized selection of items was judged difficult to use and its relevancy not well understood by the testers. Furthermore, we could only present

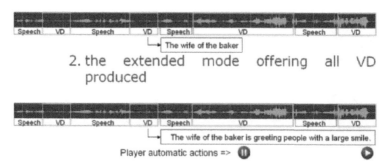

FIGURE 16.7
Graph explaining the difference between standard and extended mode of DV.

and test content which we had been given the right to modify for the experiment (since changing the sound track is a modification of the artwork and is a violation of copyright). In our web experiments, we presented seven short films from Kino with the permission of their producers. From this evaluation, we came to the conclusion that we needed a better real life understanding of individuals' varying needs. So we decided to do an *in situ* study to re-evaluate the functionality of the player and to see if there were other needs that were not covered by our first design.

In situ Study Impact

The *in situ* study aimed at assisting the viewing of audio-video production *without* DV by 10 blind and low vision individuals. In this study, the experimenter answered all of the questions from the participants to help them understand and be able to summarize the content (Chapdelaine, 2010; Chapdelaine and Jarry, 2010). We found that all of the functions provided in our initial design of the player were useful, but also that additional functions were needed to deal with sources of confusion or misunderstanding that caused a person with visual impairment to abandon listening to the content. We will briefly sum up the results of this study. Primarily, we saw that the quantity of DV needed varied substantially, depending not only on the type of content but also on the degree of visual acuity of the subject. For example, a person without any visual acuity would require more DV than a person who has the potential to distinguish human faces in a high contrast image. We also observed that specific scene conditions (low contrast images, large groups of people, etc.) could reduce the threshold of low vision individuals so that they would need as much description as blind individuals. We concluded that a function allowing the user to change the quantity of DV at any time would be highly desirable.

Furthermore, we observed that some users made remarks in a questioning tone to confirm information about the character, the scene, or the action. We concluded that the person understood what was going on but needed rapid confirmation to avoid confusion and to continue to follow the story. In the concluding interviews, many participants stated that when they were not able to have these confirmations they would often abandon the viewing with a sense of saturation. We concluded that the absence of a quick confirmation mechanism caused a cognitive overload and that some recall functionality was required to accomplish this task.

The Accessible CRIM DVDPLayer

In order to meet the requirements identified in the *in situ* study, we designed a specialized and accessible player for DVDs that could render DV for the individuals who are blind or have low vision. Our goal was to produce DV for the existing commercially available content; this allowed us to conduct a

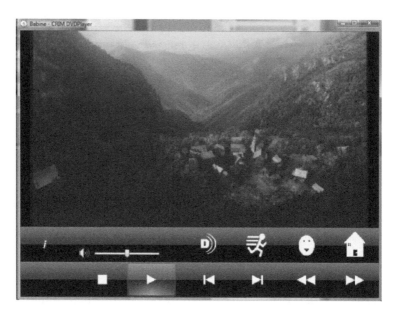

FIGURE 16.8
Screen shot of CRIM DVDPlayer.

large usability study for our player and the DV we produced. The player makes a time map of a DVD to enable the synchronization of the rendering of DV at the right moment, irrespective of whether the person requested standard or extended quantity DV. We also implemented innovative functions that give users on-demand identification of the scene, of the actors present in the scene, and of all actions in the scene available from the DV (recall functions). This information was based on the validated items of the production timeline of the VDManager. Furthermore, we implemented functions to give contextual information such as a synopsis and main actors lists where users could listen to a summary of the given film or episode of a series and also get a description of the main characters with a sample of their speech. Our goal was to test this player, called the CRIM DVDPlayer (Figure 16.8) with many participants. The player would be downloaded into the computer of the participants who could rent DVDs from the same organization where they usually get audio or Braille books, la Bibliothèque et Archives nationales du Quèbec (BAnQ).

Usability Study

We now present some of the results of the 6-months usability study where 43 participants (residents of 10 regions of Québec), in the comfort of their home and at their convenience, listened to a total of 104 DVDs. The DVDs were composed of three feature films, one television drama series, two television comedy series, one scientific documentary, one series on ecological housing construction, and an environmental news magazine program. The total viewing time for all participants was 171 h and 37 min. Some participants listened twice to each DVD, once in standard mode and once in extended mode to experience the difference. The usability study dealt with the quality of the DV and on the functionalities of the CRIM DVDPlayer. Evaluations were conducted by phone interviews and were not mandatory. Still, out of the 104 rented DVDs, only six evaluations were not completed either because the participant went on vacation or was too busy to do the interview.

Methodology

The methodology of the project was based on interaction with a website and telephone interviews. Through the website,* participants in the study were able to subscribe, get information on the project, view the list of DVDs available, and download the CRIM DVDPlayer. Once the subscription was received, a telephone interview was conducted to fill in user profile information and to provide each user with an identification number and password to download the player. Support for the loan of the DVDs was provided by the Service québécois du livre adapté (SQLA) of the BAnQ. Once the participant received the DVD and turned on the player, he or she would connect to a CRIM's server to download the related DV audio files. The player also gathers a trace to log some components of the computer (audio cards, antivirus software, existing audio and video filters, and codec) and the interactions of the participant (via keyboard or mouse click). These logs were used to assist us when a participant needed technical support and also to study the pattern of usage, detect problems, and monitor learning of the functionalities. When the DVD was returned, a telephone interview was conducted to evaluate the usability of the player and the quality of the DV.

Profile of the Participants

The group of 43 participants was composed of 23 males and 20 females with the majority of them being between 45 and 60 years of age. The age distribution can be presented in three groups: 27.9% were under 45 (distributed as followed: 4.7% less than 20, 11.6% between 21 and 35, and 11.6% between 36 and 45), 46.5% were between 46 and 60, while the remaining 25.6% were more than 61 years old. We also took into account the users' visual acuity and distinguished between subjects whose impairment was from birth or an early age (BI) and those who became impaired after the age of 16 (BE). Our group was composed of 28% blind BI, 19% blind BE, 28% low vision BI and 26% low vision BE. Most of the participants (77%) had a professional qualification or university degree. A majority of the subjects had used a screen

---

* http://www.acces-vd.crim.ca/

reader for more than 10 years (56%) and only 9% were inexperienced. The experienced screen enlarger users (i.e., those with more than 10 years experience) accounted for 26% of the subjects while the less experienced accounted for 2%. Only 3% of the subjects habitually used the accessibility functions available on their computer and 5% used no technology at all.

Looking at this distribution, we considered it a representative sample of the blind and low vision population that are long-standing computer users and are functional in the sense that they had adapted to their visual impairment for many years. Most of them had used assisted technologies for more than 10 years (56% in the case of screen readers and 26% in the case of screen enlargers for a total of 81%). A majority of participants (47%) were between 46 and 60 years of age and, since most of them had used an assisted technology for many years, they were eager to test a new technology that would give them access to culture and entertainment. We believe that the reason why a majority of the subjects were in an older age range is that they had more free time to participate in the study and fewer work or family responsibilities. The 25% of participants over 61 years old who had used assisted technologies for many years are not representative of that age group. (For many people of that age, the visual impairment would be recent and they may be in re-adaptation programs or have no previous computer experience. This could explain why they are less represented in this study.) In the future, the aging population will be more and more acquainted with technology and will eventually be more eager users of assisted technology if they become blind or visually impaired. Another aspect of the participants' profile is their consumption of audio-video content, principally coming from television. Almost 54% of them watched between 5 and 10 h of TV per week. Most of them (64%) were always alone or often alone when they watched TV. Only 35% reported using DV while listening to TV but all of those who did not do so (65%) said they did not know how to activate the DV when it was available. Indeed, 84% stated that they did not even know when it was available. (Most of the time this information is not accessibly indicated in the broadcasters' web schedules.)

Results

We will briefly present some of the results of the usability study, first about the player performance and then about our DV production. The player is set to the standard level of DV by default and 30% of the participants did not change this level. When they did so, changes were usually made in the first session (25% of the cases). On the other hand, 70% changed the description level so that 23% listened to the standard level, 33% used the extended level, and 44% mixed the levels depending on their immediate needs. All the participants who changed the level found that this operation was easily executed and they appreciated having this option. No one rated the function "more or less easy" or "difficult" and none stated that they "more or less" appreciated the function or deprecated it. The recall functions for the scene, actors, or actions were rarely used in the first session (13% of cases). Participants often discovered these functions in the first evaluation and usage increased to 55% on subsequent sessions. The recall functions were found easy to use in 97% of cases and 94% of participants appreciated having this option (while 6% appreciated having them "more or less" and none deprecated them). From the logs, we found that recall of scene identification was used 294 times, actors were recalled 575 times, and actions were recalled 351 times.

Two problems were reported during the evaluations. Many participants had problems balancing the sound volume of DV with that of the video. In 63% of cases, the comment was made that the volume of DV was generally too loud or too low. On the logging reports, we observed 5784 interactions with the volume function. This function was rated easy to use 63% of the time and was appreciated 54% of the time but clearly this problem made viewing less pleasant for some. We launched a new version of the player that would log the type of audio cards in participants' computers to study this problem further since it does not arise on all computers or on all DVDs with a given computer. The results are still being investigated to find a solution. Our second problem was related to synchronization where the DV would speak over the dialogue; this was reported by some participants but not by others. Logging the usage of processor, memory, and disk revealed some instances of saturation when the DVD was played. Further logging revealed cases where computationally demanding antivirus software had been installed. Some people had more than one antivirus installed without their knowledge. We informed these participants of the antivirus problem and this led to reduction of the number of instances of synchronization problems.

The quality of the DV was judged based on five positive questions and five negative questions. Positive questions addressed aspects such as whether the quantity of DV was adequate, clear, and relevant and whether the quality of French was good and the synthetic voice rendering satisfactory. The negative questions were asked to ensure consistency in answers and avoid creating a bias toward a favorable evaluation. These questions would target aspects such as if there were too much VD, if it was confusing, if sound effects were obscured by too much DV, if there were instances where the DV was inadequate for understanding, or if it contained irrelevant information. In 90% of the cases, the participants agreed to the positive questions, 8% more or less agreed, 2% disagreed, and 0.6% had no opinion. The answers to the negative questions were consistent with those of the positive questions. Only 10% agreed with the negative statements, 8% more or less agreed, 81% disagreed, and 0.9% had no opinion. Interestingly, the positive question that had the fewest affirmative responses concerned the synthetic voice; all the other positive questions had more than 90% affirmative responses. In the case of the synthetic voice, 72% of participants agreed that it was of good quality, 22% agreed more or less, 6% not at all, and 1% had no opinion. Almost half did not express a preference for a human voice, contrary to our expectations. Many commented that, for them, a synthetic voice of good quality is often more desirable than a human voice. We also asked participants if they would prefer having access to DVDs quickly with a synthetic voice to waiting for a version with a human voice; 73% opted for the synthetic voice in this situation.

Discussion

The participants in our study found that having the possibility to change the quantity of DV was an essential function. A similarly high proportion of users opted for extended DV or the possibility of switching from standard to extended mode as needed. The recall functions were equally popular, rated easy to use, and highly appreciated. It is evident that the functions offered by the player greatly enhanced the experience of watching a DVD. Furthermore, the quality of the DV we provided was clearly appreciated by the participants in our study with consistently high ratings on positive questions and low ratings on negative questions. It remains to explore new solutions to eliminate synchronization problem, to rethink our volume balancing process, and to evaluate French Canadian synthetic voices to provide a better DVD experience.

Conclusion

Our first words were of hope and our last ones will be so as well. We hope that the concern of governments and broadcasters will increase to fulfill the needs of blind and low vision people and make available more DV for them in all cultural media. We hope that people looking for new work opportunities will take up the challenge to become describers as education programs proliferate in the United States, the UK, and elsewhere. Finally, we encourage our fellow researchers to continue their cutting edge work in order to provide describers with guidelines to produce effective results and tools that will empower them.

Acknowledgment

The work presented in this chapter was funded by Heritage Canada through the E- Inclusion network, and the usability testing by the Office des personnes handicapées du Québec (OPHQ) and by the MDEIE (Ministry of development, economic, innovation and exportation). We are appreciative of our collaborators for their helpful suggestions and unlimited expertise. We want to express our special gratitude to Anne Jarry for her suggestions and her tireless effort to bring DV to her community of blind and low vision people. We are also very grateful to the participants in our study who so generously gave their time and insights to make this work possible. I would like to add my personal thanks to Dr. Langis Gagnon for his diligent support and good advice. Extreme thanks to David Byrns for all this graceful coding.

References

ADS 2009. Guidelines for audiodescription initial draft of May 2009. http://www.adinternational.org/ad.html

Audio Description Coalition 2010. A Brief History of Audio Description in the U.S. http://www.audiodescriptioncoalition.org/briefhistory.htm

Benecke, B. 2007. Audio Description: Phenomena of Information Sequencing. MuTra 2007—LSP Translation Scenarios: Conference Proceedings. http://www.euroconferences.info/proceedings/2007_Proceedings/2007_Benecke_Bernd.pdf

Braun, S., 2008. Audiodescription research: State of the art and beyond. *Translation Studies in the New Millennium*, Vol. 6, 14–30.

Canadian Association of Broadcasters. 2004. Closed Captioning Standards and Protocol for Canadian English Language Broadcasters. http://www.dcmp.org/caai/nadh20.pdf

Champin, P.A., Encelle, B., Evans, N., Ollagnier-Beldame, M., Prié, Y., Troncy, R. 2010. Towards collaborative annotation for video accessibility. In Proceedings of the 2010 International Cross Disciplinary Conference on Web Accessibility (W4A), Raleigh, NC, USA.

Chapdelaine, C. 2010. "In-Situ Study of Blind Individuals Listening to Audio-Visual Contents" In 12th International ACM SIGACCESS Conference on Computers and Accessibility ASSETS'10, pp. 59–66. Orlando, Florida, October 25–27, 2010.

Chapdelaine, C., Gagnon, L. 2009. Accessible Videodescription On-Demand. In Eleventh International ACM SIGACCESS ASSETS'09. Pittsburgh, PA, USA, October 26–28.

Chapdelaine, C., Jarry, A. 2010. Lessons Learned from Blind Individuals on VideoDescription, 3rd Applied Human Factors and Ergonomics AHFE International Conference, Miami.

CRTC 2009a. Broadcasting and Telecom Regulatory Policy CRTC 2009-430. http://www.crtc.gc.ca/eng/archive/2009/2009-430.htm

CRTC 2009b. Access to TV for people with visual impairments: Audio description and described video. http://www.crtc.gc.ca/eng/info_sht/b322.htm

CRTC origins and chronology. http://www.crtc.gc.ca/eng/backgrnd/brochures/b19903.htm

Douglas, G., Corcoran, C., Pavey, S. 2006. Network 1000. Opinions and circumstances of visually impaired people in Great Britain: Report based on over 1000 interviews. Birmingham: Visual Impairment Centre for Teaching and Research, School of Education, University of Birmingham mimeo.

EBU. 2006. Results from the questionnaire—The future of access to television for blind and partially sighted people in Europe, EBU European Blind Union. http://www.euroblind.org/working-areas/access-to-information/nr/63

Ely, R., Emerson, R.W., Maggiore, T., O'Connell, T., Hudson, L. 2006. Increased content knowledge of students with visual impairments as a result of extended descriptions. *Journal of Special Education Technology*, 213, 31–43.

Foucher, S., Héritier, M., Lalonde, M., Byrns, D., Chapdelaine, C., Gagnon, L. 2007. Proof-of-concept software tools for video content extraction applied to computer-assisted descriptive video, and results of consultations with producers. Technical Report, CRIM-07/04–07, 2007.

Gagnon, L., Chapdelaine, C., Byrns, D., Foucher, S., Héritier, M., Gupta, V. 2010. Computer-Vision-Assisted System for Videodescription Scripting, In 3rd workshop Computer Vision Application for Visually-Impaired CVAVI 10—A Satellite Workshop of IEEE CVPR 2010. San Francisco, CA, USA, June 13–18, 2010.

Gagnon, L., Foucher, S., Héritier, M., Lalonde, M., Byrns, D., Chapdelaine, C., Turner, J. et al. 2009. *Towards Computer-Vision Software Tools to Increase Production and Accessibility of Video Description to Visually-Impaired People*, Universal Access in the Information Society, Springer-Verlag, Vol. 8, no. 3, pp. 199–218.

Gerzymisch-Arbogast, H. 2007. Workshop Audio Description. Workshop Audio Description. Summer School. Screen Translation. Forli. http://www.translation-concepts.org/pdf/audiodescription_forli.pdf

ITC 2000. ITC Guidance on Standards for Audiodescription. http://www.ofcom.org.uk/tv/ifi/guidance/tv_access_serv/arch

Lakritz, J., Salway, A. 2006. The Semi-Automatic Generation of Audio Description from Screenplays, Dept. of Computing. *Technical Report CS-06-05*, University of Surrey.

Mathieu, S., Turner, J.M. 2007. Audiovision interactive et adaptable. Technical Report. http://hdl.handle.net/1866/1307

Morisset L., Gonant F. 2008. Charte de l'audiodescription. http://www.travailsolidarite.gouv.fr/IMG/pdf/Charte_de_l_audiodescription_30 0909.pdf

Orero, P. 2005. Audio description: Professional recognition, practice and standards in Spain. *Translation Watch Quarterly* 1: 7–18.

Peli, E., Fine, E., Labianca, A. 1996. Evaluating visual information provided by audio description. *JVIB* 90:5. 378–385.

Pettitt, B., Sharpe, K., Cooper, S. 1996. AUDETEL: Enhancing television for visually impaired people. *BJVI* 14:2. 48–52.

Piety, P. 2004. The language system of audio description: An investigation as a discursive process. *JVIB* 98:8. 453–469.

Salway, A. 2007. A Corpus-based analysis of the language of Audio Description. In *Media for All*, Díaz Cintas, Jorge, Pilar Orero and Aline Remael, eds. Rodopi B.V., Amsterdam, New York, 151–174.

Salway, A., Lehane, B., O'Connor, N. 2007. Associating Characters with Events in Films, ACM International Conference on Image and Video Retrieval, CIVR 2007.

Schmeidler, E., Kirchner, C. 2001. Adding audio-description: Does it make a difference? *JVIB* 95:4. 197–212.

Sonali, R. 2011. RNIB International AD Exchange study. *RNIB Report.* http://www.rnib.org.uk/aboutus/Research/reports/2011/AD_pdf.pdf

Szarkowska, A. 2011. Text-to-speech audio description: towards wider availability of AD. *The Journal of Specialized Translation*, 142–163. http://www.jostrans.org/issue15/art_szarkowska.php

Thomas, Jr., R. M. 1996. Gregory T. Frazier, 58, Helped Blind See Movies with Their Ears. *New York Times*, 1996. http://www.nytimes.com/1996/07/17/us/gregory-t-frazier-58-helped-blind-see-movies-with-their-ears.html

Turner, J., Mathieu, S. 2008. Audio description text for indexing films. International Cataloguing and Bibliographic Control 373, July/September, 52–56.

17

Employment, Technology, and Blind People: A Personal Perspective

Mike Cole

CONTENTS

Introduction

Ever since blind people have sought real employment the question has been: What can they do? Ever since there has been a civil rights for people with disabilities mentality in America where a remedy is in place to combat discrimination against people who cannot see or cannnot see well, a Rehabilitation agency has been active that includes blind people. So blind people wish to live independently in "real" working and middle class positions, and society has marshaled resources to bring employment about. What is missing? We ask that question, because unemployment among blind people is very high. Possession of marketable skills by blind people must be strengthened, and everyone must accept the idea and embrace it that vision, while certainly here to stay, is not the only way to vocational fulfillment, let alone getting the bills paid.

Many efforts have been mounted. Some have worked. A brief review of some jobs includes some manufacturing work. For example, in the 1930s the Wagner O'Day Act made possible assembly and light manufacturing jobs where the Federal Government purchased goods and services made by programs staffed by blind workers. Wages were low, Department of Labor standards were relaxed, but eventually, in the 1950s, social welfare with a work incentive made it possible for people to earn a subsistence wage. Through the political organizing of blind people on behalf of themselves, they sought to have the work incentives built in to welfare law so that enough money could come in that significant numbers of them could become independent. Thousands of people got work in the network of workshops under the National Industries for The Blind (National Industries for the Blind 2010). Today that system has modernized, workers earn above minimum wage, management training components have been added to the program, and the range of jobs has expanded into the service sector. Also in the 1930s the Randolph–Sheppard Act (as amended and as codified as Chapter 6A of Title 20 of the U.S.) established vending businesses operated by blind people. Most Business Enterprise Programs are sponsored and financed by State Rehabilitation programs.

Blind individuals worked in darkrooms, they tuned pianos, but more than that, they learned the whole business of piano technician work, performing major rebuilds, working for the most part as self-employed business people. They sewed, farmed, and worked in sales. Conditions improved, technology improved resulting in much greater diversity in the jobs being done by people who are blind. Now they are massage therapists, office workers, radio personalities, counselors, lawyers, teachers, and administrators. They have flocked to public employment where equal access often has real meaning. The equipment is provided, proper support is funded by the Federal Government with a relatively straightforward process for determining eligibility. Blind individuals have worked as entertainers, we all know some of the people who have achieved fame and some fortune traveling the world as major stars. They have made a go of being musicians and comics at local levels too, working with churches, volunteering their talents in the service industry. The road ahead runs toward more blind people landing jobs in the everyday labor market, blending in seamlessly with their sighted colleagues.

Since blind people have done so many things, the legal backing blind people have fought for and received from society has proven to be well justified. More people could join the ranks of the successfully employed but for some problems that persist:

- The world does not understand accessibility. For example: a Flash Player has nothing labeled. Indeed, websites, including interactive ones, simply do not work all too often.

- People who are not blind but who possess engineering skills refuse in many cases to find out from blind people what they want, what works and what does not work, resulting in creative energy wasted.

- Corporations pay lip service to developing accessible technology, but we are often left wondering if anyone was actually sincere about blind consumer preferences, since blind people are spoken with at the conclusion of the development of a product, almost never at the beginning.

- Blind people doing everyday things face difficulties receiving media time; only the mountain climbers, the super stars, or people performing public meltdowns make it on to television, or so it seems.

- Blindness is still depicted as the worst possible thing that can happen to a person.

- Blind people themselves must get the training in the adaptive skills, learn to work with synthetic speech, and perfect their ability to use Braille well. They must work to be at peace with their poor vision or no vision so they might get on about the business of life out in the world, hard as it can sometimes be.

Blind people pose a social, political, and economic problem for this society, because we insist on full participation. We, blind people, are way too smart, having received a great deal of subsidized education, to remain permanently unemployed. Technology has helped and continues to open doors to employment for blind people, but we have not thought and planned and educated and adapted our way to an employment percentage worth bragging about, though many components are now in place to bring about positive change. We perform a variety of jobs but we are unemployed at least twice as much as our sighted colleagues.

Employment Really?

To get started, we should ask ourselves: Is employment actually feasible for people with severe vision loss or total blindness? We can unequivocally say that the answer to the feasibility question is "yes." Today's reality, as employment plays out, is mixed, which is an improvement over where we have been. Social Security is designed with a relatively smooth path to benefits for newly blind people who have paid in, largely because it is assumed that blindness is synonymous with permanent unemployment. That is so much the case that State Rehabilitation programs are reimbursed in full for the money spent to rehabilitate a blind person who comes off of welfare and gets a job and holds that job for 90 days. The Government's willingness to assume that financial risk is based on a hunch that the numbers of successful rehabilitation "closures" (placements) will be relatively small. To be fair, this reimbursement is to act as an incentive for State Rehabilitation programs to work hard for people with severe disabilities and people who really need socioeconomic help.

The Law?

Yes, an employer can be complained against with the Justice Department for discrimination, and after administrative remedies are exhausted, cases can be pursued in court. Like all civil rights law, we are glad legal remedies exist, but realistically we know they will seldom be exercised. (See the Americans with Disabilities Act of 1990, as amended.)

Employment is structurally seen as less than likely. Antidiscrimination laws and regulations are on the books. Let us go a little further.

Technology for What?

Technology has made the carrying out of the tasks of essential functions of many jobs doable. Indeed, blind people often write the access programs from a perspective of real, call it personal, knowledge about what needs to be done. Technology provides alternatives to print, through provision of screen reading solutions. Today smartphones talk, regular office software often works with screen readers, barcode readers can talk, testing programs, industrial manufacturing robotics, email, word processors, spreadsheets, databases, diagnostic equipment, let alone tools that report on conditions, null points, compass directions, precise measurements: all can be used by blind people, making more jobs available than ever before. Sounds like progress, right?

Ready?

How about the blind people themselves? Are they ready to take on integrated employment?

Let us step back through these phenomena and conditions, systems, and policies to see if employment of blind and low vision people is a solved problem. Here is a hint: we find a mixed bag.

How It Was

No doubt blind people worked in the early days of The Republic. And certainly some blind people lived lives of dependence doing very little. Common sense tells us blind people answered the biological imperative, that is, we know they were parents. True educational opportunities for blind people really only moved forward, schooling significant numbers of blind people as the nineteenth century proceeded. State-Sponsored Schools for the Blind were established by the end of the century. Braille was not adopted as the standard reading and writing medium until well into the twentieth century (Irwin 1970). For those with low vision, enlarging solutions were not perfected until late in the twentieth century. And there was a small glimmer of a notion that blind people just might work and live with a degree of self-sufficiency. A blind middle class would have to wait for greater modernity and for the fruits of education to develop. In the meantime, blind people would either be taken care of by their families or they would be housed forever in dorms and workshops, receiving pin money at best.

Expectations

I mentioned the efforts of the people themselves to make their situation better, more independent. It is early twentieth century and the industrial revolution is on. You go to a State School for the Blind from the early grades through high school, maybe you are an excellent student or maybe you are an average student, but you become educated. At many State schools, crafts and piano technician work were part of the curriculum along with sewing. The founders of the schools, many of them blind go-getters, fought for a vocational option to be part of the educational plan. The advocate-driven social planning idea was that some jobs could be proven feasible by blind people so that if all else failed, they would be able to look after themselves. Given the times, early industrialization, War, Depression times, and given that there was no welfare safety net in place (far from it) we might forgive our early program planners for seeking a one-size-fits-all set of solutions.

Policy Changes

The government was finally brought to bear to open things up a bit. In 1935, the Social Security Act established legal blindness, that point where a blind person was judged to be in the protected class of people who could receive benefits based on blindness. Those benefits were small, but meaningful. For example, a franking privilege that made the distribution of Brailled and recorded material free to the nation's blind citizens in the 1930s made it possible for the blind people to read. The amount of material was small, in fact, politics crept in insisting the material be inspirational—the Government would not be party to making controversial material available—but the use of Government to do that which it was uniquely positioned to do helped blind people gain knowledge, and their expectations for a better life were helped to flourish. The New Deal and changing attitudes in the amazing 1930s moved the notion of employment forward. The Wagner O'Day Act, later amended to become the Wagner Javits O'Day Act of 1936, established a mechanism whereby the Government would purchase from a select list of products and services from agencies serving a blind population. The Government purchasing procedure exists today (National Industries for the Blind 2010). It led to the establishment of nonprofit workshops that employed the blind workers and could bid for work contracts. Rules were established to ensure that products said to be made by blind workers were in fact made by them. And while the pay was poor, the effort at making accessible jobs cracked open another door toward a more full participation in community life; at least some money could start to come in. The Randolph–Sheppard Act of 1938 went a step further. Blind people could be trained to operate food and dry stand concessions in Government buildings. The blind person would be the boss, he or she would be a business person; the actual hope was that after gaining experience, the vendor could move in to private business.*

    All three of these efforts worked toward the blind being more independent and employed. Regular integrated middle-class employment would come eventually. Today the Wagner Javits O'Day act shops report employment of 6000 blind individuals in America. The Randolph–Sheppard Act reports 2580 licensed vendors operating facilities in government buildings across the nation.

Hard Sell?

And what of discrimination? Employers are not in a rush to hire people who cannot see well. They are concerned that a blind employee could not perform the "essential functions of the job" and that expensive equipment, equipment the employer is unaware of for the most part, will have to be purchased. The blind person will get hurt, will not fit in, will not be able to get to and

---

* http://ncsab.org/

from work, will be trapped in the building in case of emergency—the fears go on and on. The fears grow out of stereotyping and ignorance; employment problems are solvable, if all pull in the same direction. Discrimination against blind people can seem perfectly reasonable, but for one basic truth: many, if not most, jobs can be done successfully and well without vision or without full vision. Blind people want to work; often they have the motivation, the skills, and the need to work; civil rights law supports equality of opportunity, and technology can render the tasks of work accessible. How then will we plan and design our way to high employment with promotions and independence for those who make the effort?

Changing the Brand

Good public education is needed, because when we look around, we do not see blind people doing everyday jobs. Oh, they are out there, but blindness is a rather low incidence disability. When an employer knows that he or she might be on shaky ground rejecting the application of a blind person out of hand, progress can be said to have been made. So the threat of being caught discriminating is the real motivator for employers. It is not much, but it removes a tendency toward an automatic set of doubts that write off employment for blind people. Too bad the public does not realize that that technical support person on the phone is totally blind. What a shame that the citizen boating on that lake does not realize that a blind attorney ran the case for water testing for the State in its oversight function. The soldier using his or her field pack has no idea that the things in the pack were tested and packed by a group of blind people. The IRS worker might very well be blind, the social security information person is blind, the dispatcher sending the tow truck or school bus might be blind, person sitting across from us on the bus might be a clerk for the Sheriff's Department, or the person who transcribed the case notes from a doctor might be blind. If people knew of the various things blind people do on a regular basis, it would surely help the employment picture by normalizing employment and blindness. We benefit from news stories of amazing blind people. Even better are stories where blind working people are regular employees seen and noticed as normal.

Blindness OK

The true and persistent force through the twentieth and into the twenty-first century has been the blind people themselves. They organized into powerful political organizations, brought lawsuits, demonstrated against discrimination and the perpetuation of stereotyping in the media. The National Federation of the Blind (NFB) and the American Council of the Blind (ACB) are the prime movers behind legislation that established rehabilitation and special education, and that advanced employment expansion. And in these days of enhanced electronic solutions to just about everything, they work tirelessly to make technology accessible, from Government services that are mandated to be accessible but are not, to website design and everyday appliances and information and search services. The fight is hard, blindness is simply not considered, it takes organization to put politicians and other policy makers on notice that we will not be kept out. Blind individuals and groups also assist technology developers, because we know best what we need. There is something else we know: businesses, producers of materials, interactive websites, software, and so on, are often highly unaware about just what makes for access by people who have poor vision or no vision; we know that we, blind people, must help in the effort. May this chapter speak the plea, bring blind people into the development process, and pay them for their knowledge. It is much better than settling lawsuits.

Amazing But

What of technological solutions? Everything sighted people do can be simulated, substituted for, and made completely accessible through blind peoples' remaining senses. So good, let us declare success and move on to the next chapter.

Wait, let us take it slow around this curve. I listened to a podcast about a young man who wanted more than anything to be a recording engineer, to do postproduction sound recording and editing work. How exciting to know that there are programs that are fully accessible to blind people using screen readers. (Those programs have been written by blind people.) Ah but wait, the program of choice in the recording industry was Pro Tools, made for Apple, fully inaccessible to PC users who are blind at the time. So this young man put himself in the woodshed for 6 months to learn the graphical presentation of the Pro Tools screen. He could get a screen reader to tell him everything about the screen as he moved around with his arrow keys, and by memorizing the screen layouts, he could work with the program. He got and held a job in his chosen field. Well, great, so recording jobs are easy right? Wrong. That which this young man had to do, no one else might ever do. It is simply too hard, software changes all the time, the making of inaccessible technologies usable through memorization and rote procedures does not increase employment, it limits it to a very few people with fantastic patience.

The System

How are a potential employee and the right technology matched up? In a reasonably well-run State, an employer is found who is willing to give our blind employee a chance. A Rehabilitation Counselor employed by the State is somewhat knowledgeable about technological solutions, or at least he or she knows where to get good information about it. Someone in the town, the region, the State has the ability to analyze the work site's set of tasks and make recommendations concerning purchases or work place accommodations that will enable our blind potential worker to fit in on the job. The Rehabilitation system has strong incentives to see to it that people are placed in jobs. It is their core reason for existing, numbers are how a Rehab Counselor distinguishes himself or herself, and remember the potential for Social Security is to reimburse the State agency for successful placements.

The would-be worker may have appropriate equipment purchased for him or her, brought on to the work site, and configured so that it will work with the employer's systems. Negotiations may occur between many individuals, like as though this hire is a project. The supervisor has no doubt gone out on a limb, unless the CEO of the company has made this hire a personal statement; could be the CEO made promises on the golf course. No matter how, the project is set in motion, each hire is a project involving much effort, because technologies are not always compatible and because not all employment issues are technology based.

Do we see how the stars must align? Do we see how things can go very right or not work at all?

Now let us look at specific aspects of work. What could blind people do that could result in blue or white collar work and that could enable them to make choices about the kind of work they could pursue? They could type, speak, sell, and develop x-rays in darkrooms. They could learn small engine repair, they could sew in production shops, weave, wind brooms, and work on assembly lines performing repetitive well-learned tasks. Briefly, they went into chiropractic work. Some did massage therapy.

What jobs could be performed without vision? This defined the efforts of social institutions that worked toward fostering employment for blind people. Surely there is more.

Adapting the Job: Adapting the Method

Managing the Print Barrier

Looking through a microscope, editing large bundles of handwritten reports and manuscripts, reviewing work orders obviously place barriers in the path of blind job seekers. Let us look at solutions that work, and let us keep in mind that adaptations come about through careful planning, advocacy, even hard-fought battles. And one other concept to keep in mind: remember the idea of the person being able to perform the "essential functions of the job?" Now add to that the notion of "reasonable accommodation to the known disability of an individual." There you have the legal fulcrum for employment opportunities for people who have severe vision loss and blindness.

Human Reader

A human reader is a person whose job it is to read for a blind employee. The Public Sector may make an assistant a regular position; a blind employee might hire his or her own reader and pay for their services out of his or her own pocket. The blind employee may be in a position to train the reader, or the reader might be sought out when something must be read, signed, or filed. A reader reads, sorts, and presents print material to be signed. A skilled reader explains the nature of a document: a list, a letter, a memo, or a bill. The reader helps the blind employee sign his or her name in the proper space. The reader presents documents and files them.

Sounds good, right? A person might be able to do a great many jobs, if there can be an assistant to help now and then. Well, but an employer might not wish to hire two people to do one job. One of the employers of choice today for blind workers is with the public sector, counties, cities, State, and Federal government. In the public sector, the power of antidiscrimination law is real and paid for by the Federal Government. An assistant might simply be someone who takes some time informally to help the blind worker, or they might be someone whose job it is to facilitate the work of a blind employee. This employed assistant might be a sign language interpreter for the deaf, a reader or a driver for someone who is blind. In the case of State Rehabilitation, often times Departments welcome blind or deaf counselors to work with blind or deaf consumers. Facilitating the work of a person who can "relate" to the issues of consumers is seen as positive, well worth the cost of providing an assistant.

What Else?

Scanning and optical character recognition (OCR) software can turn print into speech or Braille with proper hardware and software. Keep in mind that people do not automatically know how to utilize scanning and OCR technologies; they present an extra layer of equipment and software to be mastered. The Internet has brought us email. Much of what used to be hard copy on the job is now wonderfully accessible with the use of computers, sound cards, and screen readers that speak and/or produce high quality Braille. Many people can be productive using enlarging TV systems. They work with a camera, enlarging the image with auto-focus, they can change the background to make the print stand out, and they can use scanner technologies too that enable the employee to split the screen and tailor the print image to suit their vision requirements (see Chapter 4).

Solutions, But Who Pays?

Answer: The employer or the employee or the State Department of Rehabilitation. How much does adaptive technology cost? A PC may cost up to a thousand dollars, outfit it with whatever software the employer uses and then add on the assistive technology. The screen reader will cost a good thousand dollars. An OCR Software package that is blind-friendly, that is it works with speech and responds to access commands (see Chapter 10), will run another thousand dollars. A Braille display, depending on its number of Braille cells, can cost from about $2000 to $6000 or $7000. An enlarging video system (commonly called a CCTV, see Chapter 4) can cost from $1800 to $3600. All that is cheaper than an employed assistant, but when I administered a program for the State I had much of that equipment and a full time secretary, plus I shared an assistant with other blind staff members. Yes, I worked in the public sector.

Doing the Job

A blind employee makes it through the interview and the paper screening; the employer decides to take a chance or the employer is thrilled at finding someone who seems to be highly qualified. What issues remain as the employee moves from hire worker to successful worker? Here are some examples of typical issues that might come up.

- Will adaptive methods produce standard accuracy and precision?
- Will modified methods used by a blind worker be seen as feasible?
- Who develops relevant adaptations of the tasks of the job?
- How is the accessibility of workplace equipment analyzed?

Fitting in

Success on the job often rests on interpersonal relations; the people-to-people part of work is probably the most important single factor in determining whether the job will work out. Work and succeeding at work is more than the sum of the work tasks. How does our mythical blind or low vision employee become "a full team member?" That is: How is interoffice mail handled? Is there a method for getting the blind employee to sign informal things like birthday cards or is there the kind of welcoming atmosphere that adapts? What is the lunch situation like, that is, does everyone scatter in their cars? Is bringing lunch okay? How do the elevators work? A major case will develop to make high-rise building elevators accessible, but for now a person often cannot operate the interactive touch screen inaccessible controls. A blind employee might have guide dog concerns. Is there a place for the dog to stretch out? Nearby relieving areas? Good communication with fellow workers on dog issues like not feeding, like petting at specified times/conditions? And reluctant as some blind individuals may want to talk about this issue, what is the availability of help? Is it fast enough? Reliable? Consistent? Not good? Problem with asking? Some jobs require no special help for anyone, blind or sighted.

Suppose the blind employee is the supervisor. That usually means more paperwork. We wonder: Does the job require a review of documents and are those documents accessible?

What Else?

Is travel part of the job? That will probably be fine in most instances, but under what circumstances do most employees do it? Do they drive? Do they travel as a group? Are the places where the employees travel served by public transit systems? If keeping accounts is part of the job, will the blind employee have a compatible system with their colleagues? When taking notes, will the notes be scrutinized by others or are the notes strictly for the employee's own use? If writing reports is part of the job, is there an accessible method or format, does an accessible form get filled out? How much reading, filing, preparation of documents, writing letters, transcribing, or taking dictation is part of the job? Do the employees work with spreadsheets, word processors, email, contacts, and databases? Are all of the software packages usable by our blind employee?

Blind People Can and Do Work

There are abilities such as keeping inventory; clerking; negotiating; advocating; counseling; meeting quotas; meeting deadlines; participating in meetings, organizing events, trainings, meal functions; arranging travel of others; answering phones; giving technical information in writing, on the phone, in written form, in a classroom setting. Strictly speaking, all of these can be done well by someone with low vision or no vision. Spoken or unspoken, is vision required? If the answer is yes, then ask, but is vision *essential*? The blind employee might very well be able to perform the essential functions of the job, therefore under civil rights law, they must have an opportunity to compete for the job. None of the aforelisted jobs or job functions can be ruled out on the basis of blindness, not any of them. The issues that do come up can mostly be addressed through open discussion and honest communication.

Impossible, Really?

Some job tasks are inherently challenging to the point of rendering them impossible or improbable given the job modifications that would be required. Driving; reading print; working with handwritten materials; making decisions based on color; error detection; some reading of test equipment; visual sign language interpreting; painting; drawing: these tasks might in fact push the envelope. However, driving as a small part of a job might be traded for some other function. Making decisions based on color might be managed with the use of excellent color detecting equipment that speaks, saying the number of the color or the name of the color. Some quality control performed under a microscope might find a robotic solution with the blind person operating the control for the robot. Many test equipments can be adapted with visual output to speech, tactile vibratory, or using the equipment with the help of an assistant. Sign language interpretation? Surely a blind person cannot do that, it might be thought. Think again, there are systems of hand-over-hand communication that do work. Painting and drawing tasks may truly be out of reach, what with the lack of reliable feedback systems for the person performing the tasks. But in every example listed here, either the task can be traded or a way can be found to keep our person on the job. And if we are to help a blind person succeed at a job, expert help, now common sense, then again creative trial-and-error, all get around barriers and will be called upon by everyone involved.

When You Are the Boss

Since the most difficult part about being a blind employee among a sighted workforce may be establishing your personal legitimacy, working with common methods that might not all work well nonvisually, or the use of unfamiliar or unworkable technologies, the best position to hold is the Boss.

Legitimacy or, am I really doing this job? Everyone wonders at one time or another whether he or she is actually doing a good job. Even when supervisors and fellow workers give us verbal support, awards, recognition, even when you win the Busy Bee award, we have those moments when we just are not sure. A blind employee might have those moments with good reason. His or her work method might be a little different, someone has to help out now and then, reading a note, walking with him or her to a new location, say for a meeting. Well the boss may be effective or not, but the owner, the manager, the director, the CEO do what they do by and large; legitimacy comes with the title.

When I was a child I sat through my share of lectures intended to give me hope and motivate me to work harder. It was said that some jobs would forever be impossible for a blind person: driving a truck, being a machinist, and being an accountant, I remember, were used as examples of jobs I would never get. Blind people have not yet become regular teamsters, but there are blind people performing complex accounting tasks. Imagine my delight when I found out there was a blind machinist; he ran the company, built the jigs, he determined the production timelines, he negotiated the contracts (jobs), and taught the employees ways of doing things that would work for him and for them.

Much of what is talked about in this chapter are the wonderful ways technology has opened up jobs for people who are blind or have low vision. Yet, there are blind employees who choose not to use any more technology than is absolutely necessary, so maybe the only technology they use is the phone. When you are the boss, you can surround yourself with people you train up to take your dictation, read the mail, both email and regular mail, file, sort, type, copy, staple just so, fax, research, run your calendar, or drive you to meetings. In this day, even the bosses who are the most well-cared for, probably still keep a note taker (PDA), cell phone, Braille writing devices, or enlarging CCTV. And let us not disparage a boss who does not use technology; those talents and skills the company wants are what the company is paying for, and if the boss seeks to utilize the services of assistants, well, they are the boss!

Unemployment, Too High!

Studies (Nyman, 2009) show that blind individuals are more out of work than at remunerative steady secure employment. Statistics are not easy to come by for all workers. For blind people the complexity is greater. Think illness, discouraged work seeker, poor transportation, inadequate preparation, discrimination, disincentives placed in the way of employment by benefits eligibility, and note that the majority of blind people are over age 55. Consider this as well: all the methods for obtaining a job, exploring job opportunities, the sending in of dozens to hundreds of applications, may not work for blind individuals. We say, well if the newspaper is inaccessible, today there is the Internet. That is the good news, the bad news is the Internet is inaccessible all too often.

One agency for the blind finds 70% unemployment, but look further and you will see that there might be 30% of blind people actively looking, but 37% not looking; so we can say that approximately 33% of blind people are working. No matter how the statistical breakdowns are published, unemployment among people who are blind is high (American Foundation for the Blind 2010; AccessWorld 2011).

Are the Jobs the Blind People Get Special or Ordinary?

After all the talk of technology and playing fields being leveled, what are those actually getting jobs doing? Looking at an internal compilation document of all the successful placements of legally blind people in California by the California Department of Rehabilitation, we find diversity, and we also find that social forces that affect everybody also have an effect on blind workers. So here is a sampling of actual placements by the person. Then we will look at trends.

Raw Data

Accountant, administrative assistant, athletic coach, attorney, auditor, auto mechanic, bagger, Braille instructor, book keeper, business manager, cabinet maker, care provider, case manager, child care worker, chiropractor's assistant, clinical psychologist, computer programmer, computer technical support worker, contractor, copywriter, counselor, customer service representative, day care center director, dental consultant, dining room attendant, dog trainer, editor, electrician, electrical engineer, eligibility worker, elementary school teacher, employment specialist, factory helper, financial planner, film processor, general clerk, general laborer, graphic designer, greeter, hospital administrator, hotel clerk, independent living services instructor, inventory clerk, janitor, job coach, job developer, language interpreter, leasing agent, legal research assistant, legal secretary, life coach speaker, loan analyst, machine operator, massage therapist, medical transcriptionist, music teacher, nurse, nurse's assistant, occupational therapist, Pastor, personal computer disassembler, phlebotomist, preschool teacher, private investigator, production worker, professor, project manager, property rental owner/manager, psychiatrist, real estate agent, real estate broker, recording engineer, registered nurse, rehabilitation counselor, restaurant manager, Spanish teacher, sewing machine operator, social worker, stocker, switchboard operator, substance abuse counselor, teacher's aid, vending operator under the Randolph–Sheppard Act.

Well, are you shocked? Impressed? Some people may have returned to their old job, once recovery from vision loss and prevocational training was completed. Some qualified by pursuing education leading to licensing, credentialing, and so on. Remember, these are people who recently got hired. The data is for Fiscal Years 2009 and 2010. The sheer diversity of successful placements is encouraging. We found density in sales jobs, clerk jobs, massage jobs, school personnel, security officer; only one person was listed as self-employed, a somewhat counterintuitive finding. There were more teachers than anything else. Then came office worker, who could be a clerk, secretary, receptionist, or switchboard operator; no doubt technology is working for these people. Customer relations come next. That includes technical support people, sales, people who can talk, listen, and negotiate using the phone. They work as massage therapists at various levels. They also work as managers and supervisors, knowing the operation, working with staff, persuading, organizing, and taking responsibility. Many people got jobs in the computer field in one capacity or another. We saw hardware technicians, programmers, instructors, and software developers. We were pleased to see professional positions, for example, therapists, lawyers, counselors, engineers, and directors. Placements in manufacturing and what is commonly called "the Trades" was disappointing. There was only one auto mechanic, one cabinet maker, only one factory helper, and one dog trainer. There was one film processor and one graphic designer. There were only four janitors. There were just two cooks and one sewing machine operator. There was only one electrician. Manufacturing is down, blue collar is down. Most of the jobs listed in a 2-year report of 350 successful job placements indicate the presence of accessible technology. We see that blind individuals who worked hard obtaining professional credentials were able to find work in their chosen fields. And we see that many of the jobs people got are jobs all right, but shaky jobs, and when we know that the effort to land a job was often great, we are struck by a tenuousness; we can sense it. Nonetheless, in a couple of generations, blind individuals have gone from sheltered employment options, and very few of those, to a relatively open job market with developing accessible technologies, thereby expanding opportunities.

What Do the Mentors Say?

The American Foundation for The Blind has a very interesting program called Career Connect. Many strategies have been tried to enhance employment opportunities for the blind people; this effort is a good one. A database of employed individuals make themselves available to give advice and counsel people who wish to enter the field in which the mentor is employed. Mentors were invited to give their views; the following is an excerpt from the mentors' comments (American Foundation for the Blind 2007, reproduced with permission).

1. Owing to the small proportion of blind employees currently in the American workforce (one mentor is the only blind employee out of 5000), it can be hard to convince management of the importance of making software accessible in-house (via script writing) or buying accessible software.
2. The more proficient blind employees there are out there, the more conducive the overall atmosphere will be for making accommodations. That is, competent blind employees can offer valuable insights in their fields, so the more blind engineers, for example, who are working, the more influence they will have on employer decisions regarding modifications in the workplace.
3. Although there is legislation in place for equal employment access, the political reality is that there are varying degrees of compliance.
4. Improvements in technology for the majority can ironically mean less access for vision-impaired workers. For example, PDF format has saved so much space, it is now the preferred method of presenting large amounts of information—but it is not accessible. The attractive graphics added for sighted viewers can also jam up software for the blind viewer.
5. It is absolutely essential for children with vision impairments to be taught computer skills early on! The more computer-literate you are,

the more you will be able to make do with the accessibility gaps everyone encounters at work.

6. More and more manuals are being offered only in PDF formats, so even for highly educated and motivated blind workers, it can be daunting or barely possible to read necessary how-to information.

7. There are rarely enough IT staff to effectively support all employees in a given workplace, so the visually impaired employees are just one voice in a chorus of demands; this can mean the blind employees have to work more hours to make their inadequate office equipment do the job. Also, the inadequate staffing of IT people can mean they have negative attitudes toward the one blind employee they perceive to be too demanding.

8. Because of the gaps in adaptive technology and the uneven compliance of many workplaces, many blind employees report having to work longer hours than their sighted peers. Or, as in the case of a blind casino employee, she cannot give directions to hotel patrons due to the lack of a tactile map.

9. On a positive note, there are more mainstream choices all the time, and everything digital is getting cheaper.

References

AccessWorld. 2011. Special issue on Disability Employment Awareness Month. *AFB AccessWorld* 12(10).

American Foundation for the Blind. 2007. CareerConnect mentors speak out on access to technology in the workplace. http://www.afb.org/Section.asp?SectionID=44&TopicID=331&SubTopicID=105&DocumentID=3687

American Foundation for the Blind. 2010. Interpreting BLS employment data. http://www.afb.org/Section.asp?SectionID=15&SubTopicID=177

Irwin, R.B. 1970. *The War of the Dots*. American Foundation for the Blind.

National Industries for the Blind 2010. Annual Report 2010—Positioned for Success. http://www.nib.org/sites/default/files/2010AnnualReport/NIBAnnualReport_2010_7-5-11_LRes.pdf

Nyman, J. 2009. Unemployment rates and reasons dissing the blind. *Braille Monitor* 52(3). http://www.nfb.org/images/nfb/publications/bm/bm09/bm0903/bm090307.htm

Index